INTRODUCTION TO
DIAGNOSTIC
IMAGING

INTRODUCTION TO DIAGNOSTIC IMAGING

Edited by

Lee Sider, M.D.

Assistant Professor of Radiology
Northwestern University Medical School
Director, Medical Student Education
Northwestern Memorial Hospital
Chicago, Illinois

Churchill Livingstone
New York, Edinburgh, London, Melbourne   1986

Library of Congress Cataloging-in-Publication Data

Introduction to diagnostic imaging.

   Bibliography: p.
   Includes index.
   1. Diagnostic imaging.   I. Sider, Lee.
RC78.7.D53I58   1986   616.07′57   86-6866
ISBN 0-443-08421-1

Distributed in the United Kingdom by Churchill Livingstone, Robert Stevenson House, 1–3 Baxter's Place, Leith Walk, Edinburgh EH1 3AF, and by associated companies, branches, and representatives throughout the world.

Accurate indications, adverse reactions, and dosage schedules for drugs are provided in this book, but it is possible that they may change. The reader is urged to review the package information data of the manufacturers of the medications mentioned.

Acquisitions Editor: *Robert A. Hurley*
Copy Editor: *Ozzievelt Owens*
Production Designer: *Charlie Lebeda*
Production Supervisor: *Sharon D. Tuder*

Printed in the United States of America

First published in 1986

To Will, Lois, Adriane, and Steve

Contributors

Richard M. Gore, M.D.
Associate Professor of Radiology
Northwestern University Medical School
Chicago, Illinois

Ronald W. Hendrix, M.D.
Associate Professor of Radiology
Northwestern University Medical School
Chicago, Illinois

Charles Lee, M.D.
Assistant Professor of Neuroradiology
University of Kentucky College of Medicine
Lexington, Kentucky

Lee Sider, M.D.
Assistant Professor of Radiology
Northwestern University Medical School
Director, Medical Student Education
Northwestern Memorial Hospital
Chicago, Illinois

Forewords

I am pleased to see a book of this character and quality added to the list of those now available to students and young clinicians. It is well written, clinically inclusive, and beautifully illustrated. It should not be considered an introduction to radiology, for it is much more advanced in content than that suggests. I believe it will be best considered a text in clinical radiology for advanced medical students and young clinicians who will welcome it, as it provides radiologic correlation for their study of medicine, surgery, and the subspecialties. Well indexed, this book is the best I have seen for the young clinician, and bridges a gap currently existing between books designed for the younger medical student in the first two years and the reference works available to those entering training in radiology.

Lucy Frank Squire, M.D.
New York, New York

Imaging has assumed a pivotal role in the present-day diagnosis and treatment of disease. Its importance becomes immediately evident to all medical students as they begin their clinical rotations. In most medical schools, the students spend the first two years familiarizing themselves with the basics of disease processes, but have little or no introduction to the tools utilized in the diagnosis and evaluation of disease. They are then confronted by a variety of imaging techniques with which they have no knowledge. Does every patient require every one of these examinations?

At one time it was simple. There was only film radiography. With the introduction of nuclear medicine, ultrasonography, computed tomography, and more recently, magnetic resonance imaging, along with associated interventional techniques including biopsy and various drainage procedures, radiology has assumed a more important role in the diagnosis, staging, and treatment of disease. Most diseases can be demonstrated by one or more of these techniques.

In view of these developments, there is a great need for a relatively short text that will introduce the medical student to the entire spectrum of imaging techniques. Clinicians are faced not with diagnoses but with certain specific clinical problems such as dyspnea, hematuria, and headache. Because the student needs to know the role of imaging in unraveling these clinical situations, this text is problem oriented. The student should be aware of the relative merits of one imaging technique versus another in a given clinical situation; thus the need for an integrated imaging approach. The student needs guidance through the maze of imaging techniques utilized in the evaluation of clinical problems; thus the need for diagnostic algorithms. The introduction of this book includes an explanation of the physical basis of various techniques and their principle clinical applications. The text is then organized by body system, giving an integrated imaging approach to common clinical problems. I am certain that the student will find this most welcome and instructional.

It has long been my belief that a text for students would be best written by recent graduates. They are familiar with the students' viewpoint and have a perspective of imaging techniques developed during their residency training. With such a background they are able to anticipate and answer the questions, and address the concerns of medical students and trainees.

I encouraged Dr. Sider to assume responsibility for the writing of this text soon after the completion of his residency training. I am most pleased by the results. He and his fellow authors have admirably accomplished their task. They are to be congratulated for the excellence and timeliness of their work. I recommend this text to all medical students and trainees. They have much to learn about diagnostic imaging. This text is a marvelous introduction to this rapidly expanding, exciting, and seemingly limitless field.

Lee F. Rogers, M.D.
Chicago, Illinois

Preface

In recent years there has been an explosion in the technology of diagnostic imaging. The introduction of the computer into radiology has greatly enhanced our ability to study and diagnose disease. Other modalities besides the standard x-rays are commonplace in a modern radiology department. Ultrasound, computed tomography, nuclear medicine, and most recently magnetic resonance imaging have become invaluable diagnostic tools.

These rapid advances in technology make it more important than ever that new physicians have a better knowledge of the precise uses of the new modalities. An accurate understanding will lead to more efficient imaging workup for their patients.

Drs. Gore, Hendrix, Lee, and I have written *Introduction to Diagnostic Imaging* mainly for medical students. Although the majority of them will not become radiologists, they all need to understand the importance of selecting the modalities that will render the most efficient and accurate diagnosis. The book has been kept purposely at an introductory level. In examining each clinical problem, an attempt has been made to integrate all imaging modalities. We feel this format is best suited to help the new clinicians understand which modality will render the most useful information for each clinical presentation.

Each contributing author is a specialist in his area. We have all recently completed our training. The memory of our training has helped focus on the information most relevant and useful to the medical student. Hopefully, the medical student and indeed any physician who reviews images will find this book a helpful guide.

Lee Sider, M.D.

Acknowledgments

I would like to acknowledge the many people who helped make this book happen. First of all my teacher and chairman, Lee F. Rogers, who suggested the project. My partners, Carolyn Johnson, Harold Matthies, Leonid Calenoff, Earl Nudelman, Robert Vogelzang, Madeleine Fisher, Peter Weinberg, Kwang Kim, and especially Ronald Hendrix and Richard Gore for their contributions and support during the writing of this book.

A special thanks also goes to my secretary Susan Sloan who grew with me as I wrote my first book and to John Kelly who often turned aging radiographs into clear photographs.

The radiology residents and students were important in helping me design a book with the topics and studies they wanted to learn more about. Four residents, Martin Cohen, Charles Marn, Lee Dennis, and Thomas Davis, deserve special thanks for their diligent proofreading.

A final thanks goes to my parents and family to whom the book is dedicated. They believed in me and this project with unrelenting conviction.

Contents

1. Introduction to Imaging   1
Lee Sider

2. Radiology of the Chest   39
Lee Sider

3. Radiology of the Urinary Tract   85
Lee Sider

4. Radiology of the Gastrointestinal Tract   133
Richard M. Gore

5. Radiology of the Bones and Joints   183
Ronald W. Hendrix

6. Radiology of the Cardiovascular System   223
Lee Sider

7. Radiology of the Central Nervous System   251
Charles Lee and Lee Sider

Index   291

by the Navy, and were brought into more widespread use in the 1940s as sound navigation and ranging (SONAR). Their medical application began in the early 1950s, and is constantly being modified. In this procedure sound waves are sent into the body and reflected back to a receptor or absorbed to various degrees by the different body components. The intensity of the reflected waves, is used in the formation of an image on a television monitor and later on film for interpretation by the radiologist.

In 1972, Hounsfield presented at a radiology conference in Great Britain a revolutionary new imaging technique that allowed sectional views of the head and abdomen that had not previously been obtainable. This new technique utilized the conventional x-ray, in combination with computers, to construct these images. It was given the name computerized axial tomography (CT). The x-ray beam used in CT is first shaped into a fan-shaped beam as it leaves the x-ray tube. After passing through the patient, it strikes special detectors instead of exposing film, and through mathematical manipulation a cross-sectional view of the body part is constructed. Computerized tomography allows excellent differentiation of the various organs and soft tissues due to its extreme sensitivity to small contrast or density differences. The head and abdomen are no longer seen as undifferentiated spaces as they are with the conventional x-ray and film combination.

The computer processing of transmitted x-ray signals has most recently been applied to the visualization of intravascular contrast media at low concentrations. The level at which such vascular opacification is seen is considerably below that in conventional angiography, in which the contrast medium must be injected directly into the desired artery and the film exposed directly by the x-ray beam after the latter has passed through the patient. This sensitive detection of low concentrations of intravascular contrast medium permits the medium to be injected into a vein with subsequent visualization of the arteries. The process is called intravenous digital subtraction angiography (DSA). The computer processing of the x-ray signal also allows very small quantities of contrast medium to be injected directly into an artery and still produce complete opacification owing to the extreme sensitivity of DSA to low concentrations of contrast medium. This is valuable in patients with renal compromise, in whom the high concentrations of injected contrast

medium needed in conventional angiography may cause further renal embarrassment.

Through the linkage of new radioactive elements to biological materials, as well as progress in the mechanics of detecting radioactivity, nuclear medicine has grown phenomenally in the last decade. The radioactive-biologic element complex is localized to various parts of the body. The liver, for example, will localize radioactively labeled sulfur colloid, while radioactively labeled MDP (methylene dysphosphonate) will localize in bone and bypass the liver. The radioactivity is detected outside the body by specialized gamma cameras placed over the organs and areas of interest. Localized defects, which result in either too much or too little radioactivity being emitted from a usually homogenous area, are then detected as pathological.

In the past 5 years, another new modality has emerged in a role that remains unclear in terms of its impact on diagnostic radiology. Magnetic resonance imaging (MR) involves the application of a strong external magnetic field along with a radio frequency signal that subsequently produces a current in a receiving coil. The current is proportional to the density of protons in the body part being scanned, since they are the components of the atom most affected by the external magnetic field. This signal is again processed by a computer to create a tomographic slice of a body section similar to that in the CT scan. Potentially, MR may be able to provide physiologic as well as anatomic information.

X-RAYS

X-rays belong to the group of radiations called electromagnetic radiations, along with radio waves, light waves, radiant heat, and gamma radiation. X-rays are produced within an x-ray tube by an energy conversion process in which a fast-moving stream of electrons is suddenly decelerated. The electrons are generated by the heating of a tungsten filament wire that serves as the negative electrode or cathode of the tube. With extreme heating, electrons separate from the filament and are available for acceleration toward the positively charged anode, which is also made of tungsten since it has a high melting point. It is the potential difference between the anode and the cathode that results in the acceleration of the electron stream. The

1

Introduction to Imaging

Lee Sider

One of the most important roles of an introductory text in diagnostic imaging is to familiarize the clinician with the physical properties of the various imaging modalities as well as with their clinical applications. It is through such a familiarity with the physics of radiology that a more complete understanding of its uses and capabilities will be possible. This knowledge also enables the clinician to efficiently obtain the maximum possible radiologic information about a patient through selection of the proper examinations. This introductory chapter will also present terms and descriptions that are invaluable in understanding the remainder of the text, and I encourage the reader to study it carefully.

Until recently the sole tool of diagnostic radiology was the x-ray. Since its discovery by Roentgen in 1895, the x-ray has been used to examine every aspect of the human body. The different parts of the body, including fat, soft tissues (organs and muscles), and

bone, as well as air (in the lung and bowel) all absorb a portion of the x-ray beam to different degrees. The portion of the x-ray beam that passes through the patient is exposed to special film to obtain the familiar x-ray image.

Through the use of various contrast agents, delineation of different aspects of the internal anatomy, not visualized with the plain x-ray beam, is possible. The x-ray and film combination alone does not differentiate the various soft-tissue structures, since they absorb x-rays to an equal degree. Only with the introduction of barium into the stomach, small bowel, or colon, or an iodine-containing contrast material into the arteries can these and various related soft tissue structures be distinguished from surrounding fat, connective tissue, and adjacent viscera.

Ultrasound has assumed an important role in modern diagnostic radiology. Ultrasonic waves were first used in 1912 in the search for the sunken ship *Titanic*

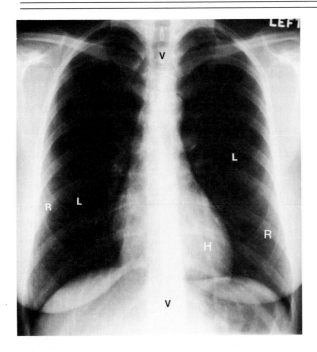

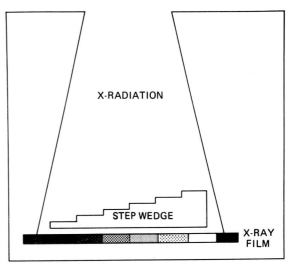

Fig. 1-6 X-ray step wedge.

Fig. 1-5 Normal chest x-ray. L = lung parenchyma, R = rib, V = vertebral body-spine, H = heart, A = aorta.

This is because the heart, being thicker, can stop more of the beam, giving it a lighter gray shade than the thinner aorta on the subsequent film. This effect of thickness is clearly demonstrated with an x-ray of a step wedge. Here a solid aluminum bar is given a staircase shape, with increasing levels of thickness. It is then exposed to an x-ray beam. The thinnest level, which contains the least amount of aluminum stops the fewest x-rays, producing the darkest shade of gray, while the thickest portion of the aluminum bar stops the most x-rays, poducing the lightest shade of gray on the film (Fig. 1-6). The orderly progression between the two extremes of thickness results in the same orderly progression of darker to lighter shades of gray on the x-ray film.

Another example of how the densities of different tissues create a meaningful x-ray image is with the plain x-ray view of the abdomen (Fig. 1-7). Fat is less dense than the surrounding soft tissues of the abdomen, stopping fewer x-rays than the liver, for example. Thus, with proper exposure techniques, one can see the black, fat-lined flank stripe outlining the out-

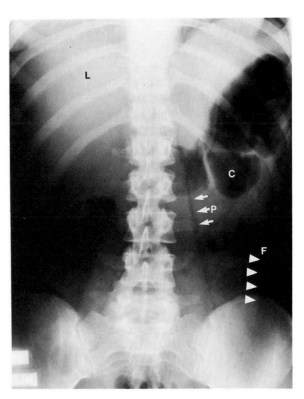

Fig. 1-7 Normal abdomen. L = liver area, F = fat of the flank stripe (arrowheads), C = air within the colon, P = fat lining the psoas muscle (arrows).

side of the abdomen against the gray liver. A second abdominal example of the effect of density is with the markedly less dense air contained within the loops of bowel. These collections of air stand out in a film as black areas within the gray appearing abdomen.

A film of the lower leg gives yet another example of how the various properties of tissue interact to yield an x-ray image (Fig. 1-8). Bone is more dense than the surrounding soft tissue, stopping more of the initial x-ray beam. In addition, the higher atomic numbers of its component elements result in the more complete absorption of the initial x-ray beam predominantly through the photoelectric effect. The compact, dense cortex of the tibia can also be differentiated from the less dense medullary portion, since it lets fewer x-rays penetrate. All of these factors interact to create an image of white bone superimposed on the gray soft tissues of the leg.

Knowledge of the normal x-ray appearance of the chest, abdomen, leg, or any body part to be examined is necessary in order to be able to recognize and diagnose an abnormality. It is a familiarity with normal anatomy that allows the radiologist to detect abnormalities. Subsequent chapters, as they divide the body into the different organ systems, will present further examples of normal anatomy and the abnormal alterations that help in the diagnosis of a disease process. An abnormal soft-tissue mass or a change in or loss of

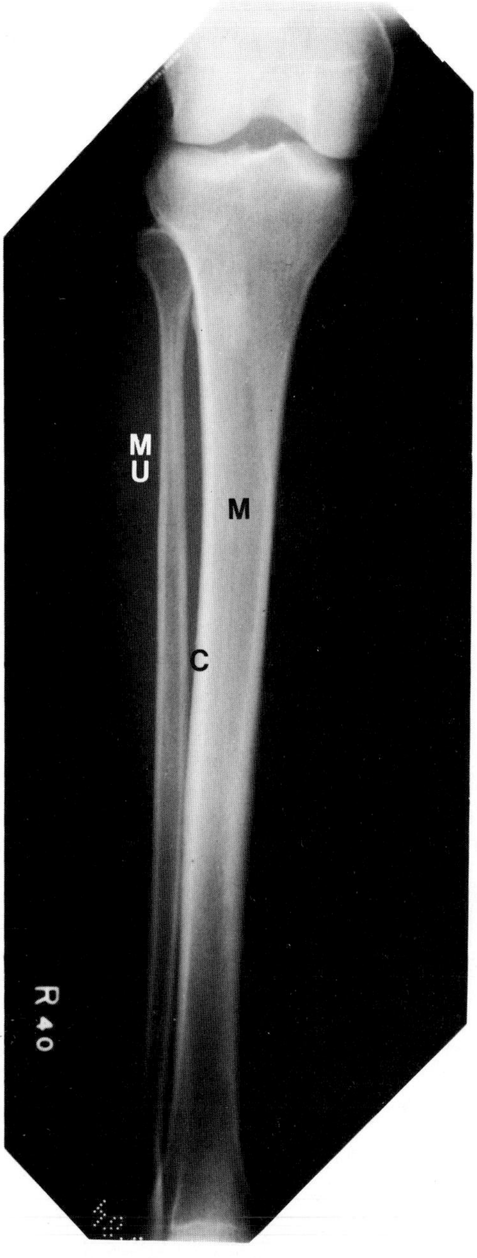

Fig. 1-8 Normal tibia and fibula. C = cortex of tibia, M = medullary portion of tibia, MU = muscle.

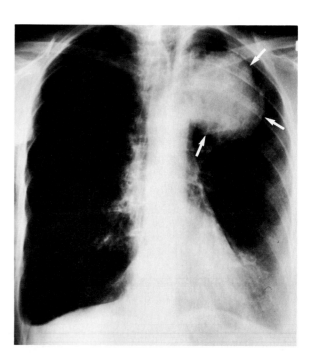

Fig. 1-9 Lung carcinoma (arrows).

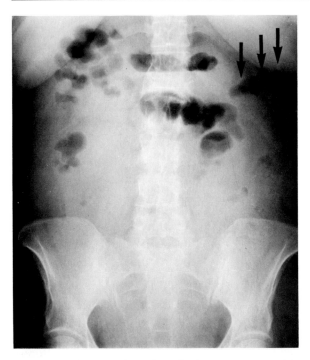

Fig. 1-10 Splenomegaly. Enlarged spleen in a patient with leukemia is manifested by an inferior displacement of the air-filled splenic flexure (arrows).

the normal anatomy signifies disease. This may, for example, consist of a solid, soft-tissue-density mass superimposed over what should be homogeneously black lung tissue, representing a lung carcinoma (Fig. 1-9). The pushing down of the normally high portion of the left colon or splenic flexure from its position just below the diaphragm may represent an enlarged spleen displacing the bowel (Fig. 1-10). The irregular outline of the neck of the femur with an abnormal angulation of the femoral head represents a fracture of the femoral neck (Fig. 1-11).

In order to obtain more information about the various soft-tissue components that have a similar density and atomic number, and which therefore cannot be differentiated on a plain x-ray film, contrast agents have been developed. In modern radiology, barium and iodine salts are in common use for this purpose. Both have almost ideal atomic numbers for an exclusive photoelectric effect and subsequent complete absorption of the x-ray beam, by comparison with surrounding soft tissues that transmit a portion of the beam. The resulting x-ray film is white where the beam has met the contrast agent.

Barium can be swallowed as a liquid suspension for an upper gastrointestinal (UGI) examination and

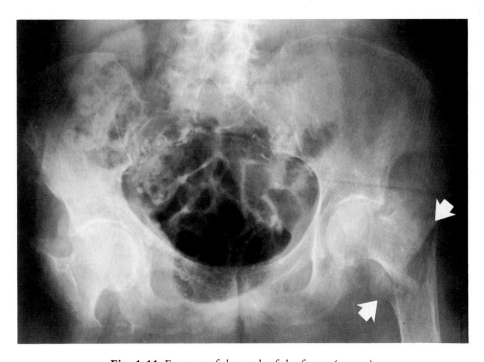

Fig. 1-11 Fracture of the neck of the femur (arrows).

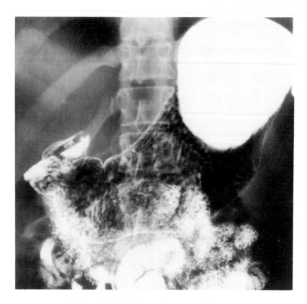

Fig. 1-12 Normal upper GI tract.

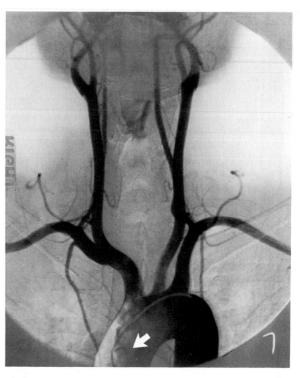

Fig. 1-13 Angiogram of aortic arch, done with a special subtraction technique that allows better visualization of the contrast-medium-filled carotid arteries without distortion by the overlying bones of the cervical spine. As a result of the subtraction technique, the contrast medium appears black and the bones are barely discernible. The catheter tip is in the ascending aorta (arrow).

coats the lining of the stomach and small bowel (Fig. 1-12). This allows the radiologist to detect various disease processes of the bowel mucosa, from ulcers to cancer. Barium can also be given rectally in order to visualize the mucosa of the rectum and colon in a lower gastrointestinal examination (LGI). The mucosal linings are not visible without the barium. It is again through a familiarity with the normal anatomy of the stomach or colon that the radiologist can detect an alteration that represents a pathologic process.

Iodine is used in two ways to differentiate and further study the various components of the soft tissues. It can be injected directly into an artery via the piercing of the skin and the placing of a tube or catheter to the desired area of study. The iodinated contrast medium is then injected through the catheter and the blood supply to the organ or extremity can be well seen in the resulting arteriogram (Fig. 1-13). This is called vascular opacification. Abnormally tortuous, enlarged, or displaced vessels or the absence of certain arteries or veins all signify an abnormality. The iodinated medium may also be injected into a peripheral vein. The blood containing this iodine salt is then filtered and concentrated by the kidney, demonstrating the various structures of the urinary system as they fill with contrast laden-urine that also appears white in the subsequent x-ray film. This is the basis for the

intravenous pyelogram or IVP (Fig. 1-14). The loss or alteration of the normal gentle branching of the collecting structures, or an extra mass of tissue on the kidney, outline or indicate an abnormality.

Fluoroscopy is the ability to visualize an x-ray image live on a television monitor. In this technique the x-rays are generated continuously instead of in a single pulse, as with a simple film-screen exposure. After they pass through the patient during fluoroscopy, the x-rays are directed to a detecting device that converts their pattern to an electronic signal for the television image, rather than being sent toward the familiar film cassette. The detecting device is a large tower, called an image intensifier (Fig. 1-15), on a moving carriage that can be placed across the patient to examine various locations in the body. It is this ability to see events as they occur on the TV monitor that allows the radiologist to watch the progress of barium during LGI, or the arteriographer to direct the course of his catheter to the proper location before injection of the contrast medium for an arteriogram.

Tomography is a process that results in the blurring of all structures outside a desired plane of interest within the patient through the use of a combination of a moving x-ray tube and x-ray film cassette. This allows the radiologist to better visualize the organ or area of interest. Tomographic sections are obtained from the simultaneous but opposite movement of the tube and x-ray film. The "pivot" point for the two opposite directions of movement is the only plane that remains in focus, since in the final image it is the only area not "moving" (Fig. 1-16). All structures above and below are perceived as being in motion and so appear blurred on the film. The further a plane is above this "pivot" plane, the greater is its perceived "movement" and so the more it appears to be blurred. For example, although it is often obscured by overlying bowel gas, the kidney usually lies in the posterior third of the abdomen. By choosing a posterior plane for the fulcrum, all structures in the anterior portion of the abdomen, such as bowel gas, are perceived as moving by the tomographic technique, and so is blurred, resulting in better visualization of the more posterior kidney and its collecting structures (Fig. 1-17). Tomography facilitates diagnosis by allowing

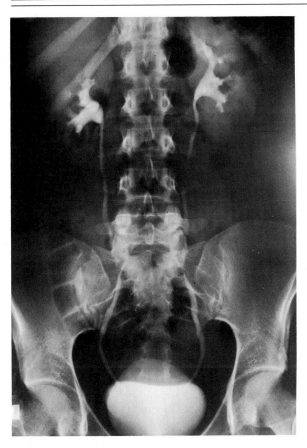

Fig. 1-14 Contrast-medium-filled collecting system in an IVP.

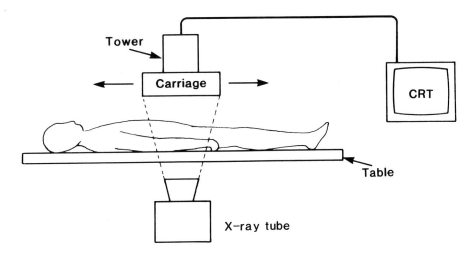

Fig. 1-15 Fluoroscopy setup.

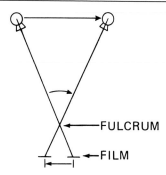

FULCRUM

FILM

Fig. 1-16 Tomography setup.

the clear definition of bony or soft tissue anatomy at any predetermined level.

ULTRASOUND

Ultrasound examination involves the use of high-energy sound waves that are beyond the range of human hearing for the imaging of body parts. The sound beam is similar to an x-ray beam in that both consist of waves of transmitted energy. The sound wave is created in the transducer head and is projected or transmitted into the patient. There it interacts with the soft tissues and is reflected, deflected, or absorbed by the different components of the patient's anatomy. Only the portion of a sound signal that is reflected back and reaches the same transducer head is detected or received for subsequent image formation (Fig. 1-18). The sound signal is converted to an electronic signal and interpreted by a computer that assigns shades of gray to returning sound waves of varying intensities. This follows the same concept as correlating the intensity of transmitted x-rays to a shade of gray in the final x-ray image. An image is subsequently made on film from the electronic signal for interpretation by the radiologist.

In ultrasound examination, the transducer is the device with which the doctor or technologist "scans" the patient. It may either look like a small power drill or be in the shape of a microphone. Oil is applied to the patient's skin to create an airtight path between

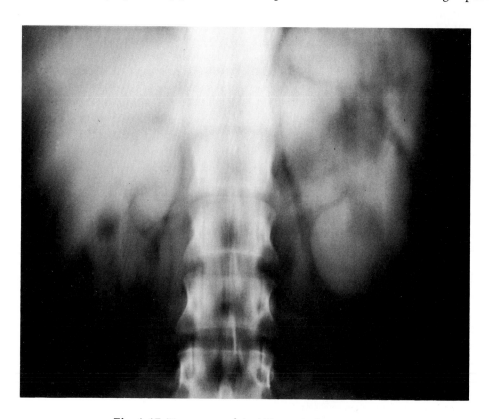

Fig. 1-17 Tomogram of the kidneys during an IVP.

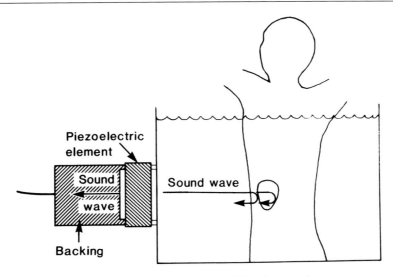

Fig. 1-18 Direction and detection of the ultrasound wave.

the transducer head and the skin. Any interposed air between the transducer and the skin interrupts the sound wave transmission into and out of the patient.

The most important component of the ultrasound transducer is its piezoelectric crystal. An electrical field is momentarily applied to the crystal by surrounding electrodes. With the application of voltage to these electrodes the crystal suddenly changes shape, and then snaps back to its original shape when the voltage is removed. The turning on and off of this momentary electrical field produces the vibration of the crystal, which, like a cymbal that has been struck a sharp blow, then generates sound waves. A backing block behind the vibrating crystal quickly dampens it to prepare it for its second function: as a detector or receiver of the echoes reflected from within the patient. The transducer spends 0.1 percent of its time sending the sound wave into the patient, and listens or receives the returning sound waves 99.9 percent of the time.

The sound that is reflected back and reaches the transducer is also detected by an alteration in the shape of the crystal. The fluctuation of the crystal shape caused by these reflected waves works in exactly the reverse manner as the sound-generation process. The momentary change in shape of the crystal creates an electronic signal that is carried away from the transducer by the same surrounding electrodes and is then fed into a computer. The returning echo is then as-

signed a shade of gray according to its strength. The stronger the echo the darker the gray.

The time needed for the ultrasound signal to return to the transducer identifies the depth from which it was reflected. The shades of gray produced in relation to depth are then displayed on a TV monitor from which the final film is generated. The image on the monitor is like a slice of tissue, which may be oriented in any direction, although transverse and longitudinal sections are usually obtained for comparison with the known and familiar normal anatomy of a body section. The ultrasonic "slice" on the TV monitor may be a static or fixed view, although newer electronics now allow a continuous or dynamic image, similar to that in x-ray fluoroscopy, allowing one to follow an action within the body. This is called real-time scanning. It permits movements within the body, such as the fetal heartbeat or tumbling of a heavy gallstone with various dependent positions to be observed.

Just as the amount of energy in x-rays that are transmitted through the patient to the x-ray film results in an image on the film, so in ultrasound does the amount of energy in sound waves that are returned or reflected back to the transducer head result in the image. Likewise too, the physical characteristics of the medium determine what percentage of an initial sound-wave beam is reflected back to the transducer to create the final image. The percentage of the initially transmitted wave that is reflected back depends

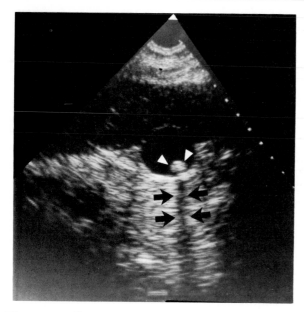

Fig. 1-19 Gallstone (arrowheads) with distal shadowing (arrows).

for example, there is a great difference in density between a gallstone and its surrounding soft tissues and the fluid bile. When a transmitted sound wave meets the gallstone amidst the soft tissues, a great deal of the sound is reflected back to the transducer from the interface of the two densities. The resulting image is an intense collection of echoes resulting in a "specular reflector" or bright collection of echos (Fig. 1-19). Since most of the initially transmitted sound waves are returned to the transducer, there are few waves left to penetrate the structures beyond the gallstone, thus preventing visualization of the deeper anatomy. This results in an absence of echoes posterior to the gallstone in the final image, and is called "shadowing," since the gallstones blocks or prevents further sound-wave transmission. Just as blocking the rays of the sun casts a shadow.

In situations in which the density difference between two tissues is less marked, a softer echo pattern results at their interface, and many sound waves continue to be transmitted, allowing visualization of the deeper structures. An example of this gentle echo collection occurs with the gallbladder wall. Which is more compact or slightly more dense than the soft tissues that are anterior to it. A soft line of echoes representing the wall is seen in the ultrasound image, since only a portion of the sound is reflected back to

on the difference in densities of the various tissue components within the body. A greater density difference between two adjacent tissues leads to more sound being reflected at their interface. Clinical examples can best demonstrate this principle. Thus,

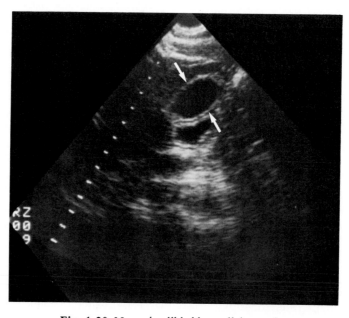

Fig. 1-20 Normal gallbladder wall (arrows).

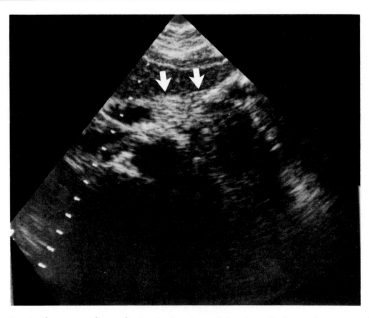

Fig. 1-21 Gas in the stomach results in shadowing of the dorsally located pancreas (arrows).

the transducer from the interface between the gallbladder wall and soft tissues. But since only a few echoes are reflected back, many sound waves are still available for deeper transmission, allowing the imaging of stuctures posterior to the gallbladder (Fig. 1-20).

In addition to being reflected and used in image formation, sound may be absorbed to different degrees by certain soft tissues. It is readily absorbed by fat, air or gas, and bone. When sound is absorbed by a tissue, there is no further transmission of the sound wave, and no visualization of the more distal anatomy. This total absorption of the sound wave produces a type of shadowing similar to the shadow of a specular reflector. A common example of absorption of the entire sound wave is by anteriorly situated bowel gas in studying the abdomen. The resultant shadowing creates a problem by preventing visualization of the posterior anatomy, such as the pancreas, as will be discussed later (Fig. 1-21).

Fluid-filled structures allow complete transmission or propagation of the sound wave, a unique characteristic of fluid that renders ultrasound very helpful in distinguishing between fluid-filled structures and those composed of solid tissues. The simple renal cyst is a good clinical example. The sound wave that initially enters the cyst is easily transmitted by the cyst fluid, with only minimal absorption or reflection. This results in a strong sound wave reaching the soft tissues behind the cyst, opposite the point of entry of the wave. The soft tissues posterior to the cyst are thus very echogenic in comparison to the more muted echos after they pass through the more solid renal tissue, which both reflects and absorbs some of the initial sound wave. In addition, the posterior wall of the cyst is well seen, since the fluid allows the unimpeded transmission of sound. This is called "back-wall enhancement." Being of a homogeneous density, with no interfaces to reflect any portion of the initial sound wave back to the transducer, the contents of a cyst demonstrates a complete absence of echoes, or are anechoic. Waves traveling through the renal parenchyma, on the other hand, meet many interfaces, resulting in the characteristic, gentle hypoechoic pattern typical of a solid organ. An anechoic pattern with back-wall enhancement and a strong posterior echo is unique to a fluid filled mass, and allows its differentiation from a solid mass. When the

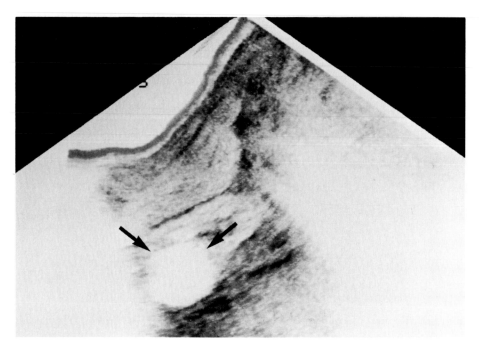

Fig. 1-22 Renal cyst (arrows).

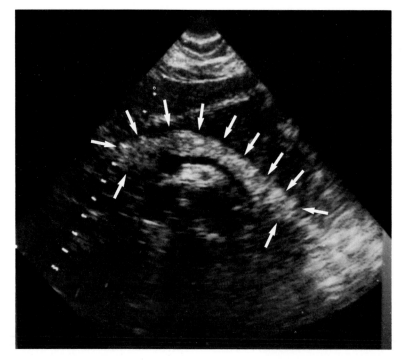

Fig. 1-23 Same patient as in Figure 1-21 after the administration of 3 cups of water. The pancreas is now well imaged (arrows).

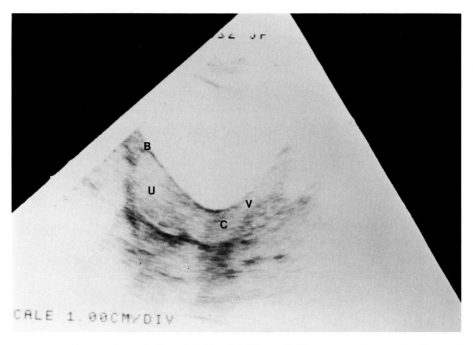

Fig. 1-24 Sagital view through the pelvis. B = bladder wall, U = uterus, C = cervix, V = vagina.

above criteria are strictly enforced, ultrasound becomes the diagnostic procedure of choice for fluid identification (Fig. 1-22).

The excellent transmission of sound through fluids can also be a mechanical aid for visualizing the deep anatomy of the abdomen and pelvis. In order to visualize the pancreas, it is often necessary to have the patient drink three cups of water in order to fill the stomach with fluid, displacing air and allowing a route for the transmission of sound waves to the retroperitoneal pancreas (Fig. 1-23). Another example is instructing a patient not to void for several hours before visualizing the deep anatomy of the pelvis (i.e., the ovaries and uterus). The fluid-filled bladder allows easy access of the sound waves to the pelvis and deeper structures (Fig. 1-24). The fluid-filled stomach or bladder is thus called a "sonic window," since it allows the clear visualization of deep anatomy that would otherwise be blocked.

The ability to identify solid structures — normal or abnormal — is based on their typical shape and location as well as on interfaces within them. For example, the normal kidney is comparatively a homogeneous organ with few macroscopic changes or interfaces within its parenchyma, and the resulting image is that of the familiar reniform shape, with gentle echoes or a hypoechoic pattern (Fig. 1-25). In contrast, the pancreas is a collection of macroscopic lobules separated by fibrous connective tissue and an extensive ductal system. Thus the pancreatic image is of a dense or hyperechoic organ in the familiar boomerang shape (Fig. 1-23). The liver is somewhat less homogeneous than the kidney, having a lobular configuration as well as an extensive ductal system. It is more homogeneous in density, with fewer interfaces than the neighboring pancreas. As a result, the liver is typically less "echogenic" (echo producing) than the pancreas but more echogenic than the neighboring right kidney (Fig. 1-26). The typical echo characteristics of an organ (hyper- or hypoechoic), in addition to its familiar shape (the reniform kidney or boomerang-shaped pancreas) and expected location, permit its easy identification.

Ultrasound may be used to detect diffuse disease as well as such a localized process as a mass. There may be a general alteration of the typical echo pattern that indicates a diffuse process involving a particular organ, and which may cause a reverse or flip-flop in

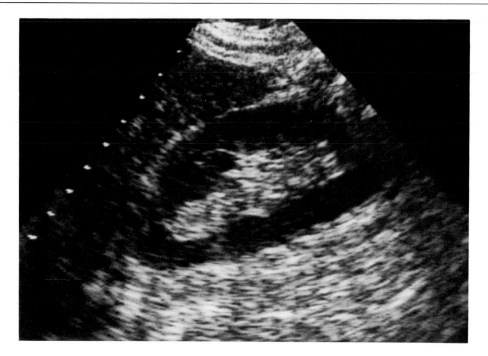

Fig. 1-25 Normal kidney.

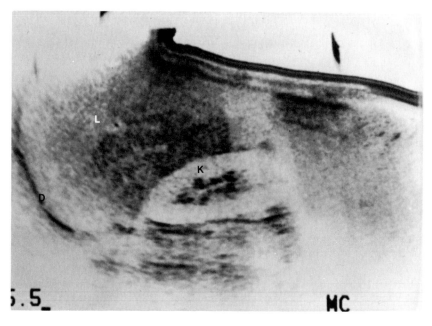

Fig. 1-26 Normal liver and right kidney relationship. L = liver, K = kidney, D = diaphragm.

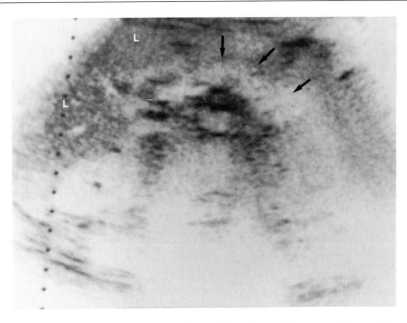

Fig. 1-27 Acute pancreatitis. The pancreas is now hypoechoic (arrows) in comparison to the normal liver (L).

the comparative echogenicity of two organs. For example, when infiltrated with the edema of acute pancreatitis, the pancreas may appear significantly less echogenic than the liver (Fig. 1-27). The edema-filled pancreas reflects back less sound because many of its interfaces are blunted by the inflammatory fluid. Another example is the abnormal hyperechogenicity of the fibrosed kidney of chronic renal failure. Here the fibrous replacement of the once relatively homogeneous renal parenchyma creates many new interfaces (Fig. 1-28). These interfaces produce more reflection of an initial sound wave, resulting in a kidney even more dense or echogenic than the usually denser neighboring liver. There has been a reverse in the relative echo density of the two organs from the normal situation, signifying a diffuse pathologic process in one of the two.

This same hyperechoic/hypoechoic behavior may be used to define a localized pathologic process as a mass. For instance, a collection of echoes is present in the upper pole of the kidney, which is different as compared to the normal, hypoechoic renal parenchyma (Fig. 1-29). The echo pattern of the normal kidney is clearly different from a localized hypoechoic mass — the typical finding in renal cell carcinoma. Additionally, a normally densely echogenic pancreas may show a focal collection of less dense echoes or a hypoechoic mass (Fig. 1-30), which is typical of a pancreatic carcinoma. Masses can also produce a combination of echo patterns. A combination anechoic/hypoechoic/hyperechoic pattern is called a complex pattern and is said to be produced by a complex mass. This typically occurs with an abscess containing areas of liquid necrosis resulting in fluid or anechoic regions. There are also areas of edema, which lead to hypoechogenicity, and dense capsules or dystrophic calcifications, leading to hyperechoic areas. An example of a complex mass is a renal carbuncle (Fig. 1-31).

The appearance of fluid in unsuspected locations can also signify a pathologic process. An example is ascites, which has the classic appearance of an anechoic collection in the dependent areas of the abdomen, such as the cul-de-sac or area between the right kidney and liver (Morrison's pouch) (Fig. 1-32). In the normal patient there is no fluid in these locations, and when even a small amount of ascitic fluid is present, it is easily detected by ultrasound.

In summary, it is the physical characteristics of the tissues being studied that produce an image in ultra-

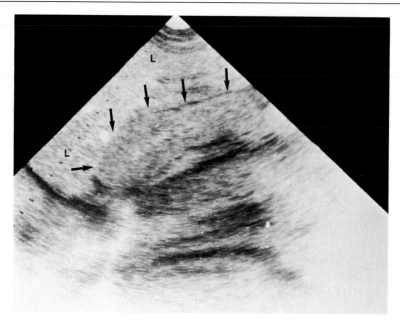

Fig. 1-28 Chronic renal failure. The kidney is now hyperechoic (arrows) in comparison to the normal liver (L).

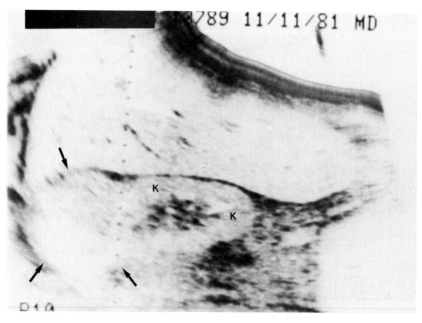

Fig. 1-29 Renal-cell carcinoma. Hypoechoic mass representing a renal-cell carcinoma (arrows) of the upper pole of the kidney (K).

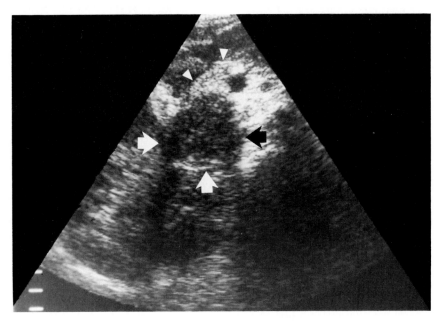

Fig. 1-30 Pancreatic carcinoma. Hypoechoic mass replacing the head of the pancreas (arrows). The normal pancreas is hyperechoic (arrowheads).

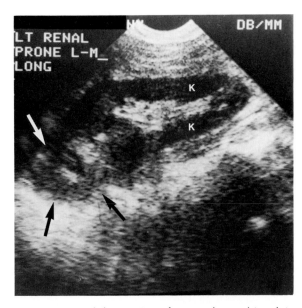

Fig. 1-31 Renal abscess. Complex mass (arrows) involving the upper pole of the left kidney (K).

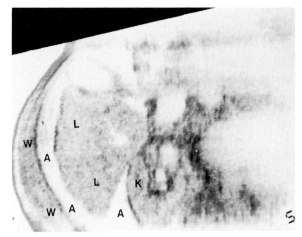

Fig. 1-32 Ascites. Massive amount of fluid (A) separates the liver (L) from the abdominal wall (W), and fluid is situated between the liver and the right kidney (K).

sound. The relative amount of sound reflected back to the transducer at the different interfaces versus the amount of the sound wave that is halted or absorbed by the tissues results in this image.

Because fluid-filled structures have no interfaces and transmit sound well, they demonstrate no echoes, with strong echoes being seen posterior to them. Occasionally, a solid structure is composed of very homogeneous material that may also give an anechoic echo pattern, but without the typical back wall enhancement, thus signifying a solid mass.

Fat, bone, and gas effectively absorb sound. These structures provide shadowing of the deep anatomy. The histologic homogeneity of a tissue determines its typical echo density. More homogeneous organs, like the kidney, generate fewer echoes and are referred to as hypoechoic. Less homogeneous organs with multiple tissue interfaces, like the pancreas, are hyperechoic.

Alterations in the normal echo relationships of adjacent organs, as well as the appearance of localized masses, signify pathologic processes. Careful attention and comparison of the adjacent anatomy are important in detecting disease in such cases.

Ultrasound can be a very sensitive but subtle imaging tool. The following table lists the disease processes in which it finds its major indications.

MAJOR INDICATIONS FOR ULTRASOUND EXAMINATION

I. Chest
  A. Pleural fluid
    1. Determination
    2. Thoracentesis
II. Cardiovascular
  A. Aorta
    1. Aneurysm
    2. Graft evaluation
  B. Echocardiography (not covered in this text)
III. Renal
  A. Mass
    1. Cyst
    2. Tumor
    3. Other (inflammatory)
    4. Follow up
  B. Hydronephrosis detection
  C. Nephrolithiasis
    1. Detection
    2. Follow up
  D. Cystic renal disease: Adult
  E. Biopsy localization
  F. Renal transplant evaluation
IV. Gastrointestinal
  A. Liver
    1. Mass
      a. Neoplasm
        1. Primary
          a. Malignant
          b. Benign
        2. Metastatic involvement
      b. Abscess
      c. Cyst
    2. Diffuse alteration-cirrhosis
  B. Pancreas
    1. Mass
      a. Solid (tumor)
      b. Fluid (pseudocyst)
    2. Pancreatitis
  C. Biliary system
    1. Cholylethiasis
    2. Ductal dilatation-jaundice
      a. Intrahepatic
      b. Extrahepatic
    3. Acute or chronic cholecystitis
    4. Carcinoma of the gallbladder
    5. Adenomyosis of the gallbladder
    6. Polyp of the gallbladder
  D. Spleen
    1. Size
    2. Trauma-infarction or hemorrhage
    3. Mass
      a. Neoplasm
      b. Cyst
V. Retroperitoneal
  A. Lymphadenopathy
VI. Pelvic
  A. Gynecologic diseases
    1. Uterus
      a. Mass-benign vs malignant
      b. IUD

(List continued.)

(List continued.)

c. Congenital anomalies
2. Ovary
   a. Mass-cystic disease or neoplastic disease
   b. Inflammatory — PID
3. Fallopian tubes
   a. Ectopic pregnancy
   b. Inflammatory
B. Obstetrics
   1. Ovarian follicle determination
   2. Fetal progress
   3. Fetal anomalies
   4. Amniocentesis
   5. Placenta evaluation
C. Ascites
D. Prostate size
E. Pelvic adenopathy
VII. General abdomen
   A. Ascites determination
   B. Abdominal wall pathology
      1. Mass
      2. Wound abscess
VIII. Genital
   A. Testicular
      1. Neoplasm
      2. Infection
      3. Varix
      4. Torsion
      5. Fluid collection
   B. Ovarian-see gynecological indication
IX. Extremity
   A. Vascular aneurysms
   B. Mass evaluation
      1. Solid
      2. Cystic
X. Neonatal-premature brain imaging

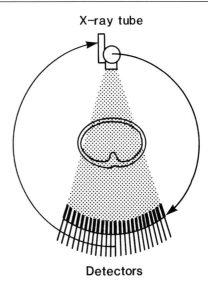

Fig. 1-33 Rotating x-ray tube within the CT gantry.

within the patient. The final image as viewed by the radiologist is derived from the computer integration of multiple exposures as an x-ray tube travels in a circle about the patient.

In modern CT scanners, this x-ray tube, like those discussed in the previous section, is mounted on a circular track, called the gantry, around an opening into which a patient is placed (Fig. 1-33). The patient lies in the gantry as the x-ray tube travels around him or her. The x-ray tube produces a series of short exposures as it changes its position along the gantry. The standard x-ray beam is shaped by the CT scanner to a specified thickness before being transmitted through the patient. In the standard x-ray tube the resulting beam fans out from the tube in a 360-degree arc, forming an imaginary cone of x-rays with the tube itself at the peak of the cone. In CT the x-ray beam is further shaped by two platelike devices that give the beam the shape of a flat fan. It is the width of this fan, as adjusted by changing the distance between these plates, that determines how thick a section of the patient will be imaged in the resulting tomographic scan.

The fan-shaped x-ray beam in CT has the same physics of tissue interaction as the ordinary x-ray. It encounters the tissues of the patient, with some being absorbed and some being transmitted through the patient. The x-rays that have passed through the patient do not expose the film directly as they do in conven-

COMPUTED TOMOGRAPHY

Computerized axial tomography, computed tomography, CAT scanning, or the now preferred CT scanning, are all terms for a computer generated tomographic image or slice through a region of interest

tional x-ray studies, but are instead projected onto very sensitive electronic detectors. These detectors are aligned directly opposite the x-ray tube, and the two devices move together in their circular paths around the gantry and patient. The detector receives all of the x-rays that pass through the patient from the rotating x-ray tube regardless of its position along the circular gantry.

The electronic detector then converts the transmitted x-ray pattern into electronic signals which are relayed to a computer for integration and subsequent formation of the tomographic slice or image. The computer constructs a tomographic image of the patient from these signals. It does this by dividing the gantry in which the patient lies into a grid-like pattern, as in graph paper, composed of a series of three-dimensional boxes. Each face of each box has a certain length and width as well as a predetermined depth (slice thickness). The two-dimensional face of the box, without depth, is called a pixel. The three dimensional unit or box is called a voxel. The depth of each box or thickness of each tomographic section is determined by the plates or collimators that form the

x-ray beam into its fan-like shape as it leaves the x-ray tube. By adjusting the collimators, from 0.15 to 2 cm of patient thickness can be imaged per slice. It is the dividing up of the patient into a series of voxels, and the recreation of this grid on the subsequent film that allows the orderly construction of the tomographic image (Fig. 1-34).

The tomographic image is formed by measuring the intensity of the transmitted radiation for each voxel in the grid after the x-ray tube has completed one rotation around the gantry. The computer then assigns a numerical value that represents the average density of that box of tissue. This averaging process is used because each box is made up of a variety of different types of tissue.

The density number that the computer assigns to each box or voxel runs on a scale from -1000 to $+1000$. The units used to represent the average tissue density are called CT numbers, and are measured in Hounsfield units (HU) after the inventor of the CT scanner. These values are based on a standard of water, which is assigned a CT number of 0. Accordingly, substances less dense than water are assigned a negative CT number. Air, for example, has a CT number of -1000. Conversely, structures that stop more x-rays than the equivalent thickness of water have a positive CT number. For example, bone may have a CT number up to $+1000$.

In summary, the computer divides the axial "slice" of the patient into a series of boxes with predetermined two- and three-dimensional measurements. By exposing these boxes to a series of x-rays about a circle or gantry, the computer then determines the average density for each box or voxel of tissue. It constructs an image by assigning an average density, or CT number, to similar locations on a reduced scale image of the gantry grid, oriented in the same way.

The initial CT image is thus a printout of a collection of numbers, each reflecting the relative density of the box of tissues that coincides with a specified location within the gantry and patient. Each voxel within the grid is then assigned a shade of gray according to its CT number, so as to produce the final image that the radiologist can interpret. Water, with its CT number of 0, is assigned a medium shade of gray. All voxels with negative CT numbers are assigned darker shades of gray that approach black the more negative their CT number becomes. All boxes with positive CT numbers are assigned lighter shades of gray than

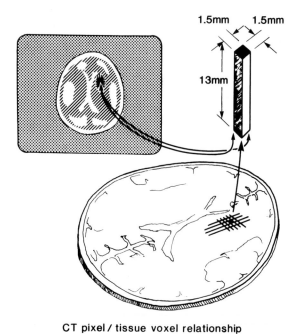

CT pixel / tissue voxel relationship

Fig. 1-34 Image construction using a grid format in CT.

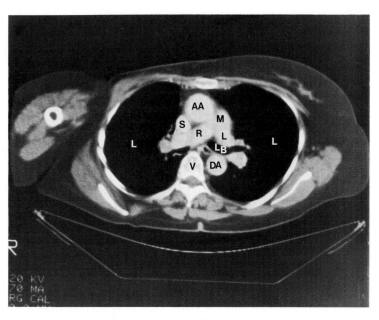

Fig. 1-35 Normal CT scan of the chest. White L = lung fields, AA = ascending aorta, DA = descending aorta, M = main pulmonary artery, R = right main pulmonary artery, black L = left main pulmonary artery, S = superior vena cava, LB = left mainstem bronchus, V = vertebral body.

water, and which approach white the more positive the CT number becomes. With computer assistance, an image has been formed that is an exact replica of a section of the patient.

Normal tissue and organ identification in the final CT image is possible on the basis of the typical CT number and its assigned shade of gray, as well as from the characteristic location and shape of the tissue. The lung is virtually a window that allows the nearly total transmission of all initial x-rays and has the lowest CT numbers, ranging from approximately -700 to -860 HU. The lungs thus appear black on the resulting image (Fig. 1-35). Fat stops less of the x-ray beam than water, but more than the aerated lungs, and has CT numbers ranging from 0 to -80 HU, depending on how much connective tissue lies within the fat. The fat is thus a darker gray than water but a lighter gray than the almost black lungs. Calcified or ossified structures have CT numbers well above 200 HU, and approach white in the resulting image. The organs of the abdomen have CT numbers ranging from 30 to 80 HU, and so are a lighter gray than water, fat, or the air-filled lungs (Fig. 1-36).

In order to diagnose a disease process, the radiologist looks for a number of different alterations. These include changes in the normal or typical CT number or density of an organ, changes in the normal relationships of the CT numbers of two organs, an abnormal mass, or an alteration or loss of normal anatomy. Examples of each of these alterations are given below.

When an organ is diffusely involved by a disease process, there may be a change in its normal density and resulting CT number. As noted earlier in the discussion of ultrasound, a section through the normal pancreas shows a thin, somewhat irregular, boomerang-shaped gland. In acute pancreatitis a fat, lumpy organ with a CT number well below what is normal for the pancreas (Fig. 1-37) is imaged. The pancreas is then said to be of lower attenuation (density) than in the normal state. This lower attenuation is secondary to the fluid infiltration in the edematous pancreas. To take another example, the normal liver has a characteristic density greater than the spleen and so appears as a lighter shade of gray than the spleen in the final CT image. In chronic alcoholism, however, there is often diffuse infiltration of the liver by fat.

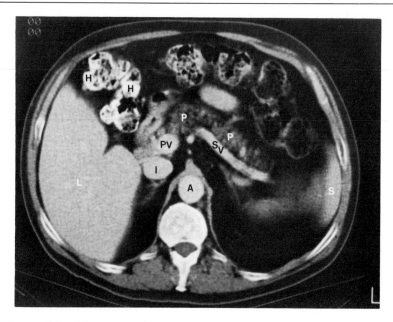

Fig. 1-36 Normal CT scan of the abdomen. L = liver, S = splenic tip, P = pancreas, H = barium in the hepatic flexure, A = aorta, SV = splenic vein, I = inferior vena cava, PV = portal vein.

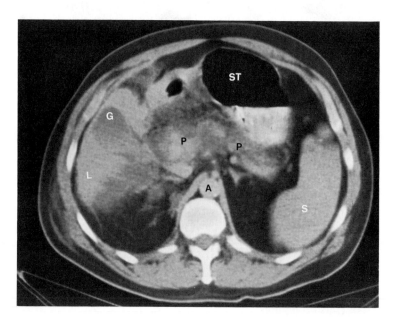

Fig. 1-37 Acute pancreatitis. P = edematous pancreas (arrowheads), L = liver, G = gallbladder, S = spleen, ST = stomach with air fluid level, A = aorta.

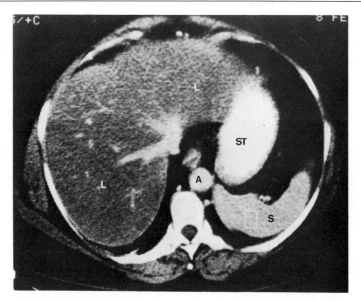

Fig. 1-38 Fatty infiltration of the liver. L = liver, S = spleen, ST = stomach filled with contrast medium, A = aorta.

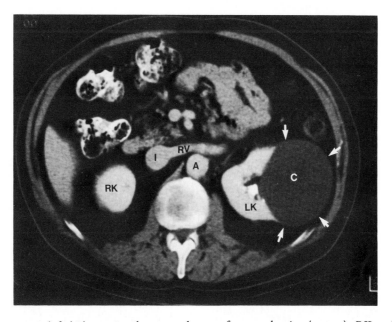

Fig. 1-39 Renal cyst. LK = left kidney, C = large renal cyst of water density (arrows), RK = tip of right kidney, A = aorta, I = inferior vena cava, RV = left renal vein entering inferior vena cava.

The liver then has an x-ray attenuation below that of the spleen and there is a reversal of the normal relationship of the densities of the two organs. The liver appears a darker gray than the spleen in the resulting image, reversing the usual situation (Fig. 1-38).

Computed tomography can also reveal an abnormal mass, and the CT number can give some clue to the nature of the tissue in the mass. In Figure 1-39, a section through the level of the kidneys demonstrate a mass projecting from the lateral boarder of the left

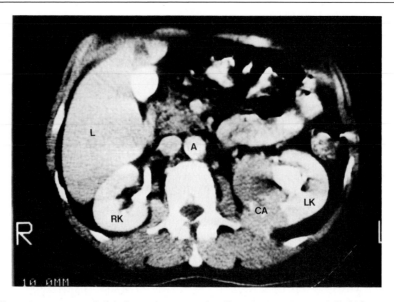

Fig. 1-40 Renal-cell carcinoma. LK = left kidney, CA = renal-cell carcinoma, RK = right kidney, L = liver, A = aorta.

kidney. When the CT number of the mass is measured it is found to be + 5, which is in the typical range for a structure of water density. The diagnosis is made of a simple renal cyst. In a different patient (Fig. 1-40) a mass is seen projecting from the left kidney. This has a CT number of + 40, which is consistent with solid tissue, and proved to be renal cell carcinoma.

Lastly, the alteration or loss of normal anatomy as a result of extra tissue accumulation also signifies an abnormal state. The aorta and inferior vena cava are typically clearly seen as two separate and discrete round structures lying anterior to the spine. In Figure 1-41A neither the aorta nor the inferior vena cava can be separated from the mass of surrounding soft tissue of the same density. The typical location and lobular appearance of this mass of tissue, which has a CT number consistent with soft tissue (+ 40 HU), indicates that it is a massive enlargement of the surrounding periaortic lymph nodes in a patient with lymphoma.

Contrast media are routinely used to better demonstrate normal and abnormal anatomy in CT images. Intravenous iodine-containing media or oral and rectal barium followed by a subsequent CT scan may aid the diagnostic process by making an abnormality more visible amidst the surrounding normal tissues or by better defining the normal tissue planes. Barium

suspensions and iodine-containing compounds are white on the CT image, as they are on a conventional direct x-ray film, in angiography, or intravenous pyelography (IVP). A section through the lymphoma patient shown in Figure 1-41A is again presented in Figure 1-41B, but this time after use of an intravenous contrast medium. The aorta appears as a separate vascular structure that can be differentiated from the surrounding mass of adenopathy. This differentiation of abnormal lymph nodes from vascular structures may be helpful if a biopsy is planned. The displacement of larger normal vessels by a mass in the abdomen or head may also indicate a disease process, and can be appreciated only after an intravenous contrast medium has been administered.

An intravenous contrast medium may also help the better identification of a tumor mass that is not clearly seen on unenhanced precontrast views. The normal parenchyma of an organ takes on a higher CT number after an iodinated intravenous contrast medium is given, since it is perfused by blood that contains the medium. Thus, normal liver appears more white in such views. If a tumor is very vascular it may enhance even more than the surrounding normal liver parenchyma making its detection easier. A richly vascular hemangioma is a good example of such a tumor (Fig. 1-42). If the tumor is of scant vascularity, as with liver

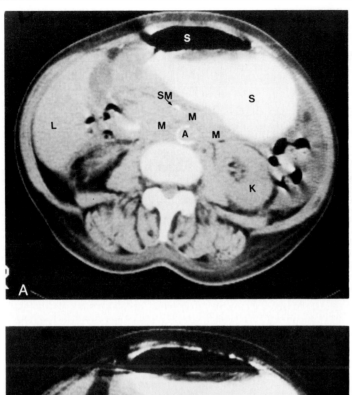

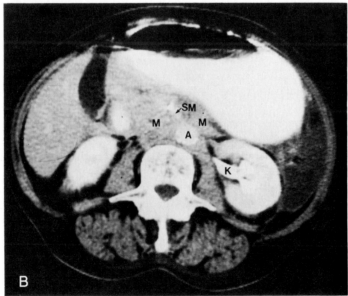

Fig. 1-41(A) Precontrast CT image, periaortic adenopathy in lymphoma. M = Soft-tissue mass of adenopathy, A = calcification within the wall of the aorta, K = left kidney, L = liver, S = stomach, SM = calcification within the wall of the superior mesenteric artery (arrow). **(B)** Postcontrast CT image, periaortic adenopathy in lymphoma. A = opacified aorta, K = contrast-medium-filled collecting system of left kidney, SM = opacified superior mesenteric density (arrow), M = adenopathy.

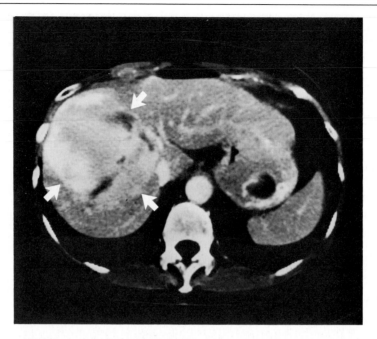

Fig. 1-42 Hemangioma. Brightly opacified portion of a vascular hemangioma (arrows) in comparison to the normal liver.

metastases from a colon carcinoma, it has a considerably lower attenuation than the normally enhancing liver parenchyma and is clearly seen after a contrast (Fig. 1-43A) medium is given, whereas on precontrast views it almost blends with the remainder of the liver (Fig. 1-43B).

Redundant loops of small bowel and colon in the abdomen can cause a great deal of confusion since they can appear as large masses of undifferentiated tissue and obscure the normal anatomy. To avoid this problem, the patient routinely is given a solution of dilute barium to drink, or an iodinated meal that appears white in the subsequent CT image. The contrast medium outlines the stomach, small bowel, and colon and allows the distinction of these normal structures and their differentiation from an abnormal mass (Fig. 1-36).

An artifact may be the greatest technical problem during the CT examination. These arise either from patient motion or high-density foreign materials. Patient motion has a devastating effect on image quality. This results mainly with the patient who cannot hold his or her breath. The time for the x-ray tube to complete one rotation around the gantry, to produce one tomographic slice, must be as short as possible so as to reduce the chance of patient breathing. The minimum time needed for one complete rotation of the x-ray tube in order to produce one tomographic section is 2 seconds. The image resulting from patient motion shows a distorted series of black and white vertical bands in all orientations, and reveals little or no diagnostic information. The density of surgical clips, bullet fragments, hip prostheses, and retained barium is considerably higher than that of any body tissue, including bone. These extremely high-density materials cause a star pattern, with its center based around the offending foreign body, and interferes with diagnosis by producing a severely distorted image (Fig. 1-44).

The machines used in CT have made many technologic advancements since their introduction. Todays CT scanners can achieve slice thicknesses as small as 0.5 mm. The thinner the slice that is imaged, the better is the resolution and sharpness of the image. The radiation dose with a complete CT examination is also the same as or lower than with conventional radiologic procedures.

The advantages of CT result from its ability to project and differentiate the soft tissues in a way not possible with standard x-ray film exposures. It can

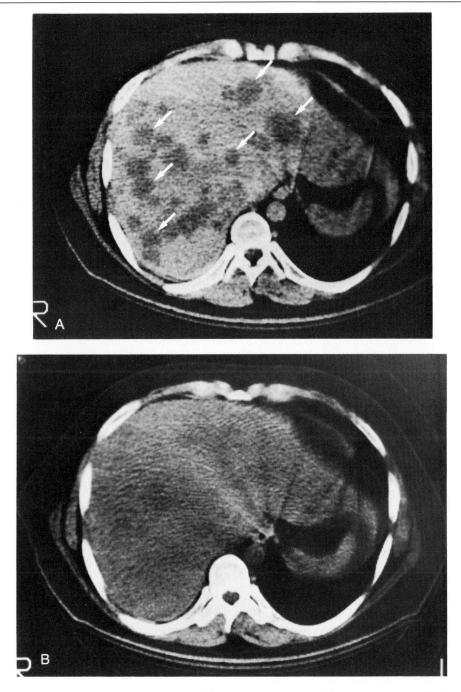

Fig. 1-43 Liver metastasis from colon carcinoma. **(A)** Postcontrast view of the same patient with the metastasis not enhancing significantly (arrows) as compared to the enhancing liver parenchyma. **(B)** Precontrast view of the abdomen.

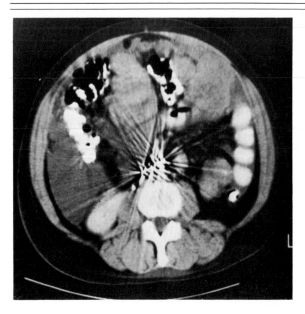

Fig. 1-44 Star artifact from surgical clips within the abdomen.

easily differentiate individual organs and tissue components, accomplishing this by revealing extremely subtle differences in tissue density. The following table lists the disease processes in which CT finds its major indications.

MAJOR INDICATIONS FOR CT
EXAMINATION

I. Head
  A. Cerebrovascular diseases
    1. Cerebral infarction
    2. Intracranial hemorrhage
    3. Trauma–subdural/epidural hematoma
  B. Intracranial tumors
  C. Hydrocephalus detection
  D. Inflammatory lesions
  E. Degenerative diseases of the CNS
    1. Brain atrophy
    2. Multiple sclerosis
    3. Postoperative or post-traumatic porencephaly

    4. Congenital hypoplasia
II. Spinal canal
  A. Herniated disk
  B. Spinal cord tumors
  C. Congenital anomalies
  D. Bony abnormalities
    1. Posterior articular degenerative disease
    2. Spinal stenosis
  E. Spinal trauma
III. Larynx
  A. Carcinoma
    1. Preoperative
    2. Recurrence
  B. Trauma
IV. Chest and mediastinum
  A. Neoplasms of the lung
    1. Primary
      a. Malignant
      b. Benign
    2. Metastases
  B. Mediastinal widening
    1. Vascular
    2. Neoplasm
    3. Lymph nodes
    4. Fat
  C. Detection of occult disease
    1. Thymoma-myasthenia gravis
    2. Lymph nodes
V. Cardiovascular
  A. Aortic dissection
  B. Aortic aneurysms
  C. Venous obstruction/thrombosis
VI. Renal
  A. Mass
    1. Neoplasm
      a. Malignant
      b. Benign
    2. Cyst
    3. Inflammatory/abscess
  B. Cystic renal disease
    1. Polycystic disease: Adult
  C. Perirenal extension
    1. Inflammatory
    2. Hemorrhage
    3. Post transplant

(List continued.)   *(List continued.)*

VII. Gastrointestinal
  A. Liver
    1. Mass
      a. Primary neoplasm
        1. Malignant
        2. Benign
      b. Metastatic involvement
      c. Abscess
      d. Cyst
  B. Pancreas
    1. Mass
      a. Neoplasm
        1. Malignant
        2. Benign
      b. Pseudocyst
    2. Pancreatitis
    3. Biopsy guidance
  C. Spleen
    1. Trauma
VIII. Adrenal
  A. Neoplasm
    1. Primary
      a. Malignant
      b. Benign
    2. Metastatic
  B. Bilateral enlargement—
     hyperplasia
IX. Retroperitoneal
  A. Lymphadenopathy
  B. Neoplasm
    1. Primary
    2. Secondary spread
  C. Extension of inflammatory process
    1. Pancreas
    2. Kidney
X. Pelvis
  A. Bladder malignancy
    1. Intrinsic
    2. Perivesical extension
  B. Prostate carcinoma—extension
  C. Pelvic lymphadenopathy
  D. Gynecologic tumor—extension
  E. Bony trauma
XI. General abdomen
  A. Tumor staging

  B. Peritoneal mass
    1. Abscess
    2. Cyst
    3. Neoplasm
XII. Musculoskeletal
  A. Tumor
    1. Malignant
    2. Benign
  B. Soft tissue mass
  C. Complex musculoskeletal anatomy
    1. Pelvis
    2. Shoulder girdle
    3. Sternum
    4. Sternoclavicular joints
    5. Accessory vertebral joints
  D. Trauma

NUCLEAR MEDICINE

The accelerated growth of nuclear medicine in the practice of diagnostic imaging has been based on the use of new radioactive pharmaceuticals that are injected into a patient's blood stream and localized to the different areas of interest. Gamma rays are emitted as the nuclei of the radioactive or excited elements in these pharmaceuticals revert to a stable ground configuration. The emission signal is detected by a new technology of receiving devices or cameras linked with computers. This combination of components allows a new flexibility and accuracy not previously possible in nuclear medicine.

A radioactive pharmaceutical contains two components: a radioactive element which is bound to a physiologic element. The nuclei of the radioactive element exist temporarily in an excited state for a finite time, which makes them useful for medical imaging; the element is called a metastable element. The feasibility of a radioactive element for medical use is based on how long its excited nuclei remain in their excited state. The time it takes for half of the atoms to revert to their stable configuration, or in other words, for the radioactivity of the element to reach half its original value, is called the half life. The radioactive elements used for clinical evaluation should have half lives long

(*List continued.*)

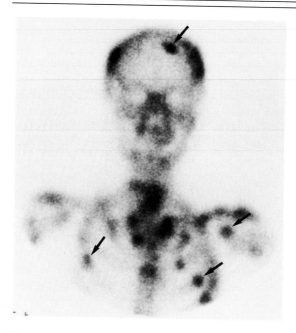

Fig. 1-47 Hot spot. Multiple metastasis to the bony skeleton (arrows) from breast carcinoma.

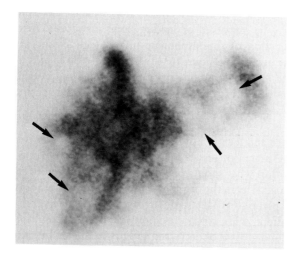

Fig. 1-48 Cold spot. Multiple metastasis to the liver (arrows) from breast carcinoma.

may yield a definitive diagnosis when combined with the patient's history.

Besides image formation, nuclear medicine studies also have the unique ability to give dynamic information about the blood supply to an organ as well as data on the functional state of the system in question. This is accomplished by linking the detecting gamma camera with a computer that can quickly collect, process, and integrate incoming signals. The computer, with its rapid processing, allows the flow of activity to be followed from the site of venous injection of the radiopharmaceutical to the right side of the heart and eventually to the aorta and various larger systemic arteries of the abdomen, extremities, or even the brain. This gives information similar to that in an angiogram. The flow studies provide gross information on vessel patency and can give quantitative information on the relative percentage of blood flow to an organ or even to part of an organ. Functional analysis also involves rapid computer processing to measure the arrival of radioactivity at a specified area, the time it takes for a given amount of activity to reach maximum levels, and the rapidity in which the activity is cleared.

An example of a nuclear medicine study of blood flow as well as organ function involves using technetium linked with dimercaptosuccinic acid (^{99m}Tc DMSA) and ^{131}I hippuran in studying the kidney. The first computer-generated images are of the angiographic flow, following the radiopharmaceutical as it progresses down the aorta to reach the renal arteries. In a normal patient, there is virtually instantaneous and symmetric renal artery visualization as the activity reaches the abdominal aorta (Fig. 1-49). Any delay in renal visualization or asymmetry in the distribution of renal flow signifies a renal artery lesion. A quantitative measurement of the blood flow symmetry can also be made to assess how much of the total flow goes to each kidney. The degree of asymmetry of the flow is given as a percentage of the total radioactivity in both kidneys. Information on the function of the kidney is available with ^{131}I hippuran. The initial arrival of activity in the kidney, the peak activity within the kidney, and its subsequent clearance are plotted on a graph in relation to time. The resulting curve, called a renogram, has a typical appearance in normal patients (see Fig. 3-6C). Any alteration from this normal curve can signal functional compromise. Not only can a diagnosis be made with this unique functional information, but the clinician can also follow the effects of medical therapy and predict subsequent problems. Functional studies can, for example, predict impending renal-transplant graft rejection before any chemical abnormalities or clinical symptoms appear.

Nuclear medical studies are very sensitive and can often find pathology before any other conventional radiographic methods. Their major drawback is their lack of specificity, since many abnormalities are not unique in appearance but are imaged simply as areas of increased or decreased activity. However, the history or clinical presentation and correlation with other radiographic study data often allows a specific and accurate diagnosis.

Among the new horizons in nuclear medical technology are positron scanning. This modality also depends on gamma ray detection, but the gamma rays are generated from different radioactive tracers than those previously discussed. Positron scanning may find use because it allows tomographic views of an organ or system. This allows sectional views similar to CT slices, thereby increasing the sensitivity and perhaps the specificity of diagnosis. The following list gives the major current indications for nuclear medical imaging.

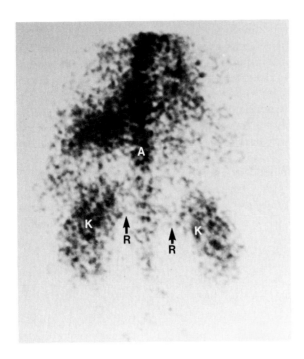

Fig. 1-49 Normal aortic angiogram in nuclear medicine. A = aortic activity, R = renal artery activity (arrows), K = kidneys.

MAJOR INDICATIONS FOR NUCLEAR MEDICINE EXAMINATIONS

I. Central nervous system
  A. Communicating hydrocephalus (indium-111)
  B. Brain (technetium-99m-glucoheptonate): Few present indications
II. Thyroid (pertechnetate or iodine-123/131)
  A. Hyperparathyroidism
    1. Graves' disease
    2. Adenoma
  B. Goiter
  C. Thyroid mass
    1. Neoplastic disease
      a. Benign
      b. Malignant
  D. Metastatic detection of known thyroid carcinoma (^{131}I)
    1. Distant—bone
    2. Local extension
  E. Therapy (^{131}I)
    1. Hyperparathyroidism
    2. Neoplastic suppression
III. Chest
  A. Detection of Pulmonary emboli
    1. Ventilation (Xenon-133)
    2. Perfusion (technetium-99m-macroaggregated albumin)
  B. Asymmetric perfusion of the two sides of the chest in pulmonary disease (^{99m}Tc-MAA)
  C. Mediastinal mass—substernal thyroid (^{123}I or pertechnetate)
IV. Cardiovascular
  A. Ischemic heart disease: Thallium stress test (thallium-201 chloride)
  B. Myocardial infarction detection (^{99m}Tc-pyrophosphate)
  C. Cardiac-wall movement abnormalities and cardiac output—gated studies (^{99m}TC-labeled RBCs)
  D. Quantitation of right-to-left cardiac shunts (^{99m}Tc-MAA)
V. Renal (^{99m}TC-dimercaptosuccinic acid and ^{131}I-orthoiodo hippuran)
  A. Renovascular hypertension

(List continued.)

B. Renal function
C. Transplant
D. Obstructive uropathy
VI. Gastrointestinal
   A. Liver/spleen (^{99m}Tc-sulfur colloid)
      1. Metastasis
      2. Diffuse alterations — cirrhosis
      3. Identifying ectopic splenic tissue
      4. Trauma
   B. Hepatobiliary imaging (^{99m}Tc-hepatobiliary iminodiacetic acid)
   C. Gastrointestinal bleeding
      1. Active (^{99m}Tc-sulfur colloid)
      2. Intermittent (^{99m}Tc-labeled RBCs)
   D. Schilling test — pernicious anemia
      1. Cobalt 58 + vitamin B12
      2. Cobalt 57 + vitamin B12 intrinsic factor
IV. General abdomen (gallium-67 citrate)
   A. Abscess
      1. Unknown location
      2. Extent or response to therapy
   B. Malignancy
      1. Unknown location of primary
      2. Extent/staging (e.g., lymphoma)
VIII. Genital (^{99m}Tc-pertechnetate)
   A. Testicular torsion
IX. Musculoskeletal (^{99m}Tc-methylene dysphosphonate)
   A. Bony metastasis
   B. Osteomyelitis
   C. Tumor extension of known bone tumor
   D. Metabolic bone disorders

MAGNETIC RESONANCE

The physics of magnetic resonance imaging (MR) is very involved and will not be presented in detail. Of more importance in this introductory text is a discussion on the benefits that MR offers over other currently available imaging modalities, its present uses, and its clinical potential for the future. The images produced in MR are generated by the radio waves that protons emit when they realign with a strong external magnetic field (Fig. 1-50). The images obtained in MR are comparable in appearance to CT images, showing a tomographic slice through the patient's head or body. They are of high resolution, like CT images, but unlike CT, MR causes no known adverse biologic effects from its magnetic field, since there is no ionizing radiation.[1]

There are many benefits of MR over CT, including multiplane image formation, excellent vascular visualization, and unique information on metabolic processes in the body. With MR a direct image can be obtained in any plane through the patient while maintaining excellent resolution. If a sagittal or coronal view is desired in CT, it must be secondarily constructed by the computer, and is thus often poor and confusing. By comparison, MR gives direct sagittal and coronal images without additional computer manipulation and reconstruction (Fig. 1-51). The image is sharp and clear and available in any plane specified by the radiologist. Blood is in constant movement and so gives a weak MR signal. In one MR format vessels and CSF spaces appear black and are clearly visualized through the surrounding soft tissues, which give a strong signal and are white. There exists a natural contrast between the two structures, and therefore is no need for administering contrast agents such as are required in CT or angiography for vascular visualization. The sharply contrasted black

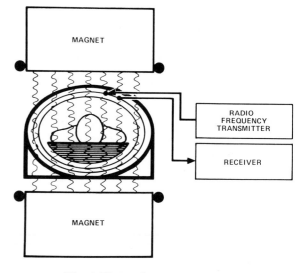

Fig. 1-50 Mechanism used in MR.

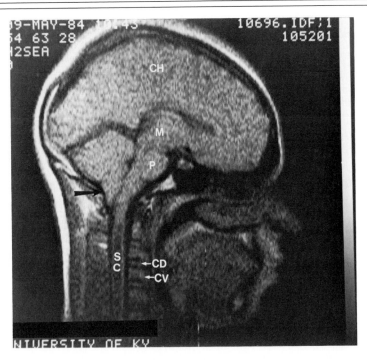

Fig. 1-51 Sagittal view of the brain in a young patient with a congenital anomaly of the cerebellum (arrow) and hydromyelia on MRI. CH = cerebral hemisphere, M = midbrain, P = pons, SC = spinal cord (dilated central canal). CV = cervical vertebral body, CD = cervical vertebral disk.

vessels and surrounding soft tissues, in combination with complete freedom in choosing the plane of section, allows noninvasive angiography.[2] The images in MR can be manipulated, reversing this black white relationship to allow information on diseased tissue. The ability of MR to provide metabolic information about normal and diseased tissue is still under intense investigation, and this technique may be able to reveal diseased tissue earlier than is now possible.[3]

The greatest application of MR has been to the central nervous system. In the brain, MR is extremely sensitive to alterations of normal tissue and may allow for earlier as well as more specific diagnosis of intracranial neoplasms (benign versus malignant) than with CT.[4] It yields good images of the posterior fossae without the artifact from the surrounding bony calvarium that is frequently seen in CT scans. Additionally, MR is useful in the detection and follow-up of demyelinating diseases. It offers the unique opportunity to directly visualize the spinal cord without the need for intrathecal contrast agents, which are needed in both CT and myelography. As a result, MR can directly show a spinal tumor or the dilated central canal in hydromyelia (Fig. 1-51). However, it has not proven useful in the evaluation of herniated disks, since it cannot adequately reveal the neural foramina or lateral recesses to show nerve-root compromise, even though the disk material itself is well imaged. Potentially, MR may find a place in the evaluation of spinal trauma and disk-space infection.

One promise of MR is in breast imaging. Here MR demonstrates a sensitivity that may be equivalent to that of mammography, but without ionizing radiation. It allows a distinction between benign and malignant processes, but cannot show the microcalcifications so typical of malignant disease, and which are the hallmarks of diagnosis in conventional mammography.[5]

Another area in which MR is proving valuable is in defining the anatomy and physiology of the cardiovascular system. It not only lacks the secondary effects of radiation and contrast media in CT and angiography, but also does not have the morbidity and mortality associated with invasive procedures such as cardiac catheterization. With MR one can clearly define such vascular pathology as an aortic aneurysm, aortic dissection, arteriovenous malformation, arterial occlusion or stenosis, atherosclerotic plaque, or the effects of tumor on adjacent vascular structures.[6] In the heart, MR with special linking to the ECG demonstrates thinning of the left ventricular wall after a myocardial infarction, left ventricular aneurysms and mural thrombi, septal hypertrophy in hypertrophic cardiomyopathy, and pericardial constriction, inflammation, and effusion.[7] It is also useful in measuring cardiac output.

The role of MR in the mediastinum is presently as an alternative to conventional tomography and CT.[8] It finds use in the differentiation of a solid mass from an abnormal or tortuous vascular mass or structure, and may also aid in characterization of the tissue-type of a tumor. Beyond this, MR is valuable for serial studies to determine a tumor's response to therapy, since radiation dose is not a factor and the study can be repeated as many times as needed without secondary adverse biologic effects.

Examination of the abdomen with MR is of only limited value at present owing to the problems of respiratory motion, cardiac motion, and bowel peristalsis. The liver and the pancreas have received the most attention. Hepatic neoplasms are easily detected, but MR has unfortunately not proved helpful in differentiating primary from metastatic neoplastic processes. Metabolic alterations of the liver, such as in cirrhosis, are well studied with MR through the metabolic data it provides. Pancreatitis and pancreatic neoplasms are also well imaged.[9]

In the pelvis, the resolving power of MR is now considered superior to that of CT. There is an abundance of fat in the retroperitoneum and pelvis that results in superb delineation of the tissue planes. The white-appearing fat is another example of MR making use of the body's natural contrast in image formation, as previously demonstrated in the vascular visualization it permits. In addition, the often complex anatomy of the pelvis is more clearly appreciated from the ability of MR to generate images in multiple planes, transverse or sagittal. The technique provides excellent views and information on the extent of neoplastic processes in the bladder, prostate, and uterus. In CT, surgical clips are frequently a problem in the

pelvis, giving a star artifact when one is trying to evaluate for recurrent tumor after radical cancer surgery. These clips produce no artifact in MR, making it useful in the follow-up of these patients.[10] Additionally, MR holds potential for clinical management in obstetrics and gynecology, since it defines the changes in the endometrium during the various phases of the menstrual cycle and pregnancy.

This brief overview of the current applications and clinical potential of MR introduces an exciting new modality in diagnostic imaging. It will take continued research and further technologic development to help realize the full potential of this new method.

REFERENCES

1. Partain CL, Price RR, Patton JA: Nuclear magnetic resonance imaging. Radiographics 4:5–10, 1984
2. Partain CL, Price RR, Patton JA: Nuclear magnetic resonance imaging. Radiographics 4:5, 1984
3. Higgins CB, Lanzer P, Stark D: Nuclear magnetic resonance imaging of the cardiovascular system. Radiographics 4:122, 1984
4. Partain CL, Price RR, Patton JA: Nuclear magnetic resonance imaging. Radiographics 4:5, 1984
5. Margulis AR: Current status of clinical magnetic resonance imaging. Radiographics 4:76, 1984
6. Yousef, SJ, Duchesneau RH, Alfidi RJ: Nuclear magnetic resonance imaging of the human breast. Radiographics 4:121, 1984
7. Herfkens RJ, Higgins CB, Hricak H, et al: Nuclear magnetic resonance imaging of the cardiovascular system. Normal and pathologic findings. Radiology 148:161–166, 1983
8. Higgins CB, Lanzer P, Stark D: Nuclear magnetic resonance imaging of the cardiovascular system. Radiographics 4:123, 1984
9. Berquist TH, Brown LR: Nuclear magnetic resonance imaging of the hilum and mediastinum. A comparison with CT and hilar tomography. Radiographics 4:155, 1984
10. Davis PL, Moss, AA, Goldberg HJ, et al: Nuclear magnetic resonance imaging of the liver and pancreas. Radiographics 4:159–169, 1984
11. Hricak H, Alpers C, Crook LE, et al: Magnetic resonance imaging of the female pelvis: Initial experience. AJR 141:1119–1128, 1983

2

Radiology of the Chest

Lee Sider

The standard chest x-ray remains the initial and often the most valuable method of investigating the chest. It is often obtained for routine screening reasons (preoperative, annual physical examination) as well as for the evaluation of suspected pulmonary or cardiovascular pathology. The standard examination consists of a frontal and lateral view of the chest.

The frontal film is obtained with the patient's chest placed against the x-ray film. The beam from the x-ray tube is directed first through the patient's back and travels anteriorly through the body to expose the film. The beam is said to travel posterior to anterior, and the resulting image is referred to as a PA view of the chest. It gives the most undistorted view of the heart and chest. Other methods of obtaining a frontal view are available when the standard positioning is not possible. The portable chest x-ray of the patient restricted to an intensive care bed is an example of such a method. Here a portably mounted x-ray tube is placed in front of the patient while the film is wedged between the patient's back and the bed. The resulting image is an anterior-to-posterior or AP view of the chest.

The anatomy seen in the frontal chest film is easy to understand (Fig. 2-1). The lungs appear as black spaces between the white ribs. Only the pulmonary arteries, veins, and bronchi are seen to course through the otherwise empty lung fields. The hila are the prominent soft-tissue shadows along the medial walls of the lung fields. The main left and right pulmonary arteries and veins are responsible for most of the density of the normal hila, and the peripheral pulmonary vessels can be followed back to their origin and termination in the hila.

The mediastinum comprises the centrally located soft tissues of the chest that lie between the left and right lung fields. The contour of the mediastinum is shaped by its anatomy. The left mediastinal border is potentially formed by four consecutive "bumps" (Fig. 2-2). The superiormost bump or prominence is from

39

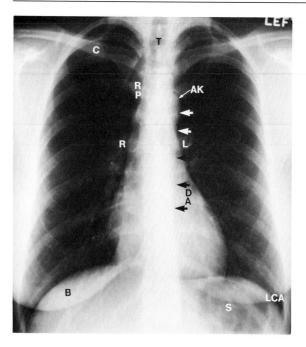

Fig. 2-1 Normal PA view of the chest. T = trachea, R = right hilum, L = left hilum, AK = aortic knob, RP = right paratracheal region (superior vena cava), DA = descending aorta (arrows), LCA = lateral costophrenic angle, C = clavicle, S = stomach bubble, B = breast shadow.

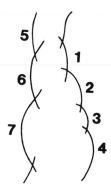

Fig. 2-2 Mediastinal anatomy. (1) Aortic knob, (2) main pulmonary artery, (3) left atrium, (4) left ventricle, (5) superior vena cava, (6) ascending aorta, (7) right atrium.

the aortic knob as the aorta changes from its ascending to a descending course. The next inferior prominence is from the main pulmonary artery as it arises from the right ventricle and before it divides into the right and left pulmonary arteries. It may both cast a prominent shadow or appear virtually nonexistent in a normal chest x-ray. The third bump is a shadow from the left atrial appendage. It is usually inapparent in the normal individual, and often gives a concave border to this portion of the left mediastinal border. The last and most prominent of the bumps is the shadow from the left ventricle. This inferiormost shadow assumes a variety of shapes and projects well into the left lung field, obscuring portions of the left lower lung from view.[1]

The right mediastinal border is made up of three potential prominences. The superiormost prominence is from the superior vena cava as it heads caudally to join with the right atrium. This bump is smooth and often concave in its contour. The shadow inferior to this is from the initial ascending portion of the aorta just after it emerges from the left ventricle.

In the normal situation it forms a gentle arc that can be traced in a continuous curve to join the left-sided aortic knob. Its predominance depends on the age of the patient (it is often dilated and tortuous in old age) as well as in diseases of the aortic valve. The inferiormost shadow is from the right atrium and forms the right heart border. It is considerably smaller than the prominent left venticle which forms the left heart border on the frontal chest film.[1] The left atrium and right ventricle are centrally located chambers that do not form a mediastinal border on the frontal film. These two chambers of the heart are better appreciated on the lateral film (see Fig. 6-1 and 6-2).

The superiormost portion of the mediastinum is occupied by the great vessels, i.e., the carotid and brachiocephalic arteries. Normally, the superior mediastinum casts a thin and straight shadow, but later in life its borders become increasingly wide and undulating as these vessels become ectatic or tortuous. The tortuous arteries extend the soft-tissue shadow laterally (Fig. 2-3).

The descending portion of the aorta can be followed as it courses inferiorly in the left and posterior portion of the chest. In younger patients it hugs the spine and courses in a straight line. Again, age causes this vessel to become tortuous, leading to a wavy and often undulating shadow of the descending aorta seen behind the heart (Fig. 2-3).

Information about the bony structures of the chest can also be obtained from the frontal chest film. The exposure techniques needed to optimally study the lung and mediastinum do not allow clear bone detail, but gross information is obtainable. The ribs, clavi-

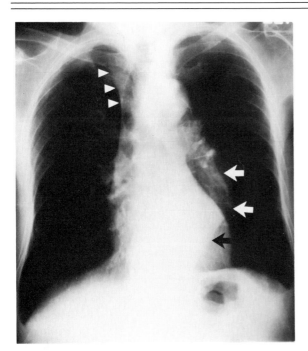

Fig. 2-3 Tortuous aorta.
History: This 78-year-old man had a long history of hypertension.
Findings: *Chest radiograph:* The superior portion of the mediastinum is widened by tortuous great vessels (arrowheads). The aorta is elongated and bows into the left side of the chest (arrows).

cles, vertebral bodies, and often the scapula and proximal humerus are included in the chest film. They can be evaluated for destructive processes, fractures, congenital deformities, postsurgical changes, and degenerative disease.

The diaphragms are the arced muscular structures that define the lower extent of the lung fields. They curve both medially and laterally, resulting in the cardiophrenic and costophrenic angles, respectively. They also curve anteriorly and posteriorly, as seen on the lateral film, to give the anterior and posterior costophrenic angles.

The lateral film helps confirm and locate a pathologic process suspected on the frontal film. The hilar anatomy is well demonstrated on the lateral film, allowing the two-dimensional view when it is combined with the frontal film. As seen on the lateral film, the hila are somewhat confusing, but familiarity with their normal appearance is helpful in confirming mediastinal adenopathy or masses (Fig. 2-4). In the lat-

eral film the right pulmonary artery and vein are anterior to the left-sided vessels. The right upper-lobe bronchus lies more superiorly than the left. An extra soft-tissue density may represent enlarged lymph nodes or another mass involving the hila.

The view of the heart on the lateral film finds the centrally located right ventricle and left atrium to be in profile. The right ventricle is anterior to the left atrium and just behind the sternum. Again, the lateral film, along with the frontal film, allows a two-dimensional view of the heart in evaluating the size of the heart's chambers.

The ascending aorta, aortic arch, and descending aorta are clearly visualized on the lateral film. The inferior vena cava casts a shadow near the diaphragm as it courses superiorly from the abdomen to join the right atrium. The thoracic spine is also clearly seen in the lateral view, and compression fractures or degen-

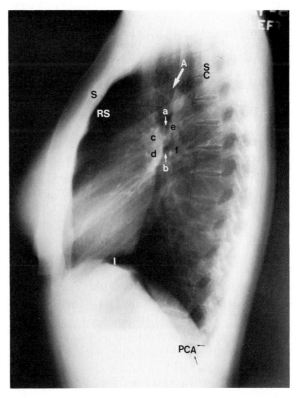

Fig. 2-4 Normal lateral view of the chest. (a) Right upper-lobe bronchus, (b) left upper-lobe bronchus, (c) right pulmonary artery, (d) right pulmonary veins, (e) left pulmonary artery, (f) left pulmonary veins. I = inferior vena cava, A = aortic arch, RS = retrosternal space; PCA = posterior costophrenic angle, S = sternum, SC = scapula.

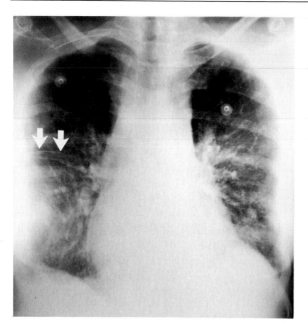 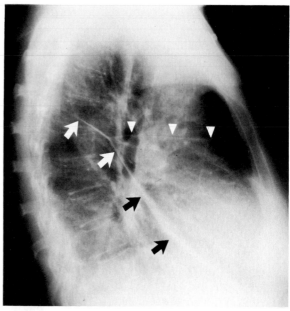

Fig. 2-5 Location of the right minor fissure. This was a 67-year-old female in congestive heart failure, with fluid trapped in the minor fissure on the frontal film (arrows).

Fig. 2-6 Location of the right minor and major fissures. This was the same patient as in Figure 2-5, with fluid trapped in both the minor fissure (arrowheads) and major fissure (arrows).

erative changes in this structure are easily demonstrated. The lateral view also results in perhaps the best view of the sternum as seen in profile.

The lungs are anatomically divided into a series of lobes defined by the major and minor fissures, which are formed by folds of the pleura. Fibrous septae that contain both peripheral pulmonary vessels and lymphatics further divide the lobes into segments. Familiarity with the lobar anatomy is important in determining the location of different pathologic processes involving the lungs. The right lung is divided by the major and minor fissures into three lobes: upper, middle and lower (Fig. 2-5 and 2-6). The major fissure has an oblique course that is best appreciated on the lateral film. It extends from the anterior portion of the diaphragm and courses superiorly and posteriorly, separating the right upper and lower lobes. The minor fissure defines the middle lobe. It extends from the midportion of the major fissure and courses in a straight anterior direction that is again best appreciated on the lateral film. The minor fissure lies in the midportion of the lung on the frontal film. The left lung has only a major fissure and is divided into an upper and lower lobe. The lingula is a subdivision of

the upper lobe and coincides anatomically with the right middle lobe.

The trachea divides into a left and a right mainstem bronchus, each of which further branches into progressively smaller bronchi. The bronchi continue to divide until they end with the smallest subunits, the alveoli. Knowledge of the bronchial anatomy helps in the localization of a tumor or foreign body for subsequent bronchoscopy or surgical resection.

Many disease processes or suspected processes involving the lung and mediastinum require further and more specific evaluation. Conventional tomography, computed tomography (CT), pulmonary angiography, nuclear medicine studies, and less utilized modalities such as digital subtraction angiography and ultrasound are among the different diagnostic tools available. Recently, transthoracic needle biopsies have involved the radiologist in obtaining tissue diagnoses of lung lesions.

Conventional tomography with its moving tube and x-ray film allows good visualization of the deep anatomy of the chest by blurring from view the more superficial structures. There are few uses of tomograms of the chest in modern radiology. If high reso-

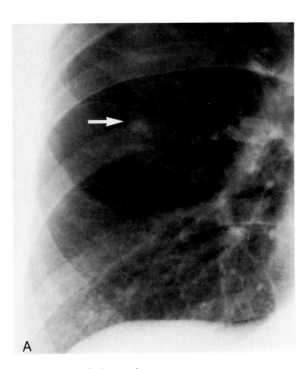

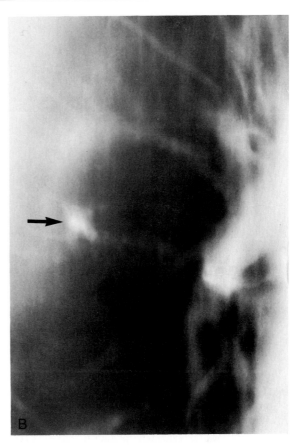

Fig. 2-7 Calcified granuloma.
History: A routine chest x-ray was done on a 74-year-old female preoperatively for cataract surgery. She did not remember having had a chest x-ray for many years previously.
Findings: **(A)** *Chest radiograph:* There is a 1-cm, ill-defined nodule in the right mid-lung field (arrow). **(B)** *Tomogram:* The nodule is densely calcified and represents a benign calcified granuloma (arrow).

lution CT is not available tomography is used to further evaluate a parenchymal nodule discovered in a routine chest x-ray. Here tomographic sections through the nodule are used to detect calcification within the nodule signifying benign disease (Fig. 2-7 A and B). The second major use of tomography is that done at a 55-degree oblique angle to evaluate the hila. The oblique orientation of the patient aligns the hilus so that it is suitable for the tomographic technique (Fig. 2-8 A and B). For this, the patient is placed in a 55-degree oblique position relative to the flat x-ray table. This view detects hilar adenopathy and the involvement of the hila by a contiguous lung mass.

Computed tomography has replaced conventional tomography in most instances, since it clearly pro-

vides information that is not obtainable with conventional studies (Fig. 2-9 A and B). Computed tomography has become the procedure of choice for evaluation of the mediastinum for involvement by intrinsic and extrinsic neoplastic and inflammatory processes. It has replaced conventional whole-lung tomography for detecting pulmonary metastatic nodules in primary malignancies with a propensity to metastasize to the chest, and for detecting other lung nodules when a single nodule is seen on the routine chest x-ray. It can accurately reveal small, obscure nodules within the lung parenchyma, especially those that are subpleural or next to the chest wall.[2] It can detect small areas of calcification in nodules that are not appreciated in conventional tomograms.[3] CT allows a more clear view of the hila as well.

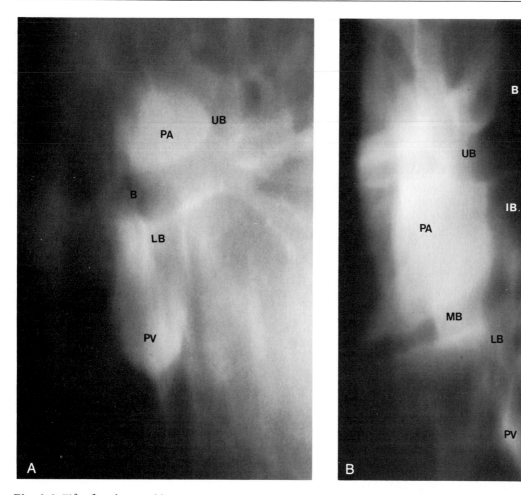

Fig. 2-8 Fifty-five-degree oblique tomograms of the hila. **(A)** Normal left hilum. PA = left pulmonary artery, PV = confluence of pulmonary veins, B = left mainstem bronchus, UB = left upper-lobe bronchus, LB = left lower-lobe bronchus. **(B)** Normal right hilum. PA = right pulmonary artery, PV = confluence of pulmonary veins, B = right mainstem bronchus, UB = right upper-lobe bronchus, IB = bronchus intermedius, MB = right middle-lobe bronchus, LB = right lower-lobe bronchus.

Nuclear medicine studies of the chest are used mainly for the initial detection of pulmonary emboli. The lung scan is a two-part examination that uses technetium-99 m macroaggregated albumin (MAA) and xenon-133 for detecting pulmonary emboli. An initial ventilation examination is done after the patient breathes xenon-133. The latter is distributed to all portions of the lung that are involved in the air-exchange process. The normal ventilation image shows two homogeneous lung fields (Fig. 2-10A). The Tc-MAA is next administered intravenously and is distributed to all portions of the lung that are being perfused by blood. It also results in homogeneous lung images in the normal patient (Fig. 2-10B).

Angiography is an invasive procedure that is today mainly performed for detecting and confirming a pulmonary embolism, and is the most specific test for the diagnosis of this lesion (Fig. 2-11). It is performed if less invasive procedures such as nuclear medicine lung scanning do not give a conclusive answer. Angiography may also be used for detecting pulmonary hypertension and congenital pulmonary vascular malformations, anomalous vessels, and sequestrations.

Transthoracic needle aspiration biopsies (TNAB)

Fig. 2-9 Normal CT scan of the chest. **(A)** Mediastinal window. The settings are made to optimize the soft tissues of the mediastinum. L = lung fields, AA = ascending aorta, DA = descending aorta, MP = main pulmonary artery, RP = right main pulmonary artery, LP = left main pulmonary artery, S = superior vena cava, B = left mainstem bronchus, V = vertebral body, RA = right arm. **(B)** Lung window. The settings are made to optimize the lung parenchyma. M = mediastinum, B = left mainstem bronchus, LH = left hilum, RH = right hilum, L = left lung fields with pulmonary vessels, CW = chest wall.

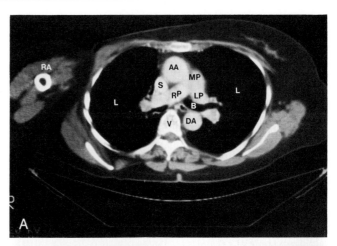

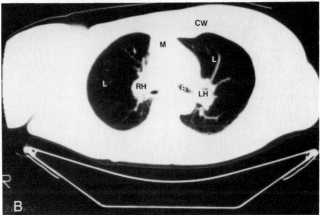

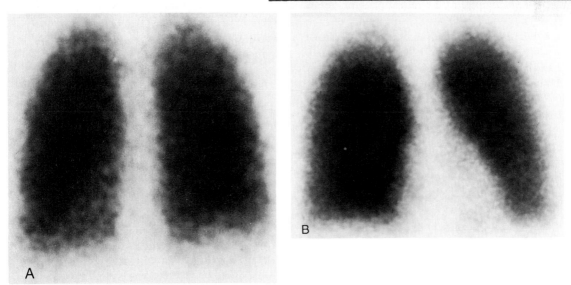

Fig. 2-10 Normal ventilation-perfusion scan. **(A)** Ventilation scan. Note the homogeneous appearance of the lungs. **(B)** Perfusion scan. There is a homogeneous appearance of the lungs. There is less activity centrally, correlating with the position of the heart.

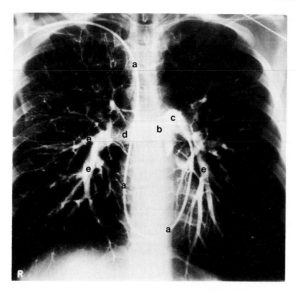

Fig. 2-11 Normal pulmonary angiogram. (a) the catheter travels through the superior vena cava, right atrium, and right ventricle, and into the main pulmonary artery. (b) Main pulmonary artery, (c) left main pulmonary artery, (d) right main pulmonary artery, (e) peripheral pulmonary arteries.

have allowed tissue diagnoses of lung nodules without the need for thoracotomy. By the introduction of a thin biopsy needle through the skin into the chest, enough tissue can often be obtained to make a diagnosis. The only significant complication is pneumothorax, which occurs in 20 percent of patients, but less than 10 percent have symptoms that require a chest tube.[4]

Ultrasound examination of the chest may be utilized for detecting and localizing pleural fluid in preparation for a thoracentesis. It can differentiate pleural fluid from pleural fibrosis and other neighboring collections of fluid (subdiaphragmatic abscesses.).

Bronchography is the opacification of the bronchial tree with the use of an oil-based, iodinated contrast medium. The medium is introduced through a tube into the left and right bronchi. This technique has been widely replaced by the fiberoptic flexible bronchoscope and CT. There are few indications for its use in today's radiology.

THE LUNG

The gross histologic anatomy of the lung is familiar, with two major components: the air sacs or alveoli and the supporting interstitial tissue. The interstitial tissue contains the pulmonary vessels and accompanying bronchi. The interstitium branches through the lungs like the branches of a tree, with the central portion or trunk of the tree coinciding with the hila of the lungs. Disease processes involving the lungs can be divided into those primarily affecting the interstitium and those resulting in the subsequent filling of the air sacs. Processes primarily involving the interstitium result from pulmonary vascular engorgement, bronchial-wall thickening, or filling of the interstitial supporting structures with edema or inflammatory fluid. The chest x-ray in interstitial disease shows a coarsening of the normally delicate linear markings in the lung, giving the chest a dirty or hazy appearance (see Fig. 2-15). This is called an interstitial or reticular pattern. Punctate collections of fluid or soft tissue may appear in the supporting network as well, resulting in 1 to 2-mm nodules superimposed on this reticular pattern (see Figs. 2-24 and 2-33). The chest x-ray is then said to have a reticulonodular pattern, which is again indicative of primarily interstitial involvement. Certain disease processes result in the edema or inflammatory fluid overflowing the interstitium and filling the usually air-filled alveolar sacs. The lung fields in the chest x-ray subsequently appear dense, solid, and white (see Fig. 2-17 and 2-19). This is called alveolar or airspace disease. This classification system helps categorize a disease process and can be used to assist in making a diagnosis as well as in describing the chest x-ray.

CLINICAL PRESENTATION: DYSPNEA (ALGORITHM 2-1)

OBSTRUCTIVE AIRWAY DISEASE

ASTHMA

Asthma is caused by a hyperactivity of the airways that results in intermittent attacks of bronchospasm and dyspnea of variable severity. The patient is asymptomatic between attacks, since the bronchospasm is completely reversible. Asthma is a common disease, seen mainly in children and usually occurring before 15 years of age.[5]

The most common chest x-ray appearance of uncomplicated asthma is that of a normal film. In more

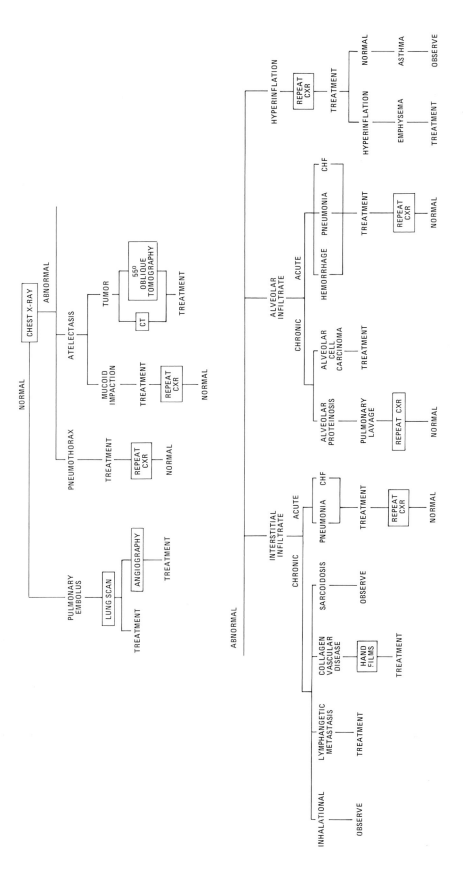

Algorithm 2-1

CLINICAL PRESENTATION: DYSPNEA

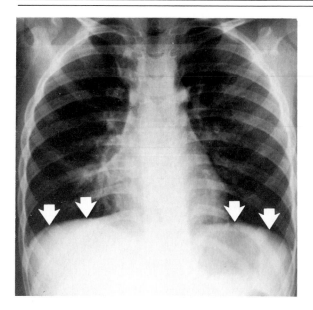

Fig. 2-12 Childhood asthma.
History: This was a 3-year-old female with severe dyspnea and wheezing. She has a history of respiratory infections.
Findings: *Chest radiograph:* There is obvious hyperexpansion of the chest with flattening of the diaphragms (arrows). There is a haziness about the perihilar areas consistent with the peribronchial cuffing of asthma.

severe attacks there may be considerable air trapping as the bronchospasm lets air enter the lungs but restricts its exit. This results in the chest x-ray appearance of overinflation or overexpansion of the lungs. The diaphragms are flattened and do not change their position with inspiration and expiration, since the trapped air keeps them depressed. There is increased space between the sternum and heart, also indicative of air trapping (Fig. 2-12).

The chest x-ray is most useful in the identification of complications in known cases of asthma. The major complications include superimposed pneumonia, secondary atelectasis from mucoid impaction, pneumothorax, and pneumomediastinum. The last presumably occurs secondarily to rupture of the alveolar sacs, with subsequent dissection of the air into the mediastinum.[6] This air appears as a lucent line outlining the mediastinum. The air may also extend into the soft tissues of the neck or into the pericardial sac (pneumopericardium) (Fig. 2-13). The chest x-ray is also useful in ruling out other conditions that cause similar presenting symptoms in previously undiagnosed cases.

BRONCHITIS

Chronic bronchitis is a mild form of chronic obstructive pulmonary disease (COPD); the more advanced stage of this is emphysema. Chronic bronchitis is defined as a chronic, productive cough without a demonstrable cause. Its attributed etiologies have included tobacco smoking, air pollution, chronic infection, a heritable disposition to bronchitis, and social class.[7]

The chest x-ray, as in asthma, is obtained to exclude other conditions that may lead to a productive cough, to search for secondary complications of bronchitis, or both. An initial diagnosis of chronic bronchitis is made clinically and not radiographically, since the chest x-ray is frequently normal. The chest x-ray may later suggest the diagnosis by revealing the prominent linear lung markings representing interstitial fibrosis (i.e., dirty chest). There are frequently dilated tubular shadows representing thickened bronchial walls.

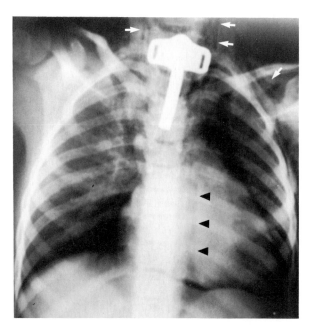

Fig. 2-13 Pneumomediastinum, status asthmaticus.
History: This was a 12-year-old female asthmatic with severe shortness of breath unrelieved by the standard medical therapy.
Findings: *Chest radiograph:* Air outlines the descending aorta (arrowheads) and extends into the soft tissues surrounding the left chest wall and neck (arrows). A tracheostomy tube has been inserted.

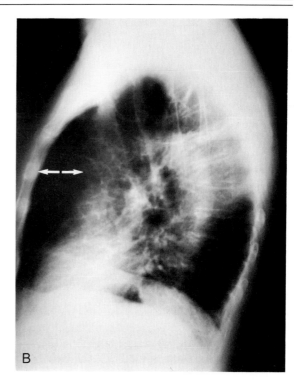

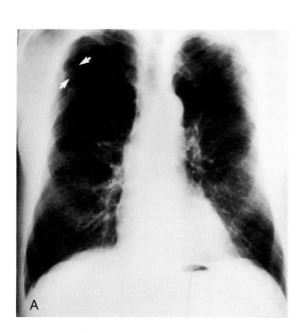

Fig. 2-14 Emphysema.
History: This was a 61-year-old male with longstanding emphysema.
Findings: **(A)** *Chest radiograph, PA view:* Blebs occupy the entire upper lung fields (arrows). The lungs are overexpanded.
(B) *Lateral view:* The diaphragms are flat and the retrosternal air space wide (arrows) as the thorax assumes a barrel shape.

EMPHYSEMA

Emphysema is defined as a chronic, unrelenting process that leads to overinflation of the lung fields with accompanying destruction of the alveolar spaces.[8] Most cases of emphysema seen in the United States are in chronic cigarette smokers.

The chest x-ray remains the primary method of evaluating the extent of involvement by emphysema. It is fairly accurate in its ability to recognize the disease.[9] The major radiographic appearances are extreme overinflation of the lung fields, oligemia (a sparsity of blood vessels), and bleb formation (Fig. 2-14 A and B). The overinflation of the lung fields is more severe than in asthma, and is manifested by flat-tening or even inversion of the domes of the diaphragms, a greatly increased width of the air space behind the sternum, accentuation of the normal thoracic kyphosis, and widely spaced, horizontally oriented ribs as the chest becomes "barrel-shaped" (see Fig. 2-37). The oligemia is manifested as a rapid tapering of the pulmonary vessels as they emerge from their origin at the hilum. Pulmonary arterial hypertension may subsequently develop and appear as a superimposed dilatation of the central main pulmonary arteries of the hila. Bullae are frequently present and appear as large air cysts that range in size from 1 cm to involvement of the entire hemithorax; they have very thin walls which are often not visible on the routine chest x-ray, and their distribution is mainly to the upper lobe.

DIFFUSE OR SEGMENTAL PARENCHYMAL LUNG DISEASE-ALVEOLAR PATTERN

Alveolar or airspace disease results from the alveolar sacs becoming filled with transudative fluid, blood, or an inflammatory exudate. Airspace diseases are usually acute in nature, such as from pulmonary edema, pneumonia, or hemorrhage. The etiologies of chronic airspace disease include alveolar proteinosis and neoplastic processes.

PULMONARY EDEMA—CARDIAC

Cardiac pulmonary edema is by far the most common cause of an acute and diffuse alveolar filling disease. Knowledge of the pathophysiology of this condition helps explain the chest x-ray changes. The failing left ventricle decompensates for a variety of reasons. It becomes an ineffective pump and leads to a backing up of pressure, first in the left ventricle and then extending into the pulmonary veins. The central pulmonary vein and later the peripheral pulmonary vessels demonstrate elevated pressures. These elevated pressures cause transudative fluid to seep from the pulmonary veins and accumulate in the surrounding interstitial space. With persistent heart failure and continued elevated pulmonary venous pressure the escaped fluid overflows the interstitium to eventually fill the alveolar sacs.

The chest x-ray changes in cardiac pulmonary edema coincide with the hemodynamic changes. First there is engorgement of the upper-lobe pulmonary veins of the hilum, as the increased central pulmonary pressure causes a redistribution or shunting of blood flow into the upper-lobe vessels. These vessels become more prominent than the lower-lobe vessels, which is a reversal of the normal state. The interstitial overflow phase or interstitial engorgement is manifested by a thickening of the normally thin interstitial network (Fig. 2-15). Thickening of these interlobular septa also produces a sign helpful in congestive heart failure: Kerley's B lines. These lines are thin, short (less than 2 cm) linear markings that lie perpendicular to the lateral border of the lower lung fields (Fig. 2-16). The chest x-ray is often more accurate than a physical examination in identifying the initial stages of pulmonary edema in which there is only interstitial engorgement in a patient with dyspnea, orthopnea, and a dry cough.

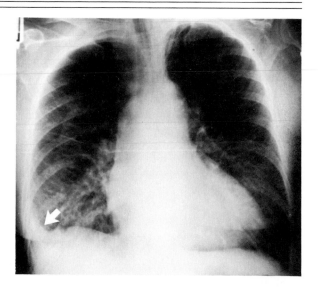

Fig. 2-15 Congestive heart failure, interstitial phase.
History: This was a 72-year-old female with frequent exacerbations of CHF.
Findings: *Chest radiograph:* There are coarse interstitial markings radiating from the hila. The upper pulmonary arteries are prominent. There is a small right pleural effusion (arrow). The heart is modestly enlarged. A nasogastric tube and central venous catheter are in place.

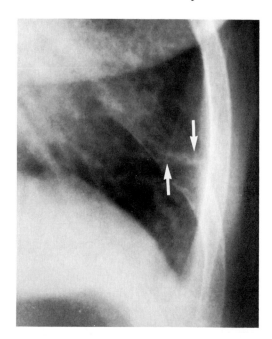

Fig. 2-16 Kerley B lines.
History: Same patient as Figure 2-15.
Findings: *Chest radiograph:* Magnified view of the lower left lung field shows the classic Kerley B lines (arrows).

Filling of the alveoli with edema fluid represents the most severe aspect of the spectrum of pulmonary edema. The airspace consolidation is concentrated symmetrically about both hila. This distribution is referred to as a "bat wing" pattern (Fig. 2-17). Clinically, patients with this pattern on a chest x-ray may be virtually without symptoms or may be extremely dyspneic or orthopneic.

Cardiac failure and the resulting pulmonary edema are accompanied by enlargement of the heart. The left ventricle is the most consistently enlarged of the cardiac chambers (Fig. 2-17). Its prominence results in a downward bulge of the left heart border on the frontal film and a posterior bulge of the heart on the lateral film (see Fig. 6-15 A and B).

Another frequent accompaniment of congestive heart failure is pleural effusion. Indeed, cardiac failure is the most common cause of such effusion.[11] The effusion is more likely to develop on the right side than on the left, but may be bilateral (see Fig. 2-15). The exuded pleural-fluid frequently works its way about the pleural reflections, leading to an accumulation of fluid in the spaces between the major and

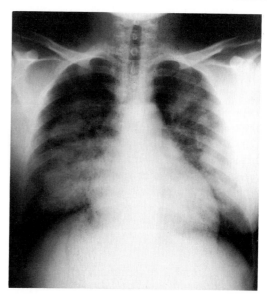

Fig. 2-17 Congestive heart failure, Alveolar pattern.
History: This was a 62-year-old female with progressive shortness of breath and swelling of the ankles.
Findings: *Chest radiograph:* There is a classic perihilar dense alveolar infiltrate. The heart is enlarged.

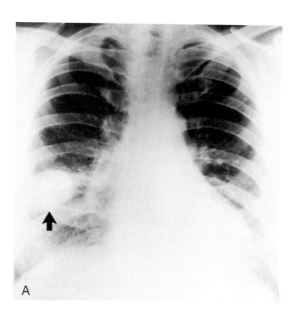

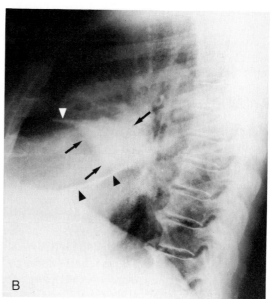

Fig. 2-18 Pseudotumor.
History: This 67-year-old male had recent congestive heart failure.
Findings: **(A)** *Chest radiograph, PA view:* A 4 cm × 6 cm mass is present in the right midlung field (arrow). The heart is enlarged but the CHF changes have otherwise resolved. **(B)** *Lateral view:* The mass on the frontal view is really ovoid, and represents fluid trapped in the minor fissure (arrows). Fluid outlines the minor (white arrowhead) and lower portions of the major fissure (black arrowhead).

minor fissures. This pocket of trapped fluid may simulate a lung mass and has been named the "phantom tumor." It has the appearance of a large mass on the frontal film although the lateral film more clearly shows an elliptical collection of trapped fluid (Fig. 2-18 A and B). Subsequent examinations show the disappearance of the fluid as the congestive heart failure resolves and the fluid is absorbed.

Both the interstitial and alveolar components of cardiac pulmonary edema clear fairly rapidly in response to adequate therapy. The chest x-ray returns completely to normal in less than 3 days in most cases.

PULMONARY EDEMA—NONCARDIAC

Many noncardiac processes result in the typical perihilar alveolar infiltrates of pulmonary edema, but with a heart of normal size. These noncardiac causes of edema include chronic renal failure, toxic inhalations (smoke), anaphylaxis (iodinated contrast medium, penicillin), narcotics, drug reactions, acute airway obstruction (foreign body), near drowning, high altitudes, fluid overload, cerebral processes (trauma, stroke, tumor), and amniotic fluid or fat emboli to the lungs.

The chest x-ray changes in such cases are very rapid, with the initial presentation being the perihilar "batwing" infiltration and a normal sized heart. The preceding interstitial changes are overshadowed by the rapidity of this process. Pleural effusions may be present.

PNEUMONIA

Certain infections of the lungs result in dyspnea, especially if they are widespread. The pneumonias classically have different appearances depending on the responsible organism and overall well-being of the patient. Certain pneumonias tend to remain more localized while others diffusely involve both lungs. Infection by some organisms produces a solid and dense alveolar-type infiltrate while others tend to cause prominently diffuse interstitial infiltrates.

Bacterial Pneumonia. Bacterial infections of the lung are classically manifested in two main patterns. *Streptococcus pneumoniae* and *Klebsiella pneumoniae* cause a filling of the alveolar sacs with inflammatory

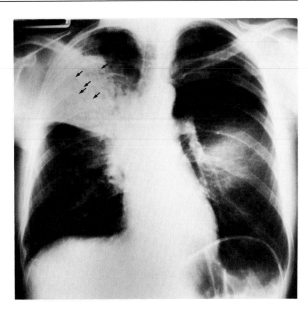

Fig. 2-19 Right upper-lobe pneumonia.
History: This 56-year-old female had a 2-week history of fever, shortness of breath and productive cough.
Findings: *Chest radiograph:* There is a dense alveolar infiltrate with obvious air bronchograms (arrows). The right mediastinal border is silhouetted by the pneumonic infiltrate, resulting in its not being discernible.

debris, resulting in a dense alveolar infiltrate termed a "lobar" or airspace pneumonia. The chest x-ray shows a whitening out of the affected portion of lung. When an infiltrate abuts the heart or diaphragm, aorta or other mediastinal structure, the normally sharp border of that structure is lost and blends with the infiltrate. This is referred to as the "silhouette sign." The loss of the normal border or haziness of the border outline is often the earliest sign of a new infiltrate (Fig. 2-19 and 2-20). The bronchi are uninvolved and remain filled with air. They appear as streaks of air density coursing through the dense white lung, and the resulting image is called an "air bronchogram" (Fig. 2-19). Before the era of antibiotic therapy, complications such as pleural effusions, empyema, and cavitation were common in bacterial pneumonia.

Staphylococcus aureus, on the other hand, incites an inflammatory process that is based in the bronchi. This results in a "bronchopneumonia" and gives the

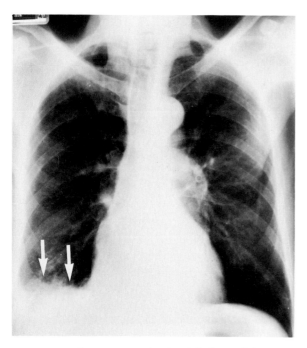

Fig. 2-20 Early pneumonia in the right lower lobe.
History: This was a 63-year-old male with fever and a productive cough.
Findings: *Chest radiograph:* There is loss of definition of the right hemidiaphragm as a result of early pneumococcal pneumonia (arrows).

chest x-ray appearance of prominent interstitial markings or may progress to a less dense "stringy" infiltrate. Air bronchograms do not occur, since the bronchi are filled with inflammatory debris instead of air. Collapse or atelectasis with secondary volume loss is a frequent accompaniment due to bronchial plugging in this disease. Cavitation, pleural effusions, and empyema are also frequent.[12] Resolution of the pneumonia is slow, with the frequent appearance of enlarging, air-filled cavities replacing the infiltrates. These are called pneumatoceles and are more frequent in children than adults (Fig. 2-21).

Aspiration Pneumonia. The aspiration of gastric contents or food is another cause of consolidation or an alveolar infiltrate. The typical distribution of these infiltrates in the lungs helps distinguish an aspiration pneumonia from a simple bacterial infection. Among the conditions predisposing to aspiration are alcoholism, recent anesthesia, head and neck surgery, mental retardation, seizure disorders, and esophageal motility disturbances.

The chest x-ray shows rapidly progressive alveolar infiltation in dependent portions of the lung. If the

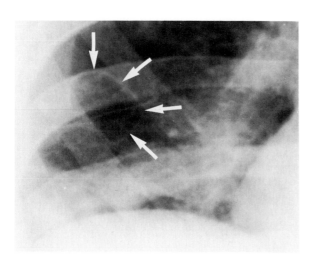

Fig. 2-21 Staphylococcal pneumonia with pneumatoceles.
History: This 26-year-old male had a previously diagnosed pneumonia that was being treated.
Findings: There is a scanty infiltrate in the base of the right lung. Pneumatoceles are present within the infiltrate (arrows).

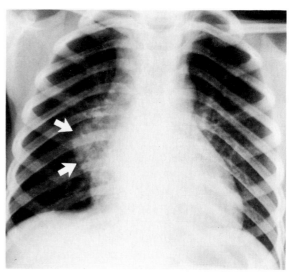

Fig. 2-22 Primary tuberculosis.
History: This was a 10-year-old female with 2 weeks of fever and night sweats.
Findings: *Chest radiograph:* There is extensive adenopathy involving the right hilum (arrows), with a scanty surrounding infiltrate.

aspiration occurs while the patient is supine, such as lying in bed, the posterior segments of the upper lobes are most frequently infiltrated. If the aspiration occurs when the patient is erect or sitting up, the lower lobes are more frequently involved. The right lung is more commonly involved than the left because of the more direct origin of the right mainstem bronchus from the trachea. The complications of aspiration pneumonia include atelectasis and abscess formation. If the patient survives, the underlying lung is often left with linear scars and pleural thickening.

Chronic aspiration pneumonia results from repeated episodes of minor aspiration while the patient is sleeping. The chest x-ray shows patchy infiltrates and atelectasis similar to the pattern seen in bronchopneumonia. Serial chest x-rays show shifting infiltration as some infiltrates resolve while others develop.

Tuberculosis. Primary tuberculosis is the initial response of the lungs to exposure of *Mycobacterium tuberculosis*. This phase of the disease is not frequently seen radiographically because few patients with primary tuberculosis have the clinical evidence of the disease that would bring them to radiologic evaluation. Symptoms, if present, are seldom striking. In the past, primary tuberculosis was seen only in children, although today it is becoming increasingly common in adults.[13]

The typical radiographic appearance of primary tuberculosis is an airspace infiltrate involving the upper lung fields. Unilateral or bilateral hilar and mediastinal adenopathy may be present. Pleural effusions and atelectasis are frequent accompaniments of these other findings (Fig. 2-22).

Postprimary or reactivation tuberculosis occurs in adults as the result of reactivation of a small focus of infection acquired in childhood or earlier in the subject's adult years. The chest x-ray demonstrates the characteristic location of the reactivated disease in the apical and posterior segments of the upper lobes or superior segment of the lower lobe of the lung. The x-ray pattern may take various forms, with segmental alveolar infiltration being the most common. Cavity formation is frequent. The walls of the cavity are smooth and thick. The infiltrate is replaced by fibrous tissue, leading to scarring in the apical and posterior lobar segments. There is a secondary volume loss as the scarring progresses with retraction of the involved

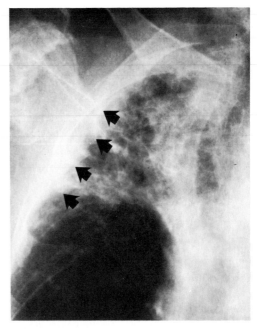

Fig. 2-23 Healed or inactive tuberculosis.
History: 82-year-old female presently in good health but was once in a "sanitarium."
Findings: *Chest radiograph:* Pleural thickening (arrows), volume loss (shift of the trachea) and fibrosis results in deformity of the right upper lung field.

segment. Elevation of the hemidiaphragm and inflation of remaining, uninvolved lung tissue occurs, filling the space left by the retracted lung segment. The hilum is also elevated as the lung shifts position (Fig. 2-23). The cavities produced by the disease may disappear. If they persist, their walls become paper thin and do not necessarily indicate active disease.

Other, less common manifestations of postprimary or reactivation tuberculosis include bronchogenic spread, miliary disease, tuberculous bronchiectasis, and tuberculoma. In bronchogenic spread the necrotic debris of the tuberculous infiltrate subsequently communicates with a bronchus, leading to a cavity plus new and distant locations of infiltration in either side of the chest. The chest x-ray shows multiple, small, ill-defined alveolar nodules that may progress to form a confluent infiltrate reminiscent of a streptococcal pneumonia. The combination of an upper-lobe cavity and disseminated, ill defined nodules is pathognomonic for tuberculosis.

Miliary tuberculosis results from the invasion of the lung by hematogenously disseminated tuberculous

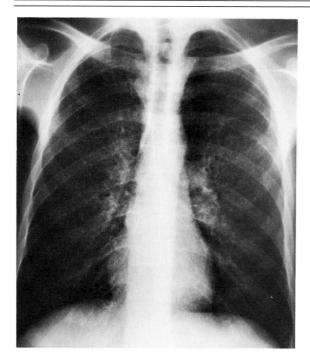

Fig. 2-24 Miliary tuberculosis.
History: This was a 27-year-old male on steroids following a renal transplant. There was a long and persistent history of tuberculosis in his family.
Findings: *Chest radiograph:* There are diffuse small nodules throughout both lung fields.

bacilli. Usually the blood-borne organisms do not invade the lungs diffusely because of an adequate host-defense mechanism. However, if the number of bacilli disseminated is great or the host-defense system in weakened, the lungs and other organs may be diffusely attacked. The initial chest x-ray shows multiple, widely distributed nodules measuring 1 mm (Fig. 2-24). These nodules are likened in appearance to "millet seeds," so giving the name miliary tuberculosis to the disease. Without appropriate chemotherapy the nodules reach 2 to 3 mm in size, with the subsequent death of the patient. With appropriate antibiotic therapy the nodules quickly clear, with no residue of the disease remaining.

Postprimary involvement of the lungs by tuberculosis may also result in the abnormally dilated and tortuous bronchi typical of bronchiectasis. This appears in the chest x-ray in the form of multiple, air-filled sacs of varying sizes. It again most commonly involves the upper segments of the lung.

The tuberculoma is a round or oval lesion most commonly found in the upper lobes. It ranges in size from 0.5 to 4.0 cm, with well-defined borders. Ninety percent of tuberculomas have surrounding nodules called "satellite" lesions.[14] Tuberculomas remain unchanged for long periods, and many calcify.

Other Pneumonias. Many other organisms cause diffuse or segmental alveolar infiltrates. The viral

Fig. 2-25 *Pneumocystis carinii* pneumonia.
History: This was a 29-year-old homosexual male with fever, malaise, and shortness of breath. Chest radiograph 5 days earlier had shown a left lower-lobe infiltrate.
Findings: *Chest radiograph,* 5 days later shows a bilateral and confluent alveolar infiltrate. An endotracheal tube is in place (arrows). The patient eventually improved, with clearance of his chest x-ray, and a diagnosis of AIDS was made.

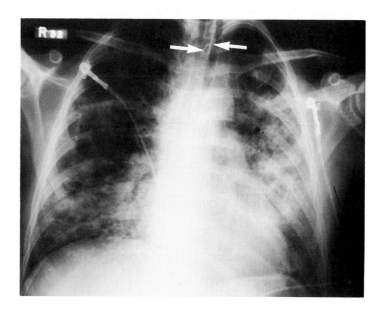

pneumonias typically result in an interstitial pattern of infiltration, although a severe infection can result in an alveolar infiltrate. The responsible viral organisms are most commonly varicella, rubeola (measles), influenza, giant cell, cytomegalovirus, Coxsackie, parainfluenza, adenovirus and respiratory syncytial viruses.[15] Various fungal infections, such as with *Histoplasma capsulatum,* can also result in alveolar infiltration. However, blastomycosis and coccidioidomycosis are infrequent sources of such infiltration.

Immunologically compromised patients are susceptible to a variety of pathogens that the healthy person easily combats. *Pneumocystis carinii* is frequently seen in male homosexuals with acquired immune deficiency syndrome (AIDS). Pneumocystis pneumonia begins as a diffuse, fine reticular pattern in the chest film that quickly progresses to a diffuse dense alveolar pattern with air bronchograms (Fig. 2-25). If the patient survives, the chest x-ray picture reverts back to a reticular pattern with eventual clearing.

PULMONARY HEMORRHAGE

The etiologies of hemorrhage into the lung parenchyma include anticoagulant therapy, trauma, Goodpasture's syndrome, bleeding disorders (hemophilia, leukemia), and massive pulmonary infarction. The chest x-ray shows a confluent, diffuse alveolar infiltrate with air bronchograms. With resolution, the infiltrate becomes increasingly inhomogenous and patchy. Recurrent bleeding episodes lead to a thickening of the interstitial septal structures and finally a fine reticular pattern indicating scarring of the lung tissue.

PULMONARY NEOPLASIA

Bronchoalveolar-Cell Carcinoma. Bronchoalveolar-cell or alveolar-cell carcinoma begins in the distal small bronchioles or alveolar walls. It accounts for 15 percent of all primary pulmonary neoplasms and its incidence appears to be rising.[16] Its growth may be slow and occur over many years.

The chest x-ray demonstrates either a localized or disseminated disease process. A peripherally located solitary nodule is seen in over 50 percent of presenting cases. The nodule is poorly defined with fluffy margins (Fig. 2-26). There may be multiple nodules local-

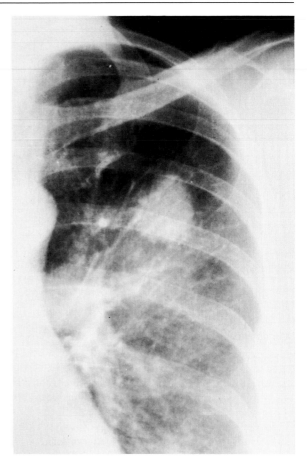

Fig. 2-26 Alveolar-cell carcinoma, solitary nodule.
History: This 59-year-old female had a routine preoperative chest x-ray for bladder repair surgery.
Findings: *Chest radiograph:* A 3-cm, ill-defined nodule with a lobulated and fluffy margin is present in the left upper-lung field.

ized to a particular portion of the lung. A segmental infiltrate reminiscent of that in bacterial disease is also identified. The disseminated forms of bronchoalveolar-cell carcinoma include those manifesting scattered bilateral fluffy nodules, those with small fine miliary involvement, and diffuse coalescent infiltrates (Fig. 2-27). Pleural effusions, mediastinal lymph node enlargement, atelectasis, and cavitation are infrequently present.

The localized nodule or infiltrate without accompanying hilar adenopathy holds a fairly good prognosis with surgical resection. Hilar lymph node involvement signifies metastasis to the mediastinum

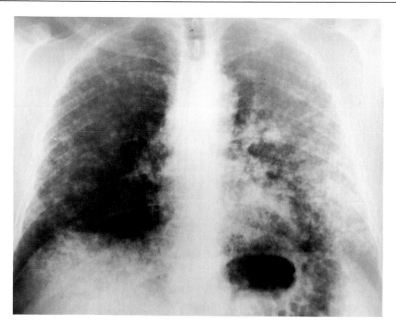

Fig. 2-27 Alveolar-cell carcinoma, disseminated.
History: This was a 56-year-old male with a long history of shortness of breath, weight loss, and hemoptysis. He always avoided medical consultation.
Findings: *Chest radiograph:* There are scattered, fluffy alveolar nodules that are coalescing to form dense infiltrates. The borders of the heart and diaphragms are ill-defined as the nodules abut and so silhouette these borders.

and carries a poor prognosis. The diffuse form of the disease also has a poor prognosis.[17]

ALVEOLAR PROTEINOSIS

Alveolar proteinosis is a disease in which the alveoli become filled with a proteinaceous material for unknown reasons. It is a relapsing disease. Even when the lungs are diffusely involved by infiltrates the patient is frequently only mildly symptomatic.

The chest x-ray shows rapidly appearing diffuse, bilateral, and confluent infiltrates with air bronchograms. The infiltrates resolve slowly, but respond quickly with dramatic clearance to pulmonary lavage.

DIFFUSE LUNG DISEASE— INTERSTITIAL PATTERN

Interstitial infiltrates unlike alveolar infiltrates are ordinarily chronically present. The common etiologies of long-standing interstitial infiltration include granulomatous disease (sarcoidosis), collagen vascular disease, metastasis from certain tumors, and inhalational irritation. The acute etiologies—congestive heart failure and infectious disease (viral, mycoplasma)—have already been discussed.

GRANULOMATOUS DISEASE— SARCOIDOSIS

Sarcoidosis is a disease of undetermined etiology, most commonly seen in the United States in the black population. There is no sex predominance, and the disease is usually first diagnosed between the ages of 20 and 40.[18] Microscopically, sarcoidosis manifests as noncaseating granulomas. The granulomas may involve any organ in the body, but in 90 percent of cases there is some chest involvement, with either mediastinal adenopathy, lung parenchymal disease, or both. The lung findings may persist unchanged for many years, but 50 percent of cases demonstrate complete resolution in 6 months to 3 years. The patient's symptoms are often unrelated to the pulmonary changes.

Many patients with sarcoidosis are asymptomatic when an abnormal chest x-ray occurs during a routine

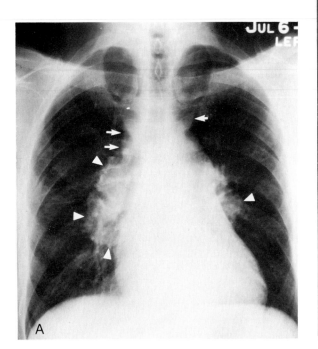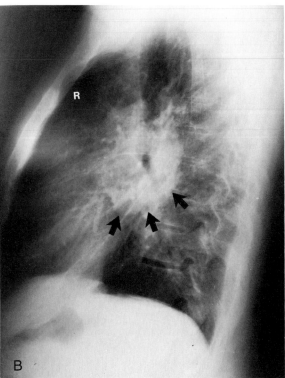

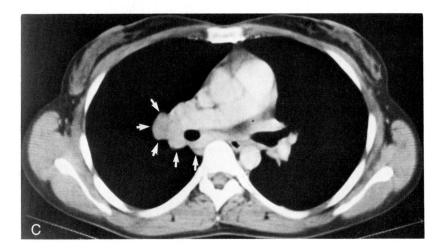

Fig. 2-28 Sarcoidosis: adenopathy.

History: This was a 29-year-old black male with a new onset of shortness of breath and fever.

Findings: (A) *Chest radiograph, PA view:* There is bilateral hilar adenopathy of equal or symmetrical proportion (arrowheads). The right paratracheal nodes are enlarged (arrows), and there is prominence of soft tissues in the left paratracheal region (arrows). The lung parenchyma is normal. **(B)** *Lateral view:* The adenopathy is confirmed about the hilum (arrows). Note there is no filling in the retrosternal air space (R) by soft tissues to indicate anterior mediastinal adenopathy. **(C)** CT — Bulky adenopathy completely surrounds the right hila and bronchus (arrows). Adenopathy is scant at the left hila at this level but was better appreciated in lower levels.

examination. There may be a resolution of the lung pathology with no change or even a worsening of the patient's symptomatology.

The findings on the chest x-ray are classified into four basic stages depending on lymph-node and lung involvement. In the first stage the chest x-ray is normal in spite of the patient's symptomatology.

The second stage is characterized by hilar and mediastinal lymph-node enlargement without lung parenchymal abnormalities, and is seen in approximately 40 percent of cases.[19] The most frequently enlarged lymph nodes are in the hilar and paratracheal areas. The nodes are bilaterally and symmetrically enlarged (Fig. 2-28 A, B, and C). The paratracheal enlargement is almost always coexistent with the hilar enlargement. From 70 to 80 percent of patients with this symmetric adenopathy eventually display a normal chest x-ray.

The third stage exhibits diffuse pulmonary involvement in one of three basic patterns. The reticulonodular pattern is a fine to heavy linear interstitial pattern superimposed over small nodules that resemble those in miliary tuberculosis (Fig. 2-29). Over 75 percent of these cases demonstrate either concurrent or prior evidence of hilar and mediastinal adenopathy. Indistinct and ill-defined nodules represent a much less common pattern of lung involvement. These nodules measure 6 to 7 mm in diameter. They may coalesce to form more confluent infiltrates resembling an infectious pneumonitis. The least common of the parenchymal lung patterns is marked by large, dense, round, well-defined nodules that simulate metastatic disease of the lungs.

Pulmonary fibrosis constitutes the fourth and end-stage involvement of the lungs. It occurs in patients in whom pulmonary changes have been present for a long time. The scarred lung exhibits linear bands of tissue that extend from the hilum, with predominant involvement of the upper lobes. The scarring is associated with blebs (air cavities), bronchiectasis, and generalized overinflation of the lung fields (Fig. 2-30).

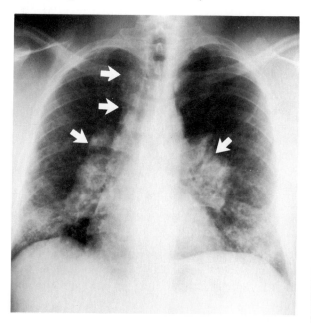

Fig. 2-29 Sarcoidosis, adenopathy and parenchymal involvement.
History: This was a 31-year-old black male with progressive sarcoidosis.
Findings: *Chest radiograph:* In addition to the symmetrical hilar and mediastinal adenopathy (arrows), there are bibasilar nodular infiltrates. The nodules are becoming more confluent.

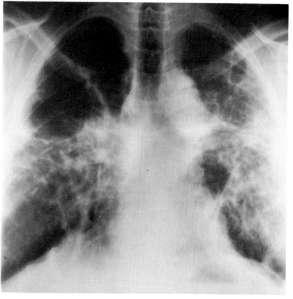

Fig. 2-30 End-stage sarcoidosis.
History: This 41-year-old black male had an 18-year history of progressive sarcoidosis.
Findings: *Chest radiograph:* Bullae have replaced the upper lobes of both lungs while fibrosis and stranding of tissue distort the remainder of the lungs.

COLLAGEN VASCULAR DISEASE

The collagen-vascular diseases that most often produce changes in the lung are rheumatoid arthritis and scleroderma. The changes result from the fibrinoid necrosis of connective tissue.

The chest x-ray changes of rheumatoid arthritis are divided into pleural effusion, diffuse interstitial fibrosis, necrobiotic nodule formation, Caplan's syndrome, and pulmonary arteritis with pulmonary hypertension. Pleural effusions represent the most common abnormality seen in the chest x-ray film. They may precede joint disease in 50 percent of cases. Most of these effusions are unilateral and are the only abnormality seen on the chest x-ray. The amount of pleural fluid may remain constant for months to years, a somewhat unique feature of rheumatoid lung disease.

The pattern of pulmonary fibrosis most often follows symptoms of joint disease. Initially there are small, generalized punctate or nodular densities that may increase in size. The nodules give way to a diffuse, medium-to-coarse interstitial pattern with predominant lower-lobe involvement. The fibrosis progresses to form diffuse, thick-walled cysts, about 5 to 8 mm in diameter, referred to as "honeycomb lung." There is an accompanying loss of lung volume. This represents true end-stage fibrosis, and may be seen as the end-stage result of various disease processes (Fig. 2-31).

The necrobiotic nodule is a rare manifestation of rheumatoid disease and is usually associated with advanced joint disease. The nodules histologically resemble the subcutaneous nodules of advanced rheumatoid disease and are found in the lungs, pleura, or pericardium. Their chest x-ray appearance is that of multiple, well-circumscribed masses ranging from 2 to 7 cm in size. These multiple nodules are easily mistaken for pulmonary metastases. They are more commonly seen near the periphery of the lungs and commonly cavitate. They may disappear and reappear in accordance with joint symptoms.

Caplan's syndrome was first described in 1953 in Welsh coal miners. It consists of rheumatoid nodules superimposed on coal miner's pneumoconiosis (silicosis). The chest x-ray changes are unrelated to the severity of the joint disease.

The last chest manifestation of rheumatoid arthritis is a severe pulmonary arteritis that leads to narrowing

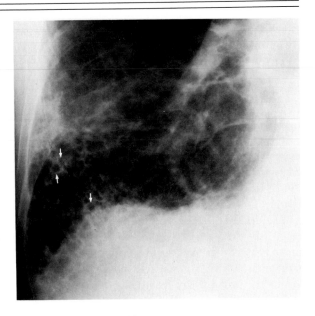

Fig. 2-31 Rheumatoid lungs.
History: This 57-year-old male had a 15-year history of rheumatoid arthritis and progressive shortness of breath.
Findings: *Chest radiograph:* Multiple air cavities have replaced the lower lung fields (arrows). They have thick walls and resemble honeycombs.

of the lumina of the pulmonary arteries. The narrowed vessels demonstrate increased intraluminal pressures that eventually result in pulmonary hypertension and cor pulmonale.

LUNG METASTASIS

Metastatic involvement of the lungs by a malignancy most often appears on the chest x-ray in the form of multiple nodules of varying sizes (Fig. 2-32). Metastatic renal cell carcinoma, gastrointestinal malignancies, bone sarcoma, and trophoblastic metastases frequently appear in the lung as multiple discrete nodules.

Less commonly, a diffuse interstitial pattern of metastasis results as the tumor invades the lymphatic vessels. The appearance in such cases is similar to that in an early interstitial pulmonary edema, with a perihilar distribution. Breast carcinoma and primary malignancies of the stomach, thyroid, pancreas, larynx, cervix, and lung frequently involve the lung via the lymphatic system, resulting in an interstitial x-ray

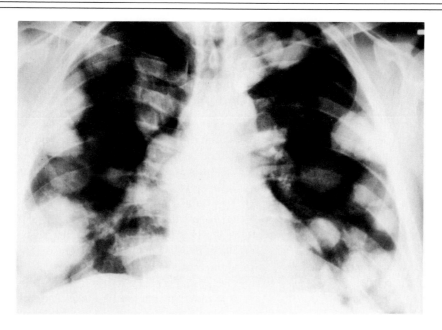

Fig. 2-32 Pulmonary metastasis.
History: This 62-year-old male was diagnosed as having colon carcinoma but was lost to follow up. He presented with a small bowel obstruction.
Findings: *Chest radiograph:* Innumerable well-defined nodules are present throughout both lung fields. The nodules are of varying sizes.

pattern. Lymphangitic metastasis results in severe dyspnea often preceding visible chest x-ray changes.

DISEASES OF INHALATIONAL ORIGIN

Many toxins within the lungs that induce secondary interstitial changes are found in polluted air in the general environment or in a work related environment. These toxins can be divided into inorganic dusts, organic dusts, toxic chemicals, and noxious gases. The most familiar diseases arising from exposure to inorganic dusts are silicosis and asbestosis.

Silicosis. Silicosis is the reaction of the lung parenchyma to free silica, which is found in a number of occupations including coal mining, stone quarrying, and sand blasting. It is seen almost exclusively in males, since they greatly predominate in these professions, and takes more than 10 years of exposure to silica to develop.

The chest x-ray in silicosis shows progression from a fine reticular pattern to a coarse fibrosis even if the exposure to silica has been terminated. Small nodules are superimposed on the reticular or interstitial pattern, leading to the familiar reticulonodular pattern. The latter pattern predominantly involves the upper lobes of the lung and is bilateral (Fig. 2-33). The nodules frequently calcify. Secondary hilar adenopathy is seen in 5 to 10 percent of cases. In these the hilar nodes may calcify about their periphery to give an appearance likened to that of an eggshell. Enlargement of mediastinal and even abdominal nodes may accompany the hilar adenopathy. These findings constitute what is termed uncomplicated silicosis. From 25 to 30 percent of all cases of the disease progress to the complicated form of silicosis.[21] The fibrotic upper lobes and enlarged nodes coalesce to form a conglomerated mass of tissue. This process, called progressive massive fibrosis (PMF), commonly occurs in the midzone or periphery of the lungs, or both. The con-

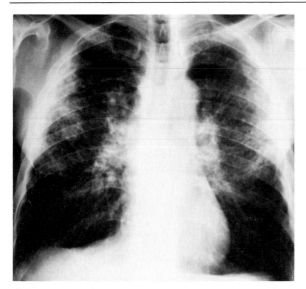

Fig. 2-33 Silicosis.
History: This was a 37-year-old male who had worked in the coal mines all of his adult life.
Finding: *Chest radiograph:* There is a coarse reticulonodular infiltrate involving both upper lung fields. The hila also appear to be enlarged.

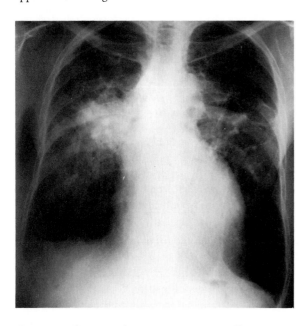

Fig. 2-34 Silicosis with progressive massive fibrosis.
History: This was a 67-year-old coal miner.
Findings: *Chest radiograph:* Bilateral masses have replaced the lung tissue of the upper lung fields. The hila are lost in the fibrotic masses and the apices are replaced by bullae.

glomerated mass, which may itself cavitate (Fig. 2-34), migrates toward the hilum, leaving large areas of bizarre, overinflated lung behind.

Asbestosis. Asbestos is among a group of minerals, including talc and mica, in common industrial use that incite an inflammatory and secondary fibrotic response in the alveolar walls and interlobular septa of the lungs. The major sources of asbestos exposure are in mining and in occupations such as insulation, textile manufacturing, construction, and ship building. Most patients with early asbestosis have no symptoms. Dyspnea is seen with the later stages of parenchymal interstitial fibrosis. Like silicosis, a long history of exposure is necessary for development of the secondary lung changes in asbestosis. Patients with asbestosis have a definite predisposition to the development of adenocarcinoma of the lung as well as to malignant mesothelioma and gastric carcinoma.

The chest x-ray often demonstrates involvement of the pleural surface with no involvement of the lung parenchyma.[21] The pleural involvement may be localized or diffuse. Localized pleural disease occurs in the form of pleural plaque formation, with the plaque being a thickened portion of the pleural lining and most frequently located along the lateral wall at the level of the mid-thorax, or on the dome of the diaphragm. Such plaques appear in the x-ray as linear thickenings of the pleural surfaces. They are usually bilateral and symmetric. Approximately 25 percent of these plaques calcify, and thus appear as dense white lines running parallel with the pleural surface (Fig. 2-35 A and B). The plaques may become more extensive, involving large portions of the pleural surface, and the condition is then termed diffuse pleural thickening. The predominant areas of involvement are the same as by the smaller pleural plaques. Pleural effusions are infrequent, and if present are usually small in volume.

The parenchymal changes in asbestosis follow a continuum, from a fine reticulation mainly in the lower lung fields to large, superimposed nodules. The combination of parenchymal and pleural changes leads to a "shaggy" appearance of the heart and diaphragm (Fig. 2-36). Lymph-node enlargement is not a feature of asbestosis.

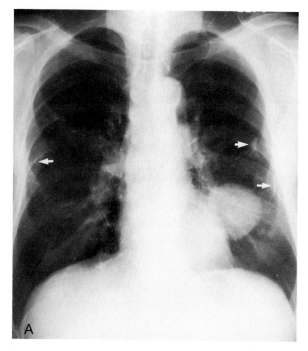

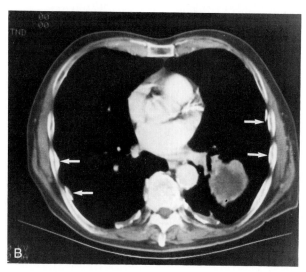

Fig. 2-35 Asbestosis and bronchogenic carcinoma.
History: This 57-year-old industrial worker had a routine chest x-ray for an insurance physical.
Findings: (A) *Chest radiograph:* Multiple pleural plaques are identified in the mid-lung fields (arrows). Some of the plaques appear calcified. In addition, a 10-cm mass is identified in the left lower-lung field. The borders of the mass are ill-defined. **(B)** *CT* scan section through the mass better demonstrates the ill-defined borders of the mass. The calcified pleural plaques are easily appreciated (arrows).

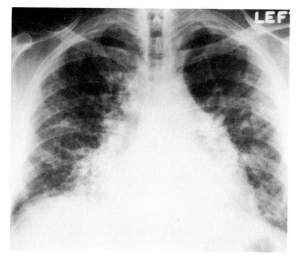

Fig. 2-36 Asbestosis.
History: This was a 62-year-old textile worker.
Findings: *Chest radiograph:* There is a coarse reticular infiltrate involving the lung bases as well as extensive pleural thickening that combine to form a "shaggy heart."

PULMONARY EMBOLI

Pulmonary emboli are blood clots obstructing branches of the pulmonary arterial system. They occur in increased incidence in complicated surgical procedures (hip surgery), bedridden patients, heart failure, postpartum, with oral contraceptive use, and with deep venous thrombosis. Only 10 to 15 percent of cases of pulmonary embolism result in secondary infarction or necrosis of the underlying lung parenchyma.[22] A high degree of clinical suspicion is needed for early diagnosis and effective therapy of this condition.

The chest x-ray is always obtained as the initial examination in a patient with dyspnea of acute onset and suspected pulmonary embolism. It functions to exclude other conditions that can lead to acute dyspnea, such as pneumothorax or a massive pleural effusion. The chest x-ray is also necessary for correlation

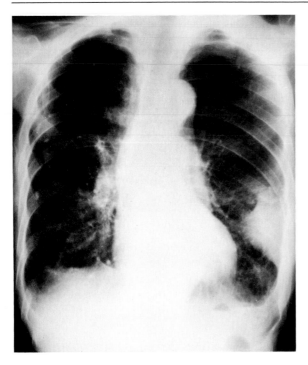

Fig. 2-37 Pulmonary emboli with infarction.
History: This was a 94-year-old male with long standing COPD who presented with acute severe respiratory distress.
Findings: *Chest radiograph:* Superimposed on the COPD changes of hyperinflation of the lungs and inverted, scalloped diaphragms is a wedge-shaped density based on the pleura. This is called a "Hampton hump."

with the subsequently done nuclear medicine ventilation/perfusion examination. The chest x-ray in cases of pulmonary embolism most frequently has a normal appearance, but certain findings may be present to suggest the diagnosis. These include oligemia, a change in pulmonary vessel size, alteration in the size and configuration of the heart, and a loss of lung volume. Oligemia is present when a section of lung is devoid of the normal vascular markings as a result of occlusion of the large central or multiple small peripheral vessels by clots. In these areas the lung appears more black in the chest x-ray, since the blood vessels are occluded. The oligemia is often accompanied by an increased size of the central pulmonary arteries as they become filled and distended with the clot. Serial examinations help in showing a progressive increase in vessel size. A loss of lung volume is best appreciated by elevation of the diaphragm. With extensive central emboli there may be acute cor pulmonale with enlargement of both the right ventricle

and main pulmonary artery segment due to a pressure back-up.

In the few cases in which the underlying lung undergoes infarction, the chest x-ray demonstrates an infiltrate from the filling of the alveoli with blood and edema fluid. Frank tissue necrosis can also add to the infiltrate. The infiltrate is wedge shaped, with the apex of the wedge pointing centrally and the base contiguous with the pleural surface. The apex of the wedge is rounded and has been described as a "hump." Air bronchograms are usually not present with the infiltrate (Fig. 2-37), although volume loss and pleural effusions are frequent accompaniments of pulmonary infarction. With a simple infarction and no tissue necrosis, the wedge-shaped infiltrate is reabsorbed in 4 to 7 days, with the chest x-ray returning to normal. When secondary tissue necrosis occurs, the clearing of the infiltrate takes 3 to 5 weeks, and often leaves permanent lung scarring and volume loss.

Following the chest x-ray, the next procedure in the work-up of a suspected pulmonary embolism is the nuclear medicine ventilation/perfusion scan (V/Q scan). With pulmonary emboli the underlying lung is usually viable and remains air filled,[22] and so demonstrates a normal, homogeneous xenon distribution (Fig. 2-38A). The second part of the V/Q scan indirectly maps the location of the emboli. The technetium-MAA injected intravenously cannot reach those segments of the pulmonary arterial system that are blocked by clots, and the perfusion scan therefore shows wedge shapes in the otherwise homogeneous lung field. Pulmonary emboli produce multiple defects that are seen on a perfusion scan and are most common in the bases of the lungs, where blood flow predominates (Fig. 2-38B). It is the classic mismatch of a normal ventilation scan with multiple segmental wedge defects on the perfusion scan that leads to the diagnosis of pulmonary embolism.

If the lung scan is inconclusive or normal, but clinical suspicion remains high, a pulmonary angiogram is performed. The angiogram is the most specific and accurate tool for the diagnosis of pulmonary embolism, but is an invasive procedure and has a definite associated morbidity and mortality. In this procedure an angiogram catheter is introduced into a peripheral arm vein at the antecubital fossa, or into the femoral vein in the groin. The catheter is then passed through the right side of the heart under fluoroscopic guidance, and injections of contrast medium are made through the catheter into the left and right pulmonary arteries. The angiogram allows direct visualiza-

matic pleural effusion (Fig. 2-42A). In both cases the fluid usually flows freely between the pleural surface and lung surface, although it may be loculated or trapped in place. Loculated fluid is often seen in inflammatory or neoplastic processes.

A decubitus view of the chest, obtained with the patient lying on the right and left side, is used to confirm the presence of a freely flowing pleural effusion versus a loculated effusion. In the decubitus position, free fluid shifts with gravity to the dependent portion of the pleural space, producing a fluid line (Fig. 2-42B). If no fluid line or level is obtained and the angle remains blunted, the fluid is either loculated by inflammatory pockets or there is no pleural effusion and the blunting is secondary to chronic pleural thickening from an old inflammatory process. Decubitus films are valuable if a thoracentesis is planned, since only free effusions will be successfully tapped. Loculated effusions result in "dry" taps.

ATELECTASIS

Atelectasis is defined as a diminished air content within the lung associated with a reduced lung volume.[25] It results from the acute obstruction of a large bronchus or multiple small bronchi. The atelectasis results from the continued absorption of oxygen from the alveolar sacs while the obstructed bronchus allows no new oxygen to be supplied. Obstruction of the larger airways is frequently the result of bronchogenic carcinoma. In fact, the finding of an atelectatic lobe or segment in an adult is first considered secondary to bronchogenic carcinoma even without visualization of a mass lesion. Other less common causes of large-airway obstruction include metastatic lesions to the bronchial walls (renal cell carcinoma, breast carcinoma, and melanoma), benign bronchial neoplasms (polyps), and foreign body aspiration. Mucus plugs in multiple smaller bronchi, as seen in asthma, chronic bronchitis, or postoperatively after the administration of respiratory depressant medications or incomplete respiratory motion, can also result in significant atelectasis. Lesions outside the bronchus can compromise the airway enough to lead to pulmonary collapse. Hilar adenopathy (from metastatic disease, sarcoidosis, tuberculosis) and left atrial enlargement are possible causes of segmental atelectasis from extrinsic bronchial compression.

The chest x-ray in atelectasis demonstrates direct and indirect signs of collapse and volume loss. When

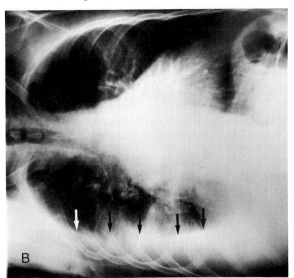

Fig. 2-42 Pleural effusion.
History: This was a 64-year-old male with known colon carcinoma and a new onset of respiratory difficulty.
Findings: (A) *Chest radiograph:* The right hemidiaphragm appears elevated. It was in normal position in a chest x-ray obtained 1 month earlier **(B)** *Radiograph with patient in right lateral decubitus position:* Pleural fluid is seen layering along the dependent lateral chest wall on the right (arrows). The fluid is trapped beneath the lung on the routine upright chest x-ray, simulating an elevated diaphragm.

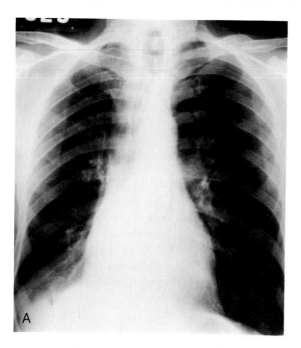

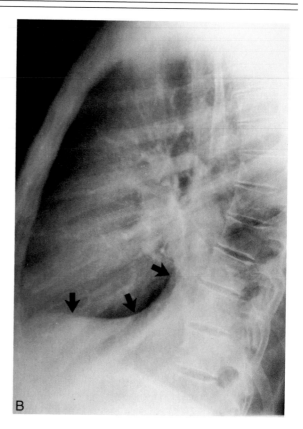

Fig. 2-43 Atelectasis.
History: This was a 63-year-old male with tachypnea a few days after a cerebrovascular accident.
Findings: **(A)** *Chest radiograph, PA view:* The border of the right hemidiaphragm is not well demarcated since it is silhouetted by a contiguous soft-tissue density. The density is homogeneous and does not have the typical appearance of a pneumonic infiltrate. **(B)** *Lateral view:* The density is from a collapsed and now airless right lower lobe. The major fissure is bowed backwards from this loss of volume (arrows). Respiratory therapy caused a mucous plug to be expectorated and the lobe re-expanded.

an entire lobe or segment collapses there is a typical wedge-shaped density that represents the airless, atelectatic segment. The location and orientation of this density are constant for the different lobes or segments. Indirect signs of collapse include crowding of the pulmonary vessels, crowding of the ribs, and elevation of the diaphragm as the lung segments lose volume. In addition, uninvolved segments and the opposite lung overexpand to help overcome the volume loss. The combination of collapse of certain segments and overinflation of others leads to a displacement or rearrangement of the normal course and location of the fissures, displacement of the hilus, and shifting of the mediastinum. The wedge-shaped density and fissure displacement are the two most consistent signs of atelectasis (Fig. 2-43 A and B, 2-44 A and B).

The workup of an atelectatic lobe or segment depends on the clinical background and anatomic involvement. In suspected cases of a central tumor, and where no mass is seen on a chest x-ray, CT is of benefit to identify an occult tumor. If a central mass is identified CT is helpful in determining the extent of involvement by tumor in order to stage the malignancy.

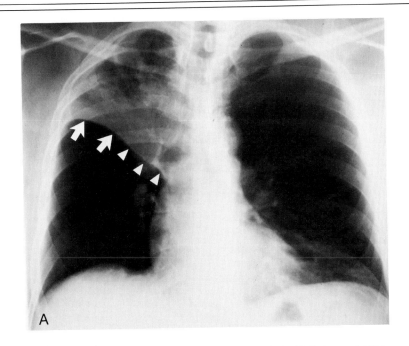

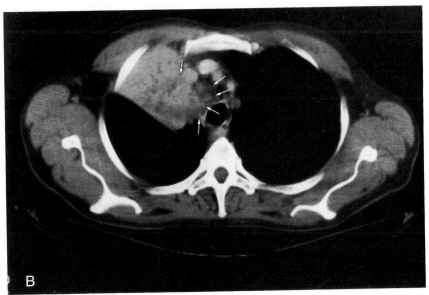

Fig. 2-44 Squamous cell carcinoma, "S" sign of Golden.
History: This was a 44-year-old male with diagnosed squamous-cell carcinoma of the lung.
Findings: **(A)** *Chest radiograph:* The mass forms the first downward arched loop of the "S" (arrowheads); the collapsed distal lung, minor fissure, forms the opposite upward loop (arrows). The mass is contiguous with the mediastinum, suggesting unresectability. **(B)** *CT scan:* The unresectability of the tumor is confirmed by discovery that the tumor is invading and infiltrating the mediastinum (arrows).

Conventional tomography is less useful. Patients with suspected mucoid impaction are treated medically and a further workup is done only if the lung does not re-expand after appropriate therapy. Foreign bodies are removed immediately by the bronchoscopist.

CLINICAL PRESENTATION: HEMOPTYSIS (ALGORITHM 2-2)

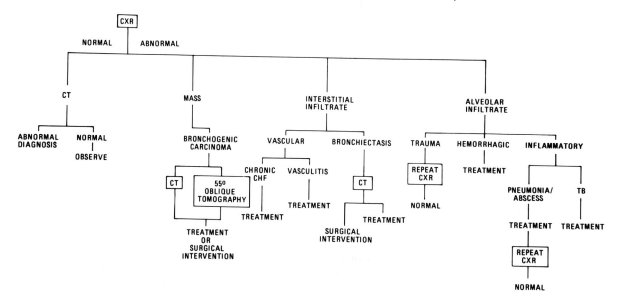

CLINICAL PRESENTATION: HEMOPTYSIS

Algorithm 2-2

INFLAMMATORY

Hemoptysis is a common feature of both chronic and acute infection involving the alveoli or bronchi. Chronic bronchitis and bronchiectasis account for 60 to 70 percent of cases and tuberculosis is seen as the cause of hemoptysis in up to 10 percent. Viral and bacterial pneumonias infrequently result in a scanty, blood-streaked sputum. A major problem in dealing with hemoptysis is in attributing it to a previously diagnosed chronic condition, such as bronchitis, which may result in missing a serious but potentially treatable neoplastic lesion. The safest approach in recurrent episodes of hemoptysis is to treat each episode as if it was the first hemoptysis and initiate a complete diagnostic evaluation.[26]

BRONCHIECTASIS

Bronchiectasis is an irreversible dilatation of the bronchial tree. It is a sequel of chronic infection, and its incidence has been greatly reduced since the introduction of antibiotics into medicine. Bronchiectasis is frequently bilateral and predominantly involves the basilar portion of the lungs. The main symptoms are a cough with a bloody, purulent sputum. A bronchiectatic segment of the lung frequently requires surgical resection to terminate the symptomatology.

The chest x-ray suggests the diagnosis by demonstrating cystic air spaces up to 2 cm in diameter, with crowding together of the remaining lung markings. An involved segment becomes scarred and virtually airless, resulting in overinflation of the neighboring segments to fill the void left by the shrunken, diseased segment.

Bronchography has always been the confirmatory examination of choice to both establish the diagnosis of bronchiectasis and to determine the extent of its involvement of the lung before surgery. It clearly demonstrates the classically dilated bronchi. Computed tomography can now be used in place of bronchography in many situations, avoiding the associated problem of introducing the oil-based contrast medium used in bronchography into a chronically infected system. Computed tomography identifies the thick-walled and dilated bronchi extending out to the periphery of the lung.[27]

MASS

BRONCHOGENIC CARCINOMA

The most important diagnosis to consider in a patient presenting with hemoptysis is bronchogenic carcinoma. The early detection of the malignancy clearly leads to an improved prognosis. The incidence of bronchogenic carcinoma is on the rise in men and even more so in women. Seventy-five percent of new cases present in the fifth and sixth decades of life. Cigarette smoking and industrial toxins (asbestos) have been found to play a significant role in the development of bronchogenic carcinoma. The current classification of histologic types of the disease is based on the World Health Organization classification. The different histologic types have different and often unique clinical and radiographic presentations and patterns. They also call for different therapeutic regimens and carry different prognoses. The most common histologic type of bronchogenic carcinoma is squamous-cell carcinoma (40 percent of cases), followed in incidence by adenocarcinoma (20 percent), small-cell or oat-cell carcinoma (20 percent), and large-cell carcinoma (15 percent).[28]

Squamous cell carcinoma is classically a centrally located intrabronchial mass lesion that is first detected on a chest x-ray through its secondary affects on the lung. The most common chest x-ray finding is a collapsed segment or lobe caused by a blockage of airflow by the centrally located intrabronchial tumor. The atelectatic or collapsed segment may be the only finding on the chest x-ray. If the tumor is large enough it may be visualized as a hilar or mediastinal mass medial to the collapsed segment. This hilar mass is ill-defined

and has spicules arising from its borders, indicating the rapid growth of this malignant tumor. The hilar mass plus the atelectatic lung segment results in the "S-sign of Golden" (Fig. 2-44 A and B). The first loop of the "S" is the tumor mass, while the oppositely oriented second loop is the collapsed segment of lung. A second common x-ray presentation is a dense infiltrate in segments of the lung distal to the intrabronchial tumor. The bronchi are unable to clear secretions past the tumor and become ideal sites for secondary bacterial infiltration. The alveolar spaces are secondarily filled with inflammatory exudate, forming the dense infiltrate. The bronchi are filled with retained secretions and exudate. There are no air bronchograms present in the infiltrates, and this is a unique feature of what is termed "postobstructive pneumonitis" (Fig. 2-45). The consolidation can improve with antibiotic therapy but frequently recurs after the therapy has been discontinued, as the intrabronchial tumor again causes a buildup of secretions and bacterial overgrowth. Cavitation is a common

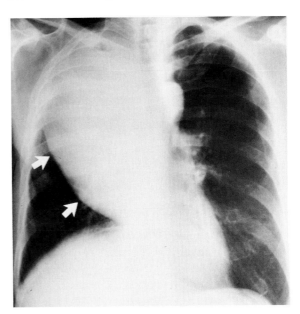

Fig. 2-45 Squamous cell carcinoma, postobstructive pneumonitis.
History: This was a 62-year-old male physician with known lung cancer.
Findings: *Chest radiograph:* The lung distal to a medially situated endobronchial tumor is totally airless, since it is filled with inflammatory debris. The minor fissure is severely bowed downwards by the space-occupying debris (arrows).

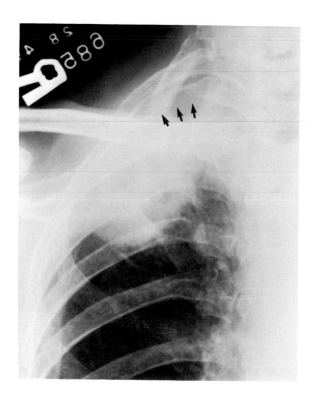

Fig. 2-46 Squamous-cell carcinoma, Pancoast tumor.
History: This 63-year-old male had prolonged chest-wall pain.
Findings: *Chest radiograph:* A dense mass occupies the apex of the right upper-lung field. Note the destroyed third rib (arrows), responsible for the patient's chest pain.

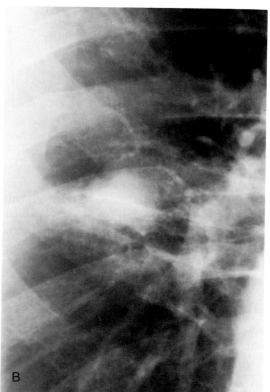

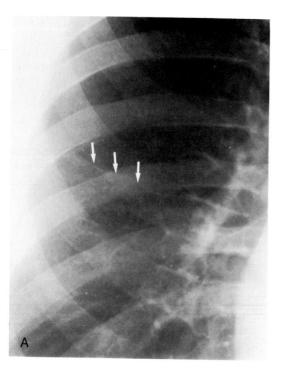

Fig. 2-47 Adenocarcinoma, scar carcinoma.
History: This 64-year-old male presented for a routine chest x-ray during a physical examination. A previous chest x-ray 4 years earlier had been reported as normal.
Findings: **(A)** *Previous chest radiograph:* A thin scar or area of fibrosis is present in the right mid-lung field. It is considered of no clinical significance (arrows). **(B)** *Current chest radiograph:* This film, obtained 4 years after the previous study, demonstrates a 3-cm nodule superimposed over the previously present benign scar.

feature of a large tumor mass of the squamous cell variety. Squamous cell tumors are the most frequent causes of the solid, dense apical masses, often with accompanying rib destruction, called "Pancoast tumors" (Fig. 2-46).

Adenocarcinoma, exclusive of the bronchoalveolar-cell carcinoma previously discussed, most commonly presents as a single peripheral nodule. The borders of the nodule are frequently loculated, shaggy, and ill-defined. The nodule is usually less than 4 cm in diameter, and if larger should suggest a tumor of a different cell type. Adenocarcinoma frequently arises from a peripherally located scar left over from a previous inflammatory process. This scar may have been present for many years with an unchanged appearance. A diagnosis of adenocarcinoma or "scar carcinoma" is suggested whenever a stable calcified granuloma or scar begins to enlarge after years of showing no change (Fig. 2-47 A and B). Adenocarcinoma often metastasizes early in its course to the hilar or mediastinal lymph nodes. Thus, a frequent presentation is a peripheral nodule with an accompanying hilar or mediastinal mass. Early metastasis to the pleura with a secondary pleural effusion, and early distal metastasis (bone) also occur with adenocarcinoma.

Small-cell or oat-cell carcinoma is primarily a centrally situated tumor that is strongly aggressive, with early metastatic spread. It most often presents as a hilar or mediastinal mass (Fig. 2-48) that represents metastatic lymph node involvement rather than the primary tumor. The tumor itself is within the bronchus and is usually not detected radiographically. Other common sites of metastatic involvement, besides the mediastinal lymph nodes, include the bone marrow and adrenal glands; infiltration into the lymphatic system of the lungs leads to the coarse reticulonodular pattern of lymphangitic metastasis.

Large-cell tumors are most often large peripheral nodules greater than 4 cm in diameter. They frequently occur in younger patients (Fig. 2-35 A and B).

The further radiographic workup of a suspected primary lung carcinoma depends on the initial chest x-ray findings or cell-type identification obtained from a sputum cytologic examination. The major tools for diagnosis include conventional tomography, computed tomography (CT) (Fig. 2-35 B and 2-44 B), and transthoracic needle aspiration biopsy (TNAB). Pulmonary arteriography, bronchography, and lung scanning have no significant place in the

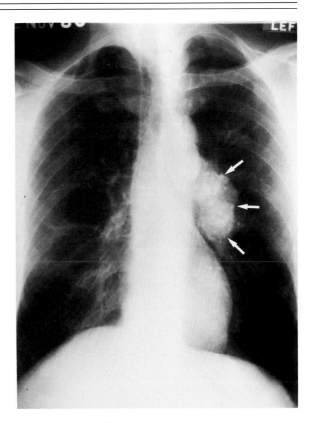

Fig. 2-48 Oat-cell carcinoma.
History: This 60-year-old male presented with dizziness and clumsiness.
Findings: *Chest radiograph:* A huge left hilar mass represents metastatic hilar adenopathy (arrows). Subsequent bronchoscopy revealed a small endobronchial tumor that proved upon biopsy to be an oat-cell carcinoma. The patient's dizziness was the result of brain metastasis.

workup of a primary lung tumor. Nuclear medicine liver and bone scans may, however, be useful in identifying metastasis once a diagnosis of lung cancer has been made.

BENIGN TUMORS

Benign neoplasms of the lung are uncommon. The most common is bronchial adenoma, which is in reality a low-grade malignancy. Bronchial adenomas are usually of the carcinoid type, and over 80 percent are centrally located within major or segmental bronchi (Fig. 2-49). The most common chest x-ray finding in cases of this tumor is identical to that in other intra-

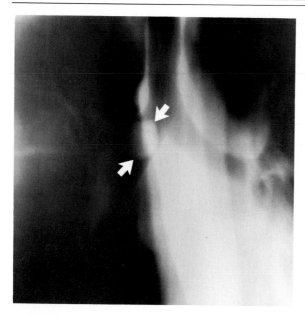

Fig. 2-49 Bronchial adenoma.
History: This 16-year-old male had progressive shortness of breath and wheezing.
Findings: *Mediastinal tomogram:* The chest x-ray suggested a mass in the right mainstem bronchus that is confirmed by conventional tomography. The lesion is well defined and attached to the superior wall of the bronchus (arrows).

bronchial lesions, constituting massive atelectasis or postobstructive pneumonitis. The less than 20 percent of bronchial adenomas that are located peripherally appear as large (average 4 cm), homogeneous, sharply circumscribed nodules in the right upper and middle lobes or lingula.[29]

Pulmonary hamartoma, another benign lesion, is a peripherally based lesion that is also well-circumscribed and solitary, but usually smaller than 4 cm in diameter. These lesions are infrequently calcified. They may grow over time, making their distinction from a bronchogenic carcinoma impossible. CT is performed to identify any calcification that would signify benign disease, but biopsy either by needle aspiration or open thoracotomy is often required for the final diagnosis.

VASCULAR DISEASES

Congestive heart failure and pulmonary embolism both may lead to hemoptysis. Mitral valvular disease results in a chronic congestive heart failure with the typically enlarged left atrium and ventricle ("mitral heart") (see Fig. 6-17). The chronically engorged interstitium eventually becomes fibrotic, leading to a dirty, coarse reticular pattern in the lung. Pulmonary vasculitis, as seen in the mixed connective-tissue disorders (rheumatoid arthritis, SLE, and others) also may lead to a prolonged hemoptysis (Fig. 2-39).

TRAUMATIC

Lung contusion or bronchial irritation by a foreign body is for obvious reasons, included in the differential diagnosis of hemoptysis. The appropriate history and a clearing of symptoms with proper therapy confirm this diagnosis.

HEMORRHAGIC

Therapy with anticoagulants or an underlying bleeding diathesis can also lead to hemorrhage into the lung parenchyma or bronchi, with secondary hemoptysis. The chest x-ray in such cases shows a dense alveolar infiltrate or consolidation. Laboratory analysis of the patient's blood confirms the diagnosis of a bleeding disorder.

CLINICAL PRESENTATION: SOLITARY PULMONARY NODULE (ALGORITHM 2-3)

Chest x-rays are obtained for a variety of screening reasons. They are routinely obtained at the start of a new job, before surgery, in chronic smokers, in persons occupationally or environmentally at risk, during annual physical examinations, in patients with respiratory symptoms, and upon admission to most hospitals. A frequent problem in such examinations is the discovery of a solitary nodule, the so-called "coin-lesion." The major concern is whether this newly discovered nodule represents a malignant or a benign process. The major differential considerations include some entities previously discussed, such as malignant and benign neoplasms, solitary granulomas (tuberculosis or histoplasmosis), single metastases, the conglomerate masses of silicosis, rounded pneumonic bacterial infiltrates, or resolving pulmonary infarctions. An abscess may present as a single nodule, with

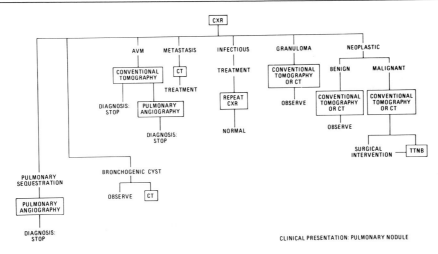

Algorithm 2-3

or without cavitation. A congenital lesion, such as an arteriovenous malformation (AVM) or pulmonary sequestration, is an infrequent cause of a solitary nodule. Lastly, bronchogenic or hydatid cysts are also included in the long differential list.

The first step in deciding whether a nodule is malignant or benign is to obtain old films of the patient's chest. If the nodule is present in a past examination and is virtually unchanged in size over a long period, it most often represents a scar or healed granuloma of old tuberculosis, and no further workup is warranted. Growth of a previously present nodule or the appearance of a new nodule should lead to the suspicion of malignancy. The classic chest x-ray findings in cases of a malignant nodule are an ill-defined, dense mass with stranding extending into the surrounding aerated lung as the tumor grows (Fig. 2-26). A conventional tomogram or CT scan is then performed to obtain a more detailed view of the nodule (Fig. 2-50). With tomography or CT, calcifications are often detected that cannot be appreciated on the plain chest x-ray. Completely calcified, central, peripheral, or punctate calcifications within the nodule signify a benign process such as a healed granuloma (Fig. 2-7 A and B).

INFECTIONS: ABSCESS

The term abscess is usually reserved for pyogenic processes. The abscess is the result of an aggressive pro-

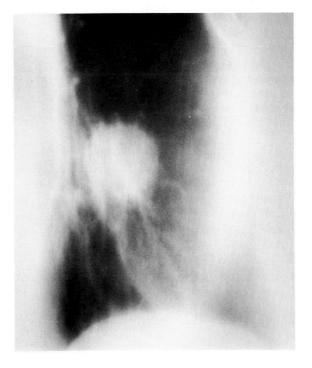

Fig. 2-50 Solitary nodule, primary bronchogenic carcinoma.
History: This was a 67-year-old female with a long history of cigarette smoking. A chest x-ray suggested a nodule behind the heart.
Findings: *Tomogram:* The borders of the nodule are irregular, with spicules radiating into the surrounding parenchyma.

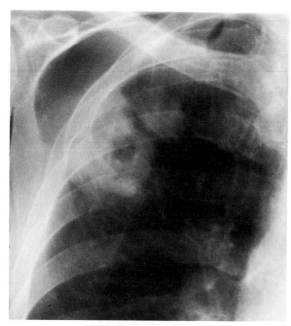

Fig. 2-51 Pulmonary abscess.
History: This 31-year-old intravenous drug abuser had a 2-week history of fever and chills.
Findings: *Chest radiograph:* An air filled cavitary mass is identified in the right upper lung field, with a surrounding infiltrate. The cavity resolved with extensive antibiotic treatment.

cess which leads to necrosis of the underlying lung. There is often evidence of a previous necrotizing pneumonia. The organisms that most commonly produce an abscess cavity include staphylococci, B-hemolytic streptococci, *Klebsiella, Pseudomonas, E. coli,* and certain anaerobes.[28]

The chest x-ray shows an ill-defined, dense nodule, often with stranding of tissue into the aerated lung from the inflammatory region surrounding the nodule. If communication with the bronchus occurs, the nodule becomes air filled and is termed a cavity. The cavity has thick walls and its inner wall is somewhat irregular (Fig. 2-51).

BRONCHOGENIC CYSTS

Bronchogenic cysts are rare congenital lesions that have a preferential distribution in the lower lobes. They often occur medially, near the mediastinum. Their chest x-ray appearance is that of a sharply circumscribed, rounded mass (Fig. 2-52). In 75 percent of cases they become infected, develop subsequent communication with the bronchial tree, and take on a resulting cystic or cavitary appearance.

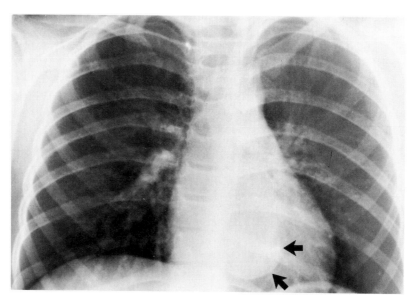

Fig. 2-52 Bronchogenic cyst.
History: This 7-year-old female had a shortness of breath and was thought to have possibly aspirated a peanut.
Findings: *Chest radiograph:* A large, well-defined circular mass is seen behind the heart (arrows). The peanut was not identified and the patient improved with supportive therapy.

ARTERIOVENOUS MALFORMATION

Arteriovenous malformations (AVMs) occur both hereditarily and spontaneously (acquired). Approximately one-third are multiple. The chest x-ray shows AVMs to be most common in the lower lobes. The classic appearance is that of a rounded, often lobular, and sharply defined nodule. Feeding vessels may be seen running into and out of the nodule, giving the appearance of "rabbit ears." The malformations range in size from under 1 cm to several centimeters in diameter.

Further workup in a case of suspected AVM includes conventional tomography, which may clearly demonstrate the feeding artery and draining vein, with the nodule being their point of communication. Angiography is required to confirm the diagnosis before any resectional surgery is performed.

PULMONARY SEQUESTRATION

A sequestration is a congenital anomaly in which a segment of lung receives its blood supply from a systemic artery instead of a pulmonary artery. Sequestrations are divided into the two varieties of intralobar and extralobar.

CLINICAL PRESENTATION: HILAR ENLARGEMENT (ALGORITHM 2-4)

The pulmonary hila are complex structures that contain the pulmonary arteries, veins, bronchi, and lymph nodes. Lymph-node enlargement, for a variety of reasons, can lead to an enlargement of the hilar shadow on the chest x-ray. The chest x-ray is also helpful in detecting accompanying abnormalities such as lung masses or infiltrates in the lungs that can help identify the cause of hilar enlargement. Again, high resolution CT allows the best visualization of the hilar anatomy, and lets one differentiate the various causes of apparent hilar enlargement, such as a single mass, multiple enlarged lymph nodes, or even a dilated pulmonary artery with no lymph-node enlargement. Computed tomography is also able to detect any coexisting mediastinal lymph-node enlargement not possible with 55-degree hilar tomography.

The causes of hilar enlargement are basically the result of three processes: a dilated pulmonary artery, metastatic or inflammatory hilar adenopathy, or a primary, contiguous bronchogenic carcinoma. One can further classify the causes of hilar enlargement into those diseases that result in unilateral hilar enlargement and those leading to bilateral hilar enlargement.

UNILATERAL HILAR ENLARGEMENT

A primary lung carcinoma may abut the hilum, leading to hilar enlargement, but more commonly the hilar enlargement results from the secondary metastatic spread of a primary lung tumor to the lymph nodes (Fig. 2-48). Distant primary malignancies (renal) may also metastasize to the hilar nodes, leading to their enlargement. Additionally, lymphoma frequently involves the hilar nodes, but usually leads to bilateral enlargement and concurrent mediastinal ade-

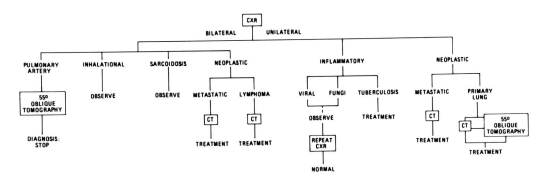

CLINICAL PRESENTATION: HILAR ADENOPATHY

Algorithm 2-4

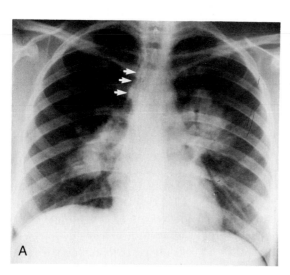

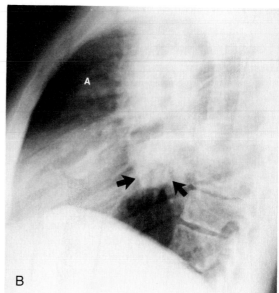

Fig. 2-53 Mediastinal lymphoma.
History: This was a 45-year-old female with known lymphoma.
Findings: (A) *Chest radiograph, PA view:* There is extensive bilateral perihilar adenopathy and contiguous extension into the lung parenchyma on the left side. The right paratracheal lymph nodes are mildly enlarged (arrows). **(B)** *Lateral view:* The hilar adenopathy is easily identified (arrows). The retrosternal airspace is partially filled in by the soft-tissue shadow of anterior mediastinal adenopathy (A).

nopathy. The most common inflammatory causes of unilateral hilar adenopathy are primary tuberculosis (Fig. 2-22), fungal infection (histoplasmosis), viral agents (measles, mononucleosis), and infrequently inhalational irritants (silicosis) and drug reactions. A pulmonary artery is often prominent but still normal, and can be mistaken for hilar disease. In this situation CT is most helpful in demonstrating the large pulmonary artery as the cause of the apparent hilar mass.

BILATERAL HILAR ENLARGEMENT

Lymphoma is the most common cause of bilateral hilar adenopathy. The involvement is usually assymmetric, with one hilum being larger than the other (Fig. 2-53 A and B). This is in contrast to sarcoidosis, the most common inflammatory etiology of hilar enlargement which classically results in symmetric enlargement (Fig. 2-28). Both lymphoma and sarcoido-

sis have mediastinal adenopathy, but the location of such involvement may help in differenting the two (sarcoidosis infrequently involves the anterior mediastinal nodes, whereas lymphoma frequently does). Inhalational irritants (silicosis) more commonly result in bilateral than unilateral hilar adenopathy (Fig. 2-33).

Pulmonary hypertension leads to bilaterally dilated pulmonary arteries and apparent hilar enlargement. Such hypertension is frequently secondary to left-sided congestive heart failure, but is also seen in chronic lung disease, pulmonary embolism, congenital heart disease (left-to-right shunts), and for idiopathic reasons. The chest x-ray appearance depends on the etiology of the hypertension. Whatever the cause, however, bilateral hilar enlargement is a common feature. The enlarged main pulmonary artery segments give rise to abnormally prominent and dilated pulmonary arteries seen radiating from the hila. These dilated arteries taper abruptly as they reach the

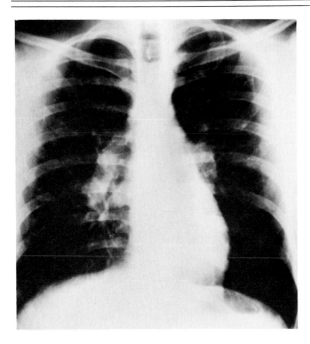

Fig. 2-54 Pulmonary hypertension.
History: Unknown.
Findings: *Chest radiograph:* Both hila are enlarged and there is a paucity of markings seen within the lung parenchyma.

peripheral portions of the lung, and virtually no vessels are seen at the lateralmost portion of the lung (Fig. 2-54). The picture has been likened to the stark appearance of a tree in the winter. The smallest branches or arteries are barely discernible in compari-

son to the thicker, more prominent central branches or pulmonary arteries. Right ventricular enlargement is frequently present. The etiology of the pulmonary hypertension may be apparent from the chest x-ray, such as the overinflated, bullous lungs of chronic obstructive lung disease or the changes of congestive heart failure.

CLINICAL PRESENTATION: MEDIASTINAL MASS (ALGORITHM 2-5)

The best way to approach an abnormal mass projecting from the mediastinum is to divide the mediastinum into three sections. The sections adopted for this text are based on the lateral view of the chest as put forward by a leading chest radiologist, Dr. Benjamin Felson[29] (Fig. 2-55). The mediastinum can be divided into anterior, middle, and posterior compartments. The anterior and middle compartments are separated by an imaginary vertical line extending along the back of the heart and in front of the trachea. The middle and posterior compartments are separated by another imaginary line connecting a point on each thoracic vertebral body 1 cm behind its anterior margin. The anterior mediastinum comprises the airspace behind the sternum and the heart and the proximalmost aortic knob. The vagus nerve, trachea, esophagus, and aortic arch lie within the middle mediastinum. The posterior mediastinum is basically

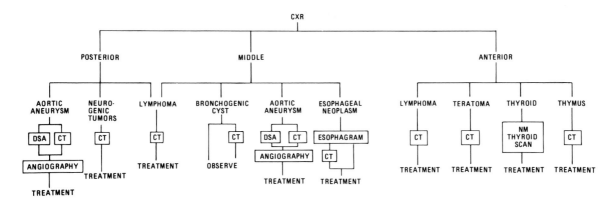

CLINICAL PRESENTATION: MEDIASTINAL MASS

Algorithm 2-5

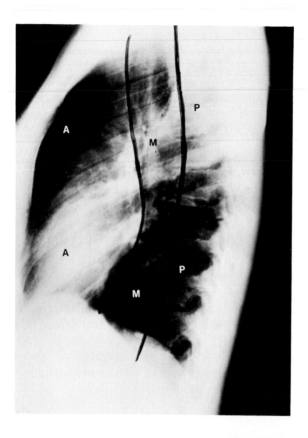

Fig. 2-55 Mediastinal divisions. A = anterior mediastinum, M = middle mediastinum, P = posterior mediastinum.

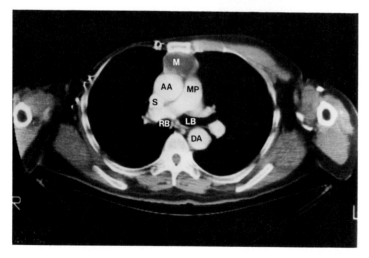

Fig. 2-56 Anterior mediastinal mass, metastatic adenopathy.

History: This 79-year-old female had had a right mastectomy for carcinoma. A chest x-ray suggested a mass projected over the spine.

Findings: *CT scan:* A section through the main pulmonary artery (MP) and ascending (AA) and descending aorta (DA) demonstrates a soft-tissue mass (M) in front of the aorta in the anterior mediastinum. A transthoracic needle biopsy confirmed metastatic breast carcinoma. S = superior vena cava, LB = left mainstem bronchus, RB = right mainstem bronchus.

comprised of the paravertebral gutter, which contains neural elements, and the descending aorta. Lymph nodes are scattered throughout all portions of the mediastinum.

ANTERIOR MEDIASTINAL MASS

The differential considerations in cases of an anterior mediastinal mass have been called the four "T's": teratoma, thymoma, ectopic or substernal thyroid extension, and terrible lymphoma (massive lymph node enlargement).

The chest x-ray appearance of an anterior mediastinal mass is a loss of aeration of the retrosternal space on the lateral radiograph. The frontal film reveals a

bulge or mass projecting on either side of the mediastinum, smoothly pushing the lung and pleura away from the mediastinum. A CT examination is performed to confirm the presence of the mass, to determine the size and extent of the mass, or to detect any calcifications or clues that may aid in making a diagnosis (Fig. 2-56).

MIDDLE MEDIASTINAL MASS

The differential diagnoses in cases of a middle mediastinal mass are mainly esophageal neoplasms (benign and malignant), aneurysm of the aorta or another great vessel, bronchogenic cyst, hiatal hernia, lymphoma, and ectopic goiter (Fig. 2-57). The CT scan is

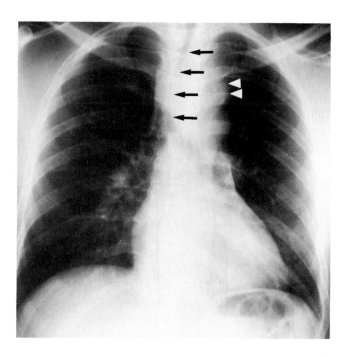

Fig. 2-57 Middle mediastinal mass, intrathoracic thyroid.
History: This 31-year-old male developed new wheezing and hemoptysis.
Findings: *Chest radiograph:* The trachea is deviated to the right and compressed by a mass (arrows). The lateral portion of the mass projects to the left of the mediastinum (arrowheads). The tracheal compression signifies that the mass lies next to the trachea and so within the middle mediastinum. Subsequent laryngoscopy and surgery revealed an enlarged thyroid that was ectopically located between the trachea and the esophagus.

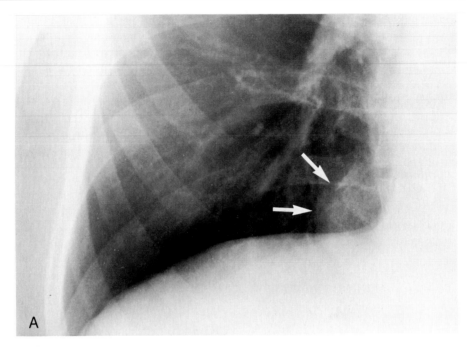

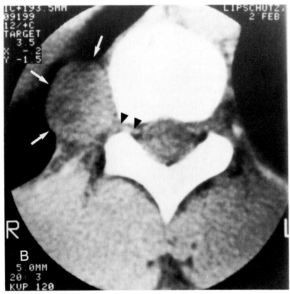

Fig. 2-58 Posterior mediastinal mass, neural tumor.
History: This was a 37-year-old male with a "pinched nerve."
Findings: **(A)** *Chest radiograph:* There is a large mass (arrows) in the lower right hemithorax. It is distinct from the diaphragm since it does not silhouette the diaphragm. **(B)** *CT scan:* The mass (arrow) arises from a nerve (arrowheads) as it exits from the spinal canal.

helpful in characterizing the mass, and can clearly distinguish an aneurysm from a solid mass. The aneurysm enhances densely after contrast-medium administration.

POSTERIOR MEDIASTINAL MASS

The differential diagnoses in cases of posterior mediastinal masses include neurogenic tumors (benign or malignant), aneurysms of the descending aorta, and lymphoma (Fig. 2-58 A and B).

REFERENCES

1. Felson B: Chest Roentgenology. WB Saunders Company, Philadelphia, 1973, p 143
2. Mukin JR, Brown LR, Croew JK, et al: Comparison of whole lung tomography and computed tomography

for detecting pulmonary nodules. AJR 131:961–984, 1978

3. Seigleman S, Settouni GA, Leo FP, et al: CT of the solitary pulmonary nodule. AJR 135:1–13, 1980

4. Mintzer RA: Chest Imaging: An Integrated Approach. Williams & Wilkins, Baltimore, 1981, p 175

5. Paré JA, Fraser RG: Synopsis of Diseases of the Chest. WB Saunders Company, Philadelphia, 1983, pp 529–530

6. Paré JA, Fraser RG: Synopsis of Diseases of the Chest. WB Saunders Company, Philadelphia, 1983, p 536

7. Cohen BH, Menkes HA, Bias WB, et al: Multiple factors in airway obstruction. Chest 77(Suppl):257, 1980

8. World Health Organization, Report of an Expert Committee: Definition and diagnosis of pulmonary diseases with special reference to chronic bronchitis and emphysema. In Chronic Cor Pulmonale, WHO Technical Report Series No. 213, 1961, pp 14–19

9. Thurlbeck WM, Henderson JA, Fraser RG: Chronic obstructive lung disease. A comparison between clinical, roentgenologic, functional and morphological criteria in chronic bronchitis, emphysema, asthma and bronchiectasis. Medicine 49:81, 1970

10. Thurlbeck WM, Simon G: Radiographic appearance of the chest in emphysema, AJR 130:429, 1978

11. Paré JA, Fraser RG: Synopsis of Diseases of the Chest. WB Saunders & Company, Philadelphia, 1983, p 682

12. Paré JA, Fraser RG: Synopsis of Diseases of the Chest. WB Saunders & Company, Philadelphia, 1983, p 271

13. Paré JA, Fraser RG: Synopsis of Diseases of the Chest. WB Saunders & Company, Philadelphia, 1983, p 292

14. Sochocky S: Tuberculoma of the lung. Am Rev Tuberc 78:403, 1958

15. Reed JC: Chest Radiology: Patterns & Differential Diagnosis. Year Book Medical Publishers, Chicago, 1981, p 200

16. Watson WL, Farpour A: Terminal bronchiolar or "alveolar cell" cancer of the lung. Two hundred sixty-five cases. Cancer 19:776, 1966

17. Tudelenham WJ, Barden RP, Campbell RE, et al: Chest Disease (Second Series) Syllabus. American College of Radiology, Chicago, 1975, pp 294–295

18. Maycock RL, Bertrand P, Morrison CE, et al: Manifestations of sarcoidosis. Analysis of 145 patients, with a review of nine series selected from the literature. Am J Med 35:67, 1963

19. Kuhs DR, McCormick VD, Greenspan RH: Pulmonary sarcoidosis. Roentgenologic analysis of 150 patients. AJR 117:777, 1973

20. Tudelenham WJ, Barden RP, Campbell RE, et al: Chest Disease (Second Series) Syllabus. American College of Radiology, Chicago, 1975, p 196

21. Reed JC: Chest Radiology: Patterns and Differential Diagnosis. Year Book Medical Publishers, Chicago, 1981, p 174

22. Freiman DG, Suyemoto J, Wessler S: Frequency of pulmonary thromboembolism in man. N Engl J Med, 272:1278, 1965

23. Inouge WY, Berggren RB, Johnson J: Spontaneous pneumothorax: Treatment and mortality. Dis Chest 51:67, 1967

24. Paré JA, Fraser RG: Synopsis of Diseases of the Chest. WB Saunders & Company, Philadelphia, 1983, p 169

25. Thorn GW, Adamo RD, Braunwald E, et al: Harrison's Principles of Internal Medicine. McGraw-Hill Book Company, New York, 1980, p 165

26. Lee JK, Sagel SS, Stanley RJ: Computed Body Tomography. Raven Press, New York, 1983, p 105

27. Paré JA, Fraser RG: Synopsis of Diseases of the Chest. WB Saunders & Company, Philadelphia, 1983, pp 401–402

28. Reed JC: Chest Radiology: Patterns and Differential Diagnosis. Year Book Medical Publishers, Chicago, 1981, p 275

29. Felson B: Chest Roentgenology. WB Saunders & Company, Philadelphia, 1973, p 416

3

Radiology of the Urinary Tract

Lee Sider

The evaluation of the kidneys and lower urinary tract is undergoing many changes in today's radiology. Most radiologists still agree that the intravenous pyelogram (IVP) should be the initial radiographic examination of the urinary tract. An initial plain film of the abdomen is often obtained to detect any abnormal calcifications in the vicinity of the kidneys, ureters, or bladder. Next is the intravenous administration of an iodine-based contrast medium that is taken up by the glomeruli. Images are obtained immediately after the injection and after some time delay to study the different phases of renal function. The immediate blush or nephrogram represents glomerular filtration (Fig. 3-1A), while the later phases in which the collecting system is visualized (ureter and bladder as well) are a function of tubular activity (Fig. 3-1B). The radiologist uses the IVP to see focal and diffuse renal parenchymal abnormalities, functional alterations, deviations from normal renal position, caly-

ceal, pelvic, ureteral, and bladder anatomic abnormalities, and different extrinsic effects on the various urinary components. Tomograms are routinely obtained to reduce the affect of overlying bowel gas. Tomography blurs all structures outside a predetermined plane which the radiographer chooses to include the main axis of the kidney (Fig. 3-1A).

Ultrasound is an important tool in renal evaluation (Fig. 3-2). A major indication for this safe and noninvasive method is to further characterize a mass seen on the screening IVP. The ultrasound examination gives valuable information about whether the mass is fluid filled or solid. The radiologist looks for an abrupt change in the echo pattern of the kidney, as well as a localized bulge or contour defect to indicate a mass. The characterization of the mass by ultrasound significantly determines further patient management. The finding of a "classic" cyst halts any further workup. Alternatively, the entire echo pattern of the kidney

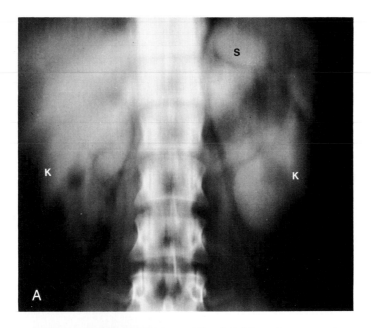

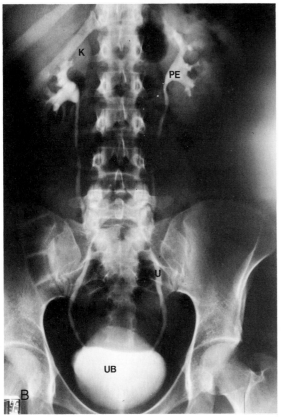

Fig. 3-1 Normal anatomy: Intravenous pyelogram (IVP). **(A)** Initial nephrogram phase obtained 30 seconds after the intravenous administration of an iodine-based contrast medium using the tomogram technique. This is the glomerular phase. S = stomach, K = kidney. **(B)** Single view of the abdomen at 5 minutes after contrast-medium administration. The entire collecting system is now filled with the processed and concentrated medium. K = kidney, PE = pelvis, U = ureter, UB = urinary bladder.

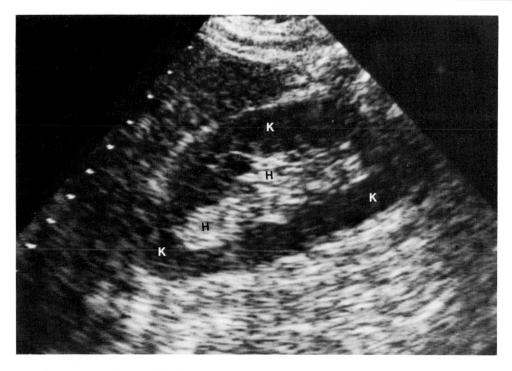

Fig. 3-2 Normal anatomy: Ultrasound (US). Longitudinal view through the long axis of the midportion of the kidney shows the natural acoustic contrast of the gentle echo character of the renal parenchyma with the harsh echo character of the fat- and fibrous-filled pelvis. K = renal parenchyma, H = renal hilum.

may be abnormal, indicating a diffuse parenchymal process.

The detection of hydronephrosis is another important indication for ultrasound. Hydronephrosis is easily detected ultrasonographically in almost any clinical setting, making ultrasound useful in the critically ill intensive-care patient. Lastly, ultrasound may reveal calculi either not seen on an IVP because they are not calcified (radiolucent) or which are too small to be seen on a plain film. Other uses of ultrasound include the examination of patients with allergies to the IVP contrast, pregnancy, poor renal function with poor renal visualization on the IVP, and renal localization prior to a biopsy or cyst drainage.

Computed tomography (CT) is rapidly becoming more useful in renal evaluation, and is eliminating the need for the more invasive procedures (Fig. 3-3A). It further characterizes a known mass by helping to determine its content (fluid, fat, or solid) and homogeneity. It clearly delineates the surrounding retroperitoneal compartment (perirenal space) that contains the kidney which cannot be seen on the IVP. Computed tomography is also useful in determining the level of a ureteral obstruction, as well as giving information about extrinsic and intrinsic bladder processes such as tumor extent and invasion (Fig. 3-3B).

Retrograde pyelography is less used as newer modalities become more important and the quality of IVPs improve (Fig. 3-4). It is valuable when clear opacification of the ureters and calyces is required and not obtained during an intravenous urogram owing to a poorly functioning kidney. Thus its main uses are in

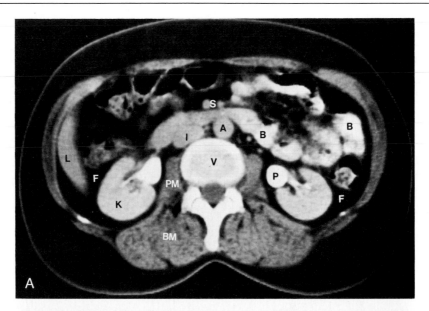

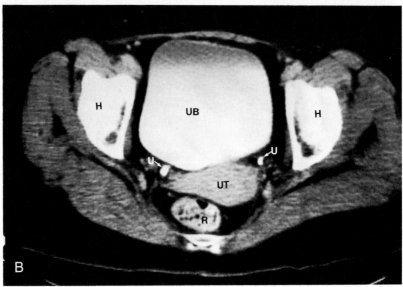

Fig. 3-3 Normal anatomy: Computerized tomography. **(A)** The first slice is a view through the kidneys after the intravenous administration of contrast medium. There is also orally administered contrast medium in the loops of the bowel. K = kidney, P = pelvis of kidney filled with excreted contrast medium, I = inferior vena cava, A = aorta, V = vertebral body, B = bowel loops filled with orally given contrast medium, L = liver tip, PM = psoas muscles, BM = back muscles, S = superior mesenteric artery and vein, F = retroperitoneal fat surrounding the kidney. **(B)** This lower slice is through a section in the female pelvis showing the urinary bladder. UB = contrast-filled urinary bladder, U = ureters before they enter the bladder, H = hips, UT = uterus, R = rectum.

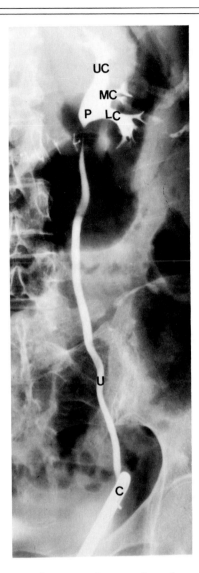

Fig. 3-4 Normal anatomy: Retrograde pyelogram. A single view demonstrates the catheter in the distal ureter. The upper, middle, and lower collecting systems are well defined. C = catheter, U = ureter, P = pelvis, UC = upper collecting system, MC = middle collecting system, LC = lower collecting system.

the evaluation of calyceal abnormalities such as papillary necrosis, transitional cell tumors, and in detection of the level of ureteral obstruction.

Renal angiography is an invasive procedure that is clearly less utilized today than in the past (Fig. 3-5). It gives information about diseases of the main renal artery for the evaluation of hypertension. Selective catheterization of a renal artery allows the evaluation

of a mass seen first with other imaging modalities. It can often differentiate a benign from a malignant neoplasm, and can also be used to stage a malignancy by injection of contrast medium into the superior mesenteric artery, celiac axis, and venous structures.

Cystography allows the investigation of intrinsic abnormalities of the bladder, such as tumors, calculi, and blood clots. However, cystoscopy, done by the urologist, has eliminated the need for this examination in most clinical situations. The determination of vesicoureteral reflux as well as urethral anatomy are current indications for voiding cystography. The bladder is filled with contrast medium via a Foley

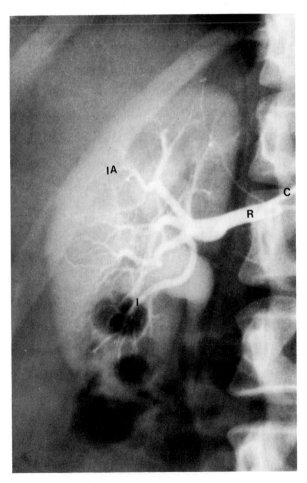

Fig. 3-5 Normal anatomy: Renal angiogram. The angiographic catheter tip has been selectively directed into the right main renal artery from its location in the aorta. There is clear delineation of the vessels of the kidney. R = main renal artery, I = interlobar arteries, IA = interlobular arteries, C = catheter.

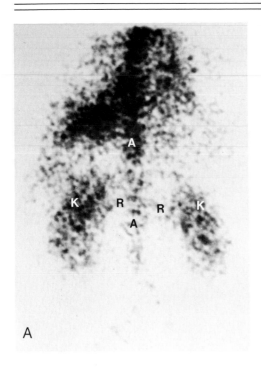

A

catheter. Then under fluoroscopic guidance the patient is instructed to void. This is called antegrade, voiding, or micturition cystourethrography. If a more complete study of the urethra is required, a retrograde investigation may be performed with a catheter in the urethral meatus, thus allowing a consistently complete view of the entire urethra. This is often necessary in male adults with dysuria, urinary tract infection, trauma, hematuria, and stress incontinence.

In recent years the field of interventional radiology has made a great impact on the diagnosis and treatment of urinary tract disease (Fig. 3-22). A percutaneous nephrostomy, involving puncture of the renal pelvis from the skin, allows the antegrade or forward opacification of the pelvis and ureter. The nephrostomy is also used to establish an avenue of drainage in an obstructed pelvis for patients who are acutely septic or azotemic. This allows a route for renal stone retrieval without the need for surgery. The localization

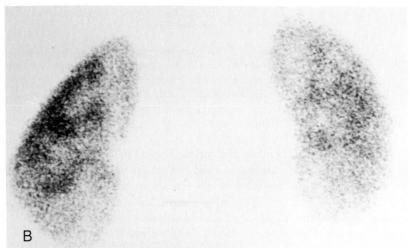

B

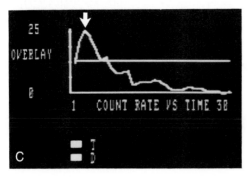

C

Fig. 3-6 Normal anatomy: Nuclear medicine renal scan. **(A)** Technetium-DMSA angiogram. A = aorta, R = renal arteries, K = kidney. **(B)** Technetium-DMSA; 2-hour-delay view. **(C)** Normal renogram curve, initial peak (arrow).

of the kidney for puncture is accomplished via the intravenous administration of contrast medium or with the aid of ultrasound.

Other invasive techniques include therapeutic renal infarction in patients with renal neoplasms, ateriovenous fistulas, and bleeding from the kidney. This either terminates the bleeding or facilitates subsequent surgery on very vascular tumors by reducing the tumor blood supply. The main thrombosing agents used are a synthetic material called Gelfoam, clotted autologous blood, bits of autologous skeletal muscle, or a small coiled wire placed in the main renal artery. Cyst puncture is an old procedure used for the diagnosis and treatment of renal cysts. It is less utilized today, since the management of renal cysts has become more conservative.

Anatomic and functional studies are possible with the intravenous administration of radioactive iodine- and technetium-containing compounds. A technetium nuclide is used to label one of various compounds that demonstrate different degrees of renal filtration, excretion, and cortical binding. Today, dimercaptosuccinic acid (DMSA) is the favored agent in many institutions. An initial series of images is obtained after injection of the radioactive compound into a peripheral arm vein. This initial blood-flow or angiogram phase allows visualization of the aorta and blood flow to the kidneys (Fig. 3-6A). Images obtained 2 hours later show the radionuclide bound to the renal cortex, giving a gross morphologic view (Fig. 3-6B). Functional analysis of the kidney is accomplished with the subsequent injection of ^{131}I-hippuran. By counting the activity over the kidneys in relation to time, the curve known as a renogram is generated (Fig. 3-6C). The initial peak indicates glomerular filtration, while the subsequent decline represents excretion of the medium (i.e., function). The combination of the two studies is valuable in transplant complications, preoperative evaluation before a nephrectomy, renovascular hypertension, obstructive uropathy, and renal parenchymal disorders.

One of the most recent tools in the evaluation of renovascular hypertension is digital subtraction angiography (DSA). With the injection of contrast medium into a peripheral antecubital vein one can obtain adequate main renal artery opacification with computer assistance (Fig. 3-7). This is now considered a good method of screening for hypertension of a vascular etiology, replacing the less sensitive timed intra-

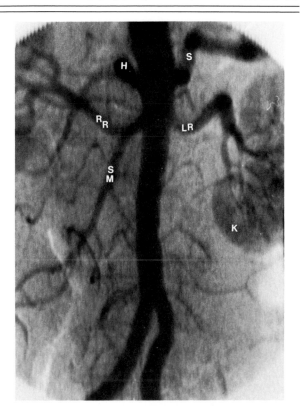

Fig. 3-7 Normal anatomy: Digital subtraction angiography (DSA). This single view of the aorta clearly demonstrates the vascular anatomy of the abdomen. H = hepatic artery, S = splenic artery, RR = right renal artery, LR = left renal artery, SM = superior mesenteric artery, K = kidney.

venous pyelogram. Digital subtraction angiography can also be used to evaluate post-transplant patients for subsequent renal artery stenosis. Additionally, it may provide a relatively noninvasive mechanism for studying the renal arteries of potential donors.

Evaluation of the female pelvis for gynecologic disease and obstetric progress is universally initially done with ultrasound (see Fig. 1-24). It is an excellent screening procedure for everything from detecting pelvic inflammatory disease to the characterization of ovarian neoplasms, and provides a safe mechanism for following the development of the fetus. The ultrasound examination is also easily and quickly performed without subjecting the patient to ionizing radiation. Further evaluation of pelvic disease is possible with a CT scan, and less importantly today with an IVP, barium enema, and other less specific or less sensitive examinations.

CLINICAL PRESENTATION: HEMATURIA (ALGORITHM 3-1)

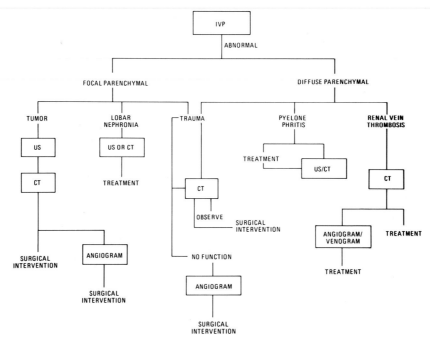

CLINICAL PRESENTATION: HEMATURIA

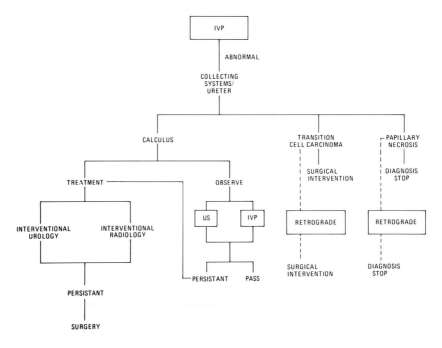

CLINICAL PRESENTATION: HEMATURIA

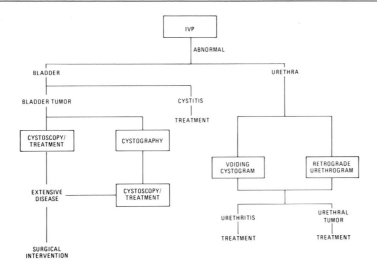

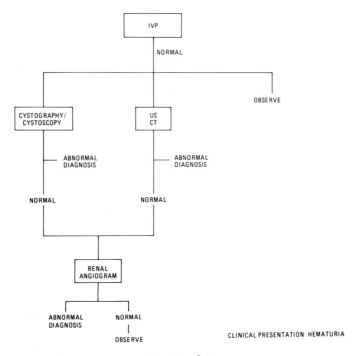

Algorithm 3-1

INFECTIONS

ACUTE PYELONEPHRITIS

Acute pyelonephritis is a common problem; however, most patients with this condition never have urograms (IVP) during the acute episode since approximately only one-quarter have abnormal IVPs.[3]

The diagnosis of acute pyelonephritis is usually made clinically. The disease is caused by bacterial invasion of the renal parenchyma, usually by *E. coli.* The nephrogram of the IVP is usually of diminished density, inhomogeneous, and of longer duration than that

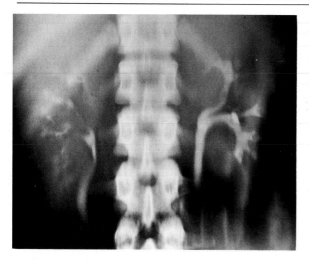

Fig. 3-8 Acute pyelonephritis: Uncomplicated.
History: This 21-year-old female presented with intense flank pain for 2 weeks.
Findings: *IVP:* The tomogram from the IVP shows compression and some distortion of the collecting system on the right by an edema-filled kidney. The left side is normal and uninvolved.

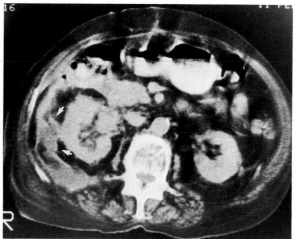

Fig. 3-9 Acute pyelonephritis with secondary perinephric extension.
History: This 42-year-old female had a 2-month history of right flank pain and fever that persisted after antibiotic therapy.
Findings: *CT scan:* The right kidney is enlarged with a perinephric fluid collection (arrows) that represents a localized abscess adjacent to the kidney. The normal left side demonstrates the clear-fat-containing perirenal space, without the abnormal water-density collections.

on the normal side. The affected kidney may be enlarged. There is a delay in the appearance of contrast medium in the calyces, which are compressed and distorted because of the inflammation of the surrounding renal parenchyma (Fig. 3-8). Infrequently there may be a localized mass with isolated segmental involvement. This has come to be known as lobar nephronia, and with the subsequent imaging modalities is difficult to differentiate from a tumor.

The ultrasound examination is also frequently normal in cases of acute pyelonephritis, although a slightly enlarged kidney with decreased renal parenchymal echoes and increased echoes from the pelvis has been observed. The major indication for ultrasound is in seeking complications such as pyonephrosis, a renal carbuncle or perinephric (retroperitoneal) abscess.[4]

The CT may again be normal with diffuse disease, or may show a patchy inhomogeneous enhancement similar to that seen on the excretory urogram. Computed tomography is most valuable for the detection and follow-up of any complications, as discussed under ultrasound (Fig. 3-9). The angiogram is often normal and not indicated. If done for other reasons it may show stretching and narrowing of the intrarenal vessels.

CHRONIC PYELONEPHRITIS

Chronic pyelonephritis results in a small and irregularly scarred kidney. This disease usually has its beginning in childhood. It may be unilateral or bilateral. When bilateral, the kidneys are asymmetric in the severity of their involvement. Factors predisposing to chronic pyelonephritis include urinary tract infection and vesicoureteral reflux. The disease is focal, resulting in a single or in multiple scattered scars that produce well-defined indentations of the renal outline, ranging from a few millimeters to several centimeters in depth. The underlying calyces are deformed and blunted as a result of pyramidal destruction and resulting fibrosis.

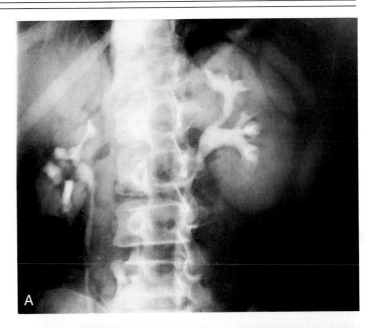

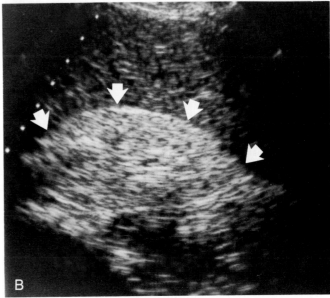

Fig. 3-10 Chronic pyelonephritis.
History: This 11-year-old female had a known reflux from the bladder into the right ureter.
Findings: (A) *IVP:* The right kidney is considerably smaller than the normal left kidney. The calyces are also blunted and distorted. **(B)** *US scan:* A longitudinal view of the kidney demonstrates it to be more echogenic (arrows) than the anteriorly situated liver. This is a reverse of the normal echo relationship.

Imaging is usually not indicated in cases of chronic pyelonephritis. The IVP, angiogram, ultrasound examination, and CT scan are used mainly to follow complications such as deteriorating renal function or a new onset of hematuria. If there is adequate renal function, the IVP demonstrates the small irregular kidneys with an inhomogeneous blush due to non-functional areas. The calyces are blunted under the scarred cortex (Fig. 3-10A).

The ultrasound examination confirms the secondary fibrosis of chronic disease by demonstrating small, irregular, hyperechoic kidneys. The increased echoes signify the unorganized fibrosis of the once homogeneous kidney (Fig. 3-10B). Masses or fluid collections surrounding the fibrotic regions may signal secondary complications such as perinephric abscess formation.

The CT scan will show effects similar to those in the urogram, with areas of nonfunctional scarring, calyceal deformity, and an overall reduction in renal size. Computed tomography is the best means for characterizing a mass or perinephric extension, and is used when these are clinically suspected.

The angiogram will demonstrate a small main artery with loss of the normal peripheral branching of the small renal interlobar arteries. The vessels are crowded together due to the small size of the kidney.

RENAL-VEIN THROMBOSIS

Renal-vein thrombosis may present in a number of ways, depending on the degree and rapidity of venous obstruction. Patients with this condition may demonstrate gross hematuria, severe flank pain, fever, and hemorrhagic shock. With acute and complete thrombosis, the kidney becomes enlarged and functionless. Secondary renal rupture, with massive retroperitoneal hemorrhage or total renal infarction, may occur.

The IVP shows renal enlargement, usually unilateral, with absent or diminished blush on the nephrogram. The enlargement may be massive and may progress within 2 months following a subsequent renal infarction to give a small, smooth, nonfunctioning kidney. If the calyces are visualized they are

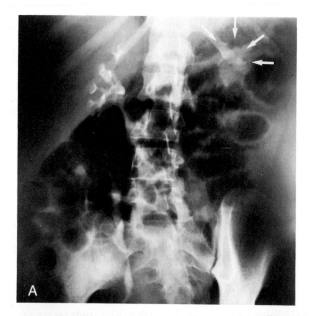

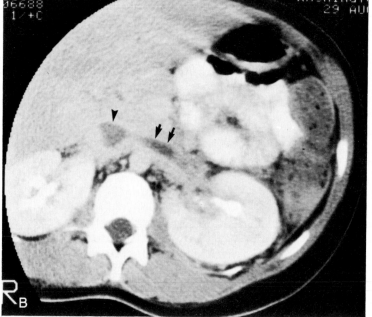

Fig. 3-11 Renal-vein thrombosis.
History: This 29-year-old black female complained of flank pain 3 days after a cesarian section. A subsequent urinalysis showed hematuria.
Findings: (A) *IVP:* Only left-upper-pole collecting system is appreciated on the 15-minute abdominal film (arrows). The left kidney, in addition, appears enlarged. **(B)** *CT scan:* The low density clot (arrows) extends through the renal vein into the inferior vena cava (arrowhead). The whiter-appearing, contrast-laden blood can be noted to form a ring around the stationary clot as it moves through the inferior vena cava .

stretched and separated by the congested parenchyma, simulating polycystic disease with its multiple parenchymal cysts (Fig. 3-11 A and see Fig. 3-31).

The ultrasound examination is nonspecific, demonstrating reduced cortical echogenicity, as in other diseases that result in renal vascular congestion and edema. It is indicated to further characterize the poorly functioning kidney and to detect any retroperitoneal hemorrhage.

The CT scan may often image the actual renal vein thrombosis as well as any inferior vena caval extension, thus leading to a definitive diagnosis. The individual veins are enlarged and may show a low-density clot bathed by the enhanced surrounding blood when contrast medium is administered into the partially thrombosed veins (Fig. 3-11B). This also implies that some residual function remains, since completely obstructed systems will show no change with contrast-medium administration, since the kidney is without function. There are prominent collateral vessels. However, CT finds its major use as the best detector of the complications of renal-vein thrombosis. It is more sensitive and specific than IVP or ultrasound.

Angiography shows narrowing, elongation, and separation of the intrarenal arteries due to parenchymal edema. Collateral venous flow may be seen as early as 1 day after the time of obstruction, with maximum development within several weeks.

Venography may be needed for a definitive diagnosis of renal-vein thrombosis in confusing clinical situations. Inferior vena caval injection of contrast medium, with the catheter below the renal veins, is initially done to evaluate any caval extension. If the cava is spared, a careful renal-vein catheterization to visualize the clots is attempted. Altough this is the most direct method for visualizing clots, it has several disadvantages and possible dangers, such as the fragmentation of emboli from an existing renal-vein clot, and lodging of the emboli in the pulmonary artery.

With gradual (chronic) block, the kidney may maintain normal function and show little or no congestion if the secondary collateral flow develops at the same rate as the occlusion. In this situation the kidney may appear normal with the various imaging modalities, or may show varying degrees of enlargement and reduced function. With the development of bypassing collateral vessels there may be notching of the ureter and collecting system as the surrounding ureteral veins enlarge.

PAPILLARY NECROSIS

Papillary necrosis, like renal-vein thrombosis, may cause hematuria, either microscopic or gross. There is a female predominance of this condition, which occurs most commonly between the ages of 40 and 60 years. Other signs and symptoms include flank pain, dysuria, urgency, fever and chills, and pyuria. The three most common etiologies are diabetes mellitus, analgesic abuse (most commonly of phenacetin), and sickle-cell anemia.

On IVP, the earliest finding is a loss of sharpness of the calyceal outline, referred to as calyceal "smudging" (Fig. 3-12). This is due to poor excretion of contrast medium from the diseased pyramid. The pyramids subsequently become ischemic and separate from the renal parenchyma. Contrast medium then surrounds the separated, sloughed-off pyramidial tissue in a circular fashion, giving rise to the "ring sign." The separated segment may cause obstruction and renal colic. With healing the calyx becomes smoothly convex, simulating a hydronephrotic collecting system (Fig. 3-12). Isolated calyces are involved in papillary necrosis, as opposed to the generalized calyceal dilatation of hydronephrosis. With severe disease the smooth cortical surface may be lost and the secondary scarring results in a lumpy and lubulated kidney. These cortical or surface changes are most commonly seen with analgesic nephropathy. This and the other IVP findings described here are diagnostic for papillary necrosis.

Retrograde pyelography may help in better visualizing the deformed calyces, but is usually not necessary (Fig. 3-13). The other imaging modalities are not of particular benefit in the diagnosis of papillary necrosis.

TUMORS

RENAL-CELL CARCINOMA

Renal-cell carcinoma must always be considered in any adult who presents with hematuria. It is three times more frequent in men than in women, and most often occurs in those over the age of 40 years. More than 60 percent of patients with renal cell carcinoma present with gross hematuria, with other symptoms including flank pain and fever. Over 30 percent of these tumors are discovered during studies performed for unrelated reasons.[5] Renal-cell carcinoma fre-

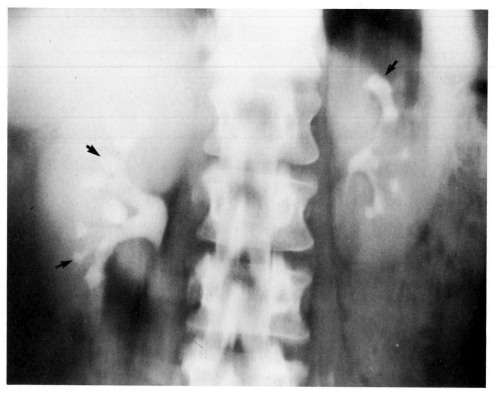

Fig. 3-12 Papillary mecrosis.
History: Recurrent urinary tract infections with microscopic hematuria in a 47-year-old male analgesic-drug abuser.
Findings: *IVP:* There is blunting and smudging (arrows) of all the calyces of both kidneys.

quently metastasizes to the lungs and also to bone, the periaortic lymph-cell nodes, liver, adrenal glands, and brain. In less than 10 percent of cases both kidneys may be involved. The tumor may also secrete various hormones, leading to paraneoplastic syndromes.

Malignant neoplasms of the kidney cause expansion leading to an elongation of renal size or a localized mass.[6] The latter may cause movement of the renal axis from its normal, slightly oblique orientation, with the kidney coming to lie in a more vertical or more horizontal plane depending on the location of the mass (Fig. 3-14 A and B). The initial nephrogram may demonstrate the mass with a blush that coincides with the arterial blood flow phase. The normal, evenly branched collecting systems are bizarrely distorted. The pelvis is also frequently distorted, and masses may be seen within it from tumor invasion. Localized ureteral or calyceal compression may lead to generalized or isolated hydronephrosis, respec-

tively. Approximately 10 percent of renal-cell adenocarcinomas will contain calcification. This may be amorphous (cloud-like), punctate, wavy, or curvilinear. Nonperipheral calcified masses are frequently malignant.

An ultrasound examination is the next study done in the evaluation of a mass seen on the IVP. It demonstrates the solid nature of the mass with an acoustic texture that is greater or less than that of the normal renal parenchyma (Fig. 3-15). Necrotic lesions have fluid collections that result in anechoic and hypoechoic areas. There may be areas of shadowing from calcification. Staging, for the evaluation for metastasis and tumor extension, is done by scanning the liver (for metastasis), retroperitoneum (for adenopathy), adrenals (for metastasis), and renal veins and inferior vena cava (for tumor extension).

Computed tomography is rapidly replacing angiography for the definitive diagnosis and staging of

Fig. 3-13 Papillary necrosis.
History: Previous episodes of colicky abdominal pain and microscopic hematuria in a 58-year-old diabetic female.
Findings: *Retrograde pyelogram:* The collecting structures demonstrate large filling defects in the opacified deformed and clubbed calyces. The filling defects proved to be portions of sloughed calyces.

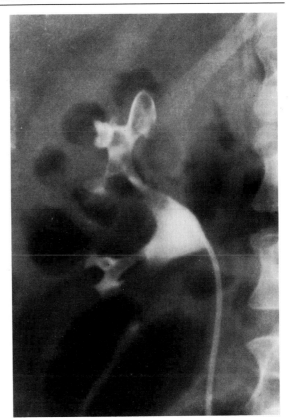

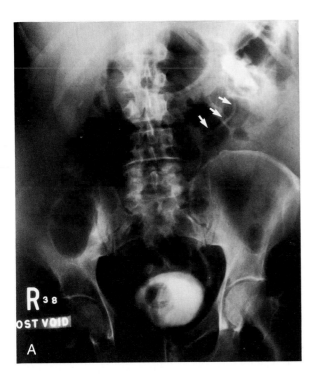

Fig. 3-14 Renal-cell carcinoma.
History: This 69-year-old male presented with a painless hematuria.
Findings: (A) *IVP:* The plain view of the abdomen 15 minutes after contrast-medium administration shows the left kidney to have an abnormal axis. The lower pole lies more laterally than normal, resulting in an almost horizontal lie of the kidney. In addition, there is lateral deviation of the most proximal portion of the left ureter (arrows). These findings suggest a mass medial to the left kidney. **(B)** *CT scan:* A subsequent CT clearly shows the mass (arrows) along with some dystrophic calcifications within the left renal mass that was not appreciated on the x-ray view (arrowheads). The mass has spread to involve the deep muscles of the back.

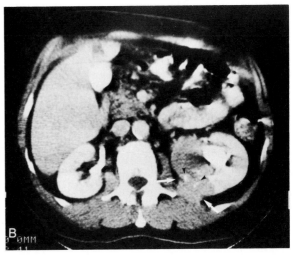

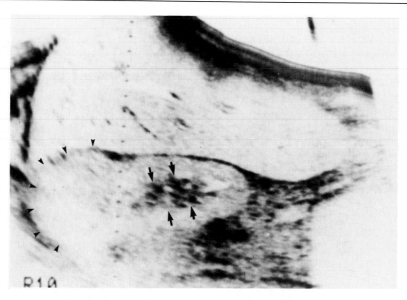

Fig. 3-15 Renal-cell carcinoma.
History: This 71-year-old male presented with metastatic nodules on his chest x-ray. Subsequent laboratory values revealed a microscopic hematuria.
Findings: *US scan:* There is a hypoechoic mass arising from the upper pole of the right kidney (arrowheads). The dense collecting-system echoes are well seen (arrows).

renal adenocarcinoma. It is usually performed after an ultrasound examination indicates a solid or mixed fluid/solid mass. The CT scan allows a more precise diagnosis than the ultrasound examination. The criteria for a diagnosis of renal-cell carcinoma include the visualization of a heterogenous mass with attenuation values close to those of the normal renal parenchyma in precontrast studies. The initial enhancement is greater than that of the normal parenchyma (arterial phase, bolus technique) but at equilibrium is less than that of the renal parenchyma surrounding the lesion. The interface between normal kidney and tumor tissue is unsharp, since a tumor capsule usually does not exist.

Staging of the tumor is also accomplished with CT (Fig. 3-14B). Surrounding lymph nodes greater than 1 cm in diameter suggest malignant spread. Tumor extension beyond the confines of the kidney is suggested by the stranding or webbing of tissue into the surrounding, low-attenuation, fat-containing perirenal space. Tumor extension into the renal vein and inferior vena cava is also revealed by CT and is a poor prognostic sign. Calcifications are easily detected. Additionally, CT is useful for postsurgical follow-up,

such as for a recurrence of tumor in the operative site.

Occasionally, ultrasound and CT cannot lead to a definitive diagnosis, and angiography will be required. Most renal adenocarcinomas are hypervascular. One characteristically sees an enlarged renal artery, chaotically distributed intrarenal vessels of irregular size, small aneurysmal "lakes," and arteriovenous communications leading to early venous opacification while the arterial structures continue to be visualized (Fig. 3-16A). Surrounding veins and arteries (capsular, intercostal, lumbar, adrenal, inferior phrenic, and gonadal) may be enlarged, since renal-cell tumors require additional blood supply and drainage. Metastatic deposits and invading transitional-cell carcinomas are usually hypovascular and thus not confused with renal-cell carcinoma. The tumor may be embolized with Gelfoam or some other substance known to decrease the vascularity of the tumor for subsequent surgery (Fig. 3-16B).

TRANSITIONAL-CELL CARCINOMA

Transitional-cell carcinoma is the most common tumor of the renal pelvis. It is often seen simulta-

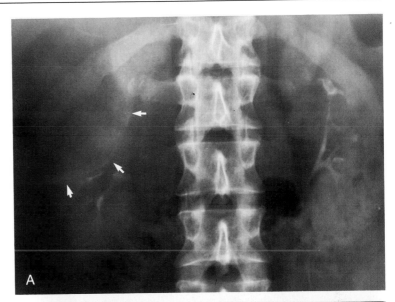

Fig. 3-18 Angiomyolipoma.
History: This 36-year-old male presented with gross hematuria and a palpable right flank mass.
Findings: (A) *IVP:* There is deformity of the upper-pole collecting systems by a large mass. No definite fatty component is appreciated (arrows). **(B)** *CT scan:* A large mass with a low density center (arrows) is seen replacing the upper pole of the kidney. The CT number of the low density center is −18, and correlates with fat.

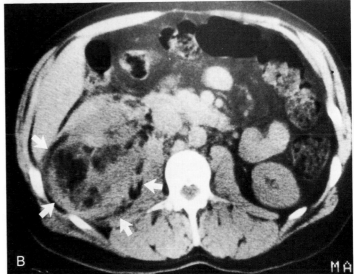

Fig. 3-19 Angiomyolipoma.
History: This 41-year-old female had a palpable right-upper-quadrant mass.
Findings: *US scan:* A very echogenic mass replaces the normal upper pole of the right kidney (arrows). The hyperechogenicity comes from the fatty component of an angiomyolipoma.

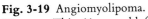
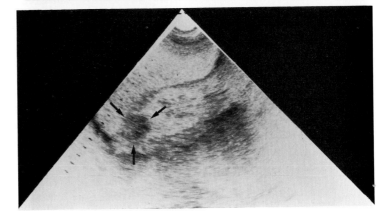

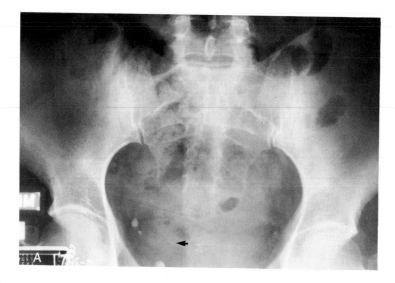

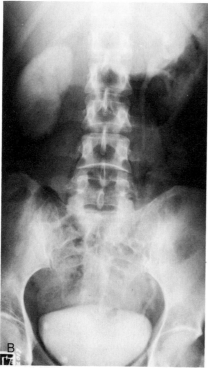
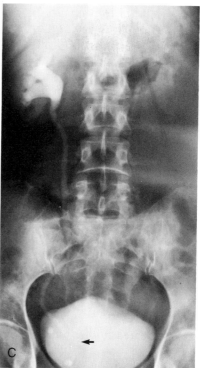

Fig. 3-20 Renal-stone disease.

History: This 25-year-old female presented to the emergency room with a 2-hour history of sudden and severe right-flank pain. She developed gross hematuria once in the ER.

Findings: (A) *IVP:* The precontrast-enhanced preliminary view of the pelvis demonstrates multiple, rounded calcifications in the lateral portion of the pelvis. These are calcifications called phleboliths within the pelvic vein. There is a single calcification just to the right of the coccyx (arrow) that can be suspected as a stone in the lower portion of the ureter. **(B)** The abdominal film obtained 30 minutes after the intravenous administration of contrast medium shows a persistent nephrogram blush on the right, without visualization of the collecting systems or right ureter. The left side is functioning normally. The stage has progressed from the initial nephrogram and contrast medium is now filling the collecting systems and ureter. **(C)** The last film of the abdomen, obtained 2 hours after contrast-medium injection, finally shows the hydronephrotic blunted calyces of the right kidney. The right ureter is filled with contrast medium to the level of the previously noted calcification (arrow). This combination of findings is confirmatory of an obstructed distal right ureter from a calcified renal stone just before the ureter enters the bladder, a common location. The normal left kidney is drained of most of the contrast medium in this 2-hour film.

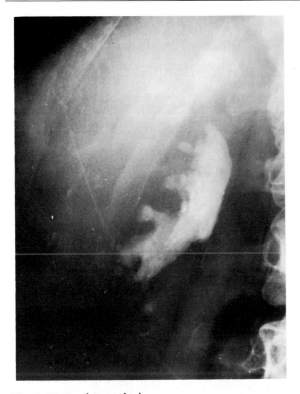

Fig. 3-21 Staghorn calculus.
History: This 57-year-old female had a recurrent urinary tract infections.
Findings: *Plain radiograph:* A large and dense calcification is present and conforms to the shape of the right collecting system. It represents a staghorn calculus within the pelvis and calyces.

structed or partially obstructed collecting system. The affected kidney may be diffusely enlarged from the obstructing stone and resulting hydronephrosis. The initial nephrogram is delayed and becomes progressively dense when compared to that on the normal side. The normal side shows the rapid appearance of the calyces and pelvis; the side with the stone demonstrates a negative defect in which the dilated calyces —not yet opacified— are surrounded by the opacified renal parenchyma. This is called a "negative nephrogram" (Fig. 3-20B). Delayed films of up to 24 hours are often needed to visualize the hydronephrotic collecting system and the point of obstruction. The ureter is dilated to the level of the completely obstructing stone, with no visualization distal to this (Fig. 3-20C). If the stone is only partially obstructive, the calyceal system is less hydronephrotic, with contrast medium passing distal to the stone and a ureter of normal caliber seen below this level. If the stone is

within the calyces or pelvis and not obstructive, the IVP is normal except for possible calcification on the preliminary film. It is not uncommon for the IVP to be therapeutic as well as diagnostic. There is an osmotic diuresis that occurs with the infusion of contrast medium and which often causes the stone to be carried down the ureter and even to the bladder, so relieving the obstruction and renal colic. Subsequent IVPs, after passage of the stone, may be normal or may show a continued partial obstruction or narrowing from an inflamed or scarred ureter.

Ultrasound and CT will identify the hydronephrosis and may also show the stone and level of obstruction. Ultrasound is very successful in revealing caly-

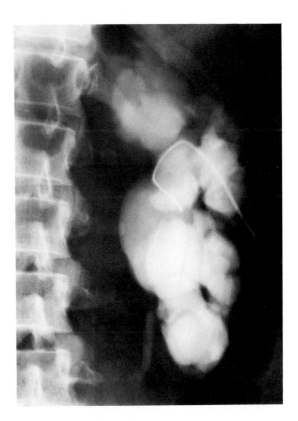

Fig. 3-22 Acute obstruction.
History: This 33-year-old female had known kidney stones and progressive left-flank pain and sepsis.
Findings: *Nephrostomy:* Through a puncture over the flank after renal localization with ultrasound, a catheter is introduced into a dilated, hydronephrotic collecting system. Contrast medium has been introduced into the renal pelvis to define the anatomy. The obstructing stone was retrieved and the patient did not require surgical intervention.

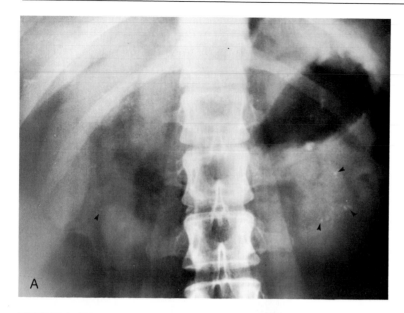

A

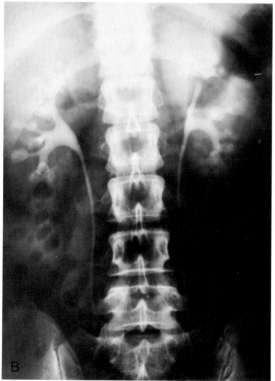

B

Fig. 3-23 Nephrocalcinosis: Medullary sponge kidney.

History: This 40-year-old female had recurrent episodes of renal colic and hematuria.

Findings: (A) *IVP:* The plain film of the abdomen, before contrast-medium administration, shows multiple punctate calcifications distributed in an arc pattern about the midportion of both kidneys (arrowheads). **(B)** The 15-minute film, after contrast-medium administration, finds the calcifications to be within the abnormally dilated collecting tubules that drain into the calyces. The dilated collecting tubules as filled with contrast medium appear as striations and are said to have a "paintbrush" appearance projecting from the otherwise normally shaped calyces.

ceal and pelvic stones, and is particularly useful for stones that are not calcified and thus not visualized on the preliminary IVP film.

Nuclear medicine studies can quantitate the secondary deterioration of renal function from the obstructive uropathy. The ^{131}I-hippuran scan will show the delayed appearance and persistent accumulation of radioactivity, similar to what is seen in the nephrogram on IVP. As renal function deteriorates there is less perfusion of the kidney. This is detected in the initial technetium-99m blood-flow study or angiogram phase. Lasix (furosemide) can be used to identify whether diuresis will allow some radioactivity to bypass the obstruction. These isotope studies can also be used to follow the effects of therapy or surgery on subsequent renal function.[9]

Modern invasive uroradiology and urology offer nonsurgical methods for treating urinary calculi. The stone may be reached via a cystoscope or a nephrostomy into the hydronephrotic collecting system (Fig. 3-22). It is then trapped in a basket or broken up via the use of sound waves, a form of ultrasound. If these methods are unsuccessful, surgical intervention is necessary. A new form of treatment is the ultrasound bath or lithotripsy which breaks a large stone into smaller fragments for easy passage.

A calcification within the renal parenchyma proper is termed nephrocalcinosis. Such calcifications may arise in a number of hypercalcemic or hypercalciuric states, including hyperparathyroidism, renal tubular acidosis, bony metastasis, multiple myeloma, and immobilization. Other causes of nephrocalcinosis, not due to elevated calcium levels, include medullary sponge kidney, hyperoxaluria, and chronic glomerulonephritis. The calcifications occur in the papillae and scattered throughout the medullary portion of the kidney.

The extent of renal parenchymal calcification is highly variable. In most cases there are a few scattered, punctate densitites. The calcifications of renal tubular acidosis are characteristic in being very dense and extensively distributed in the medullary portion of the kidney. Medullary sponge kidney, yet another cause of nephrocalcinosis, resembles a simple nephrocalcinosis as seen on preliminary films, (Fig. 3-23A), but the postinfusion study also shows dilatation of the collecting tubules, giving a "paintbrush" appearance to the surrounding calyces (Fig. 3-23B).

A third type of calcification is dystrophic calcification, occurring in renal infections, neoplasms, cyst walls, vessel walls, and vascular anomalies (Fig. 3-24).

RENAL TRAUMA

Significant renal trauma virtually always presents with some degree of hematuria. It is usually of the blunt type secondary to a motor-vehicle accident. Conservative, nonoperative management is becoming the rule for such trauma and IVP and CT are therefore important in assessing the degree of injury. If the trauma is of the penetrating variety, rapid man-agement is required, with a minimum of radiologic evaluation.[10] Three degrees of renal trauma will be considered, as based on findings at intravenous urography.[11] They are minor injury, major injury, and catastrophic injury.

Minor injury refers to contusion without disruption of the calyceal system and without a break in the renal capsule. On IVP the renal outline is normal. An intrarenal hematoma causes a localized negative defect in the nephrogram, as well as distortion of the surrounding calyces. Secondary renal edema may lead to a generally diminished nephrogram with a delayed appearance of the calyceal system. There are often clots in the collecting-system structures, appearing as negative filling defects.

If the intravenous urogram is technically satisfactory and normal, there is little need for CT. However, an abnormal IVP or clinically unstable patient (with persistent hematuria or a declining hematocrit) requires a CT examination. The findings on CT for minor injury will be the same as on IVP, with better visualization of the intrarenal hematoma.[12,13]

A hematoma surrounding the kidneys, or the extravasation of contrast medium, indicates major kidney injury. The hematoma may be restricted to the capsule that covers the kidney (subcapsular) or, in the case of a lacerated capsule, may extend into the surrounding perirenal space. The findings on IVP in

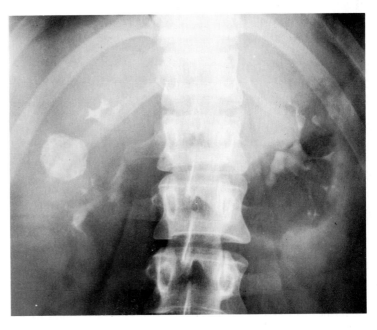

Fig. 3-24 Dystrophic calcification: Renal abscess.
History: This 37-year-old female had a past history of pyuria treated with antibiotics.
Findings: *IVP:* View of the kidneys 15 minutes after intravenous contrast-medium administration shows an amorphous, rounded, but irregular area of calcification within the right kidney.

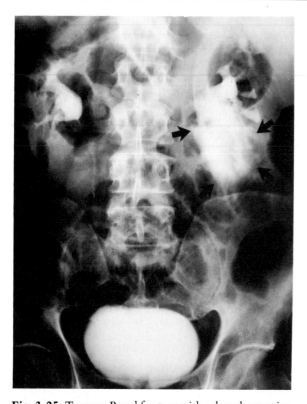

Fig. 3-25 Trauma: Renal fracture with calyceal extension.
History: This 59-year-old male had gross hematuria and a left flank mass following a motor-vehicle accident.
Findings: *IVP:* A single view of the abdomen after the administration of contrast medium shows extravasation of the contrast medium about the lower pole of the left kidney (arrows). There are mild hydronephrotic changes in the left collecting systems.

cases of perirenal hematoma are deviation of the normal renal axis or upper ureter. The renal outline is obscured by the surrounding blood, and the kidney appears large. With laceration of the collecting system one can see the extravasation of contrast medium with or without parenchymal damage. The medium is seen outside the collecting system, and may be localized about the injured calyces or extend into the perirenal (retroperitoneal) space (Fig. 3-25). The extravasated contrast medium may also extend into the lower retroperitoneum, outlining the ureters. This extracalyceal contrast medium will be easily seen in tomographic sections. The amount of leakage varies with the extent of the injury. The extravasation is self-limited and will cease in a few hours to days. The kidney will often heal with little or no radiographic change.

The CT scan will most accurately demonstrate the presence and extent of a subcapsular (without capsular injury) (Fig. 3-26) or perirenal (with capsular laceration) hematoma. It is also better able to reveal minute extravasations of contrast medium since it is more sensitive to contrast differences than is the IVP. The CT scan is frequently obtained after significant trauma, or with an unstable patient or abnormal IVP.

The last category is that of catastrophic injury. This includes the shattered kidney, tearing of the ureter or vessels in the renal hilus, or infarction. The shattered kidney shows marked deformity of the calyces, with loss of pelvic architecture. There is gross extravasation of contrast medium from the kidney if the latter is

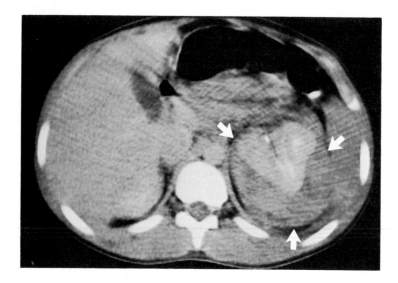

Fig. 3-26 Post-traumatic subcapsular hematoma.
History: This 21-year-old male suffered a "minor" injury while playing football and presented with painless hematuria.
Finding: *CT scan:* The left kidney blushes, indicating some remaining function as it is surrounded and elevated by the crescentic-shaped collection of blood (arrows). This smooth collection of blood is typical for a subcapsular hematoma.

functional. Massive perirenal hemorrhage is also present. In cases of avulsion of the ureter renal function is preserved, with a gross leakage of contrast medium from the site of injury. With avulsion or thrombosis of the renal artery there is no excretion of contrast medium since the kidney is totally without blood flow and function.

The CT scan will demonstrate a nonfunctioning kidney that may be deformed in its outline if fractured or shattered. With an avulsed ureter the extravasated contrast medium is easily detected in the surrounding retroperitoneum. The CT scan will also display other, associated abdominal injuries in the liver or spleen.

Nuclear medicine studies may be used to determine whether or not renal function is present. They can be used when the IVP or CT is technically unsatisfactory or for a patient with a history of allergy to iodinated contrast media. There may be isolated areas of parenchymal dysfunction in such studies, in accord with a contusion to a totally nonfunctioning kidney, as seen with an avulsed renal artery. Extravasation of radionuclide may also be detected in nuclear medicine studies, with activity diffusely scattered in the retroperitoneal tissues about the kidney and ureter.

With the availability of CT, angiography is less utilized today than it once was. It is used mainly to diagnose complete arterial occlusion in patients with unstable vital signs.

DISEASES OF THE BLADDER AND URETHRA

The last category of diseases that may cause hematuria are those of the lower urinary tract. Cystitis is usually associated with dysuria and frequency. Most cases occur in adult women, but the condition may also be seen in older men and young girls, and are caused by gram negative bacilli, usually *E. coli*. In men, cystitis is usually secondary to the obstruction caused by benign prostatic hypertrophy.

In general, urography has only a limited role in the diagnosis of cystitis. Cystoscopic examination is the main method of diagnosis. In severe cystitis an IVP or cystogram will show irregularities of the bladder mucosa from edema. The bladder is often small and contracted from chronic inflammation.

Tumors of the urinary bladder are also principally evaluated with cystoscopy. The IVP is indicated to demonstrate ureteral obstruction from a known

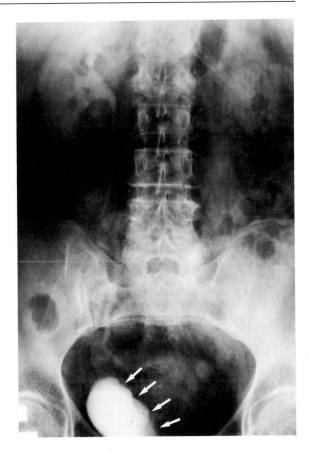

Fig. 3-27 Bladder carcinoma.
History: This 68-year-old female had a painless hematuria that was diagnosed as due to a transitional cell carcinoma of the bladder at cystoscopy.
Findings: *IVP:* A 30-minute delayed view after intravenous contrast medium was given shows a lobulated mass involving the entire left side of the bladder (arrows). The left kidney is small and functionless from the prolonged obstruction of the left ureter by the bladder tumor.

tumor, although it often reveals a clinically unsuspected tumor in an examination done for other reasons. Tumors of the bladder are of varying grades of malignancy and varying stages of infiltration of the bladder wall, as discussed previously for transitional-cell neoplasms. Ninety percent of these tumors are of uroepithelial origin, and occur most commonly on the posterior and lateral bladder walls. The peak age of their occurrence is from 50 to 80 years.

On IVP and cystography, tumors of the bladder give an irregular, fixed filling defect. The ureter may be blocked, leading to a secondary hydronephrosis

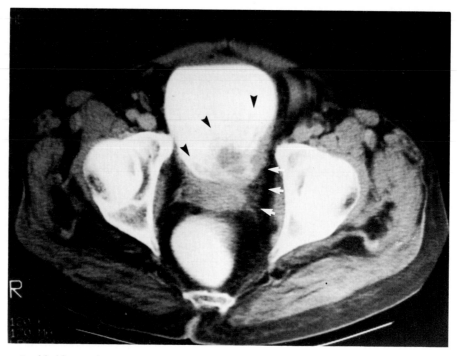

Fig. 3-28 Extensive bladder carcinoma.
History: This 71-year-old male with longstanding carcinoma of the bladder had refused previous surgical intervention.
Findings: *CT scan:* There is a large irregular mass involving the entire left half of the bladder (arrowheads) with extension into the posterior soft tissues (arrows).

(Fig. 3-27). Spread to the pelvic lymph nodes can cause deviation of the bladder and pelvic portion of the ureter. Ultrasound demonstrates an irregular mass affixed to the bladder wall, as well as the secondary hydronephrosis, if present.

Computed tomography has made the staging of bladder tumors a much easier task, and has basically eliminated the need for angiography. The tumor appears as a sessile or pedunculated mass projecting into the bladder cavity. There may be focal or diffuse wall thickening, with tumor invasion of the wall. This is easily confused with cystitis. The bladder should be filled with contrast medium during the CT scan to determine its wall thickness. The CT scan easily shows any extension into the surrounding perivesicular fat, adjacent organs, or lymph nodes. Loss of the normally well-defined borders of the bladder, as well as a definite mass projecting from the bladder, signify perivesicular extension (Fig. 3-28).

CLINICAL PRESENTATION: HYPERTENSION (ALGORITHM 3-2)

Hypertension is a common problem in the United States, affecting about 15 percent of the population. It hastens atherosclerotic disease as well as potentiating myocardial damage, congestive heart failure, cerebral hemorrhage, and renal failure. The overwhelming majority of cases are classified as essential hypertension with no demonstrable cause. It is estimated that only 6 percent of all cases of hypertension have a curable cause, with a renovascular etiology making up two-thirds of these cases. As a result, most patients with hypertension are treated medically, without any radiologic evaluation. Patients who should be studied include those with severe diastolic hypertension (over 115 mmHg), those under 40 years of age with diastolic pressures greater than 105 mmHg; those over

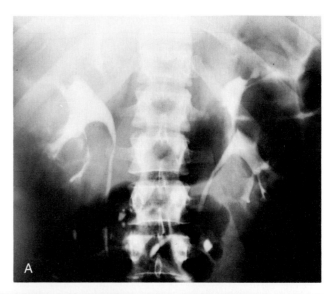

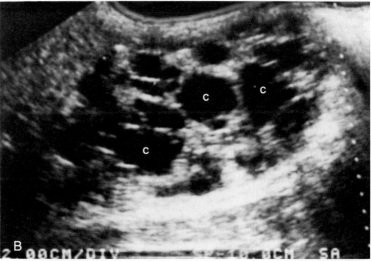

Fig. 3-31 Adult polycystic disease.
History: This 24-year-old male with known polycystic disease presented with progressive severe hypertension.
Findings: (A) *IVP:* A 15 minute post-contrast view of the abdomen shows the kidneys to be enlarged bilaterally. The calyces are bizarre in their configuration. **(B)** *US scan:* A longitudinal scan reveals the fluid content of these masses. The masses or cysts (c) have no internal echoes, and transmit sound well, as demonstrated by strong sound waves reaching the soft tissues opposite their point of entry. **(C)** *CT scan:* A section through the kidneys and liver shows that the normal renal parenchyma has been replaced by multiple cysts (c) of varying sizes that have CT values near water density. Some contrast medium can be seen in the displaced and distorted pelvis and collecting structures (arrowheads), indicating some function. In addition, multiple low-density cysts are present in the liver (arrows).

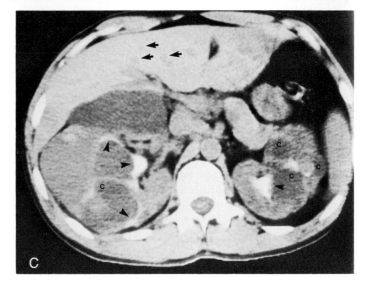

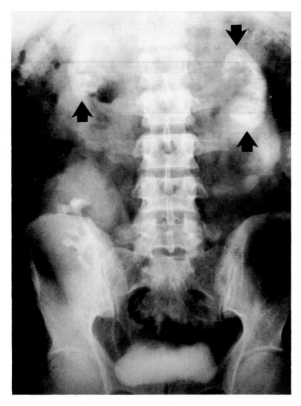

Fig. 3-32 End-stage renal disease.

History: This 40-year-old female with a long history of oxalosis had a renal transplant.

Findings: *IVP:* 15-minute film after the intravenous administration of contrast medium shows the small, native kidneys to be diffusely calcified and without discernable function (arrows). A functioning renal transplant lies in the right pelvis.

on the cause. When the failure is from chronic bilateral pyelonephritis or interstitial nephritis, the kidneys are bilaterally small and often smooth. In renal failure from obstructive causes (progessive hydronephrosis) the kidneys are large. In other progressive renal processes such as polycystic disease, amyloidosis, tuberculosis, lymphoma, and nephrocalcinosis the kidney size is variable.[20]

The IVP may be used to evaluate the cause of the renal failure, but is no longer routinely performed for most renal parenchymal diseases. However, urography is believed not to be detrimental to the function of an already damaged kidney. The patient should be well hydrated before the examination. Higher doses of contrast medium as well as tomography may be required for visualization of the kidneys, which in chronic glomerulonephritis or interstitial nephritis are small, smooth, and involved bilaterally. The collecting systems are often not seen, again due to poor function, but are intact and normal (Fig. 3-32). This is in contrast to atrophic pyelonephritis, in which the kidneys will be irregularly small and the calyces will be blunted under the thinned and scarred cortex. In cases of bilateral obstruction the kidney will be smoothly enlarged with dilated hydronephrotic collecting systems.

Retrograde studies may be useful for defining whether the collecting systems are normal or blunted. It may also reveal a point of obstruction in obstructive uropathy, but is not routinely used in the evaluation of renal failure.

Ultrasound probably finds it greatest use in patients with failed kidneys, for localization of the kidney for renal biopsy. The kidney itself is again small and will be hyperechoic as fibrosis replaces normal renal tissue. Ultrasound does not depend on the function of the kidney, nor does it affect the remaining functioning renal units (see Fig. 1-28). Computed tomography has no unique features in renal failure. Angiography is generally not indicated, but shows tapering of the main renal arteries, small intrarenal arteries, and a prolonged nephrogram.

Nuclear medicine studies may be useful in renal failure since they frequently succeed in revealing the kidneys when the standard IVP fails to do so. The nuclear medicine study is sensitive to even minimal degrees of function. The ^{131}I-hippuran scan appears to be best suited for this purpose. It can give information about whether the azotemia is prerenal, renal, or postrenal. It may also be used to follow the kidney response to medical management, by documenting improving function.

RENAL INFARCTION

Segmental infarction of the kidney may, like renal failure, also produce hypertension. Complete or chronic infarction of kidney is rarely associated with hypertension if the other kidney has adequate function. The causes of infarction include emboli from a distant source, such as an atherosclerotic plaque, thrombosis, or traumatic avulsion of the main artery or one of its major divisions.

The IVP in acute segmental or partial infarction shows a decreased or absent nephrogram of the in-

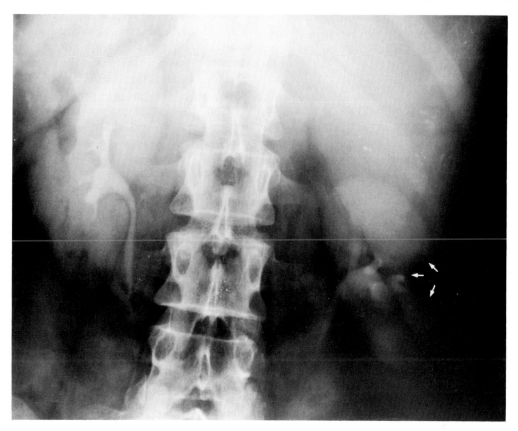

Fig. 3-33 Renal infarction.
History: This 50-year-old female with known rheumatic heart disease presented with recurrent flank pain and hematuria.
Findings: *IVP:* The 15-minute view of the kidneys after contrast-medium infusion demonstrates a small left kidney with a large wedge-type defect (arrows). The underlying calyces appear grossly normal.

volved area, which is often wedged shaped. The parenchyma eventually becomes thin. The calyces remain normal (Fig. 3-33). The infarcted area often recovers most of its function.[21]

In the majority of cases, the angiogram fails to demonstrate the actual thrombus or embolus. The selective injection of contrast medium into the renal artery demonstrates a lack of opacification of the involved arcuate and interlobar vessels. The nephrogram phase again demonstrates a nonfunctioning segment. The chronic phase appears as a depressed zone of avascularity or hypovascularity.

Retrograde studies may be useful for differentiating a segmental infarction from an area of atrophic pyelo-nephritis. In the former condition the calyces are usually normal under the cortical depression. By contrast, the calyx below the cortical depression in chronic pyelonephritis appears dilated or clubbed.

Nuclear medicine flow studies may give a quantitative analysis of relative blood flow distribution by showing the activity in different portions of the kidney. This may be helpful in cases of poorly functioning kidneys that opacify only faintly on IVP.

The globally or completely infarcted kidney is shrunken, with no opacification on the IVP and a normal pelvocalyceal system on retrograde pyelography. A decrease in renal size can be detected within 2 weeks after the onset of the infarction, and reaches its maximum by 5 weeks. The angiogram fails to demonstrate any opacification of the intrarenal or main renal arteries.

CLINICAL PRESENTATION: THE RENAL MASS (ALGORITHM 3-3)

There are many ways in which patients present for the workup of a renal mass. Often a renal mass is detected in the asymptomatic patient in an IVP done for other reasons, or is palpated during a routine physical examination. The differential considerations include renal-cell carcinoma, which needs to be considered in all cases of a mass, simple cysts, inflammatory masses, and benign neoplasms. Renal-cell carcinoma, benign neoplasms, and inflammatory lesions are discussed in other sections of this chapter and will not be presented here.

SIMPLE CYST

The most common isolated renal mass is the simple renal cyst. It accounts for over 60 percent of all renal masses.[22] Such cysts are solitary or multiple, and result in a surface bulge on the kidney. They are postulated to be a process of aging, since their number and size increase with age.[25] The cysts are most often unilocular, but can be separated by membranes into chambers that may or may not communicate. The cyst fluid is serous, and not urine. It has a typical chemical composition. In rare instances a renal-cell carcinoma occurs within the wall of the cyst. Much more common is the coexistence of a cyst and a renal carcinoma in the same kidney.

The IVP demonstrates a focal expansion of the renal outline. The nephrogram contains a negative defect since the cyst is avascular. The bordering cortex of the kidney is pushed outwards at the margin of the cyst because the cyst is a slow growing lesion. This produces a "beak" or "claw" sign, which is not pathognomonic for a cyst but suggests a slow-growing lesion (Fig. 3-34). The cyst may be completely intraparenchymal and is then diagnosed solely from a smooth displacement of the collecting system — an orderly displacement that is in contrast to the shaggy, bizarre configuration of the collecting system seen with renal-cell carcinoma.

Ultrasound is very important in the diagnosis of the simple renal cyst. With strict adherence to certain criteria the diagnosis of a simple cyst with this tech-

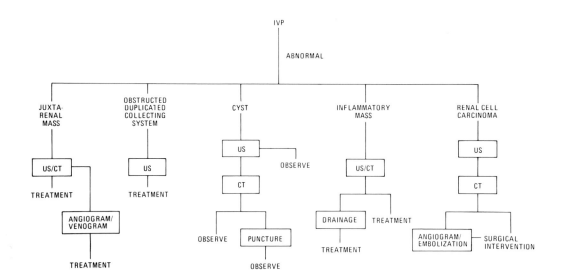

CLINICAL PRESENTATION: RENAL MASS

Algorithm 3-3

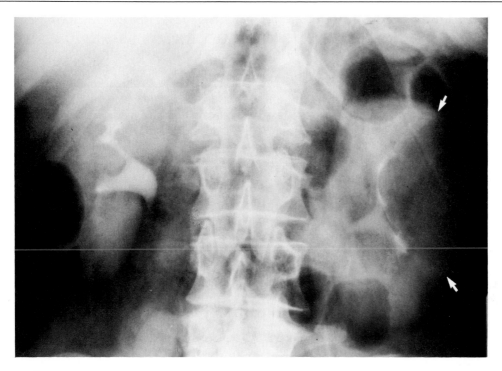

Fig. 3-34 Renal cyst.
History: This 71-year-old male had symptoms of hesitancy and frequency. An IVP was done obtained to evaluate his prostate for benign prostatic hypertrophy.
Findings: *IVP:* There is a large mass off the lateral portion of the left kidney. It appears less dense than the normally blushing renal parenchyma. There is a sharp demarcation between the renal parenchyma called the "claw-sign" (arrows), as it gives way to the cyst. There is smooth and orderly deviation of the calyces caused by the mass.

nique is almost completely assured. These criteria include a completely echo-free mass, a well-defined cyst wall, no internal echoes or septation, and good penetration of the sound through the fluid-filled mass (fluid is an excellent medium for sound transmission), giving an abundance of echoes on the opposite side of the mass (Fig. 3-35). In the event that all of the above criteria are met, the diagnosis is made and no further workup is needed. If any of the above characteristics are not present, further evaluation is necessary.

Computed tomography has now become the means of imaging a cyst in the event of a questionable ultrasound examination. The CT features of a benign renal cyst are a homogeneous, near-water density lesion, no contrast enhancement, no detectable wall to the cyst, and a smooth, well-defined interface with the renal parenchyma (Fig. 1-39). The use of CT numbers to compare materials of different unknown densities

with known standards, such as the zero of water, has not proved absolutely reliable in practice. A renal cyst may have CT numbers in the range of 0 to 20 HU.

If the lesion does not satisfy all of the ultrasound and CT criteria for a simple cyst, or if hematuria was the presenting complaint, further evaluation is needed. Angiography will demonstrate an avascular mass, with smoothly displaced surrounding vessels. The correct diagnosis can be made angiographically in over 90 percent of cases.

The percutaneous puncture of a cyst is infrequently done as an early diagnostic procedure. For percutaneous puncture, the cyst is first localized with ultrasound. In a simple cyst the fluid is clear and low in fat and lactic dehydrogenase. Contrast medium and air may be injected into the cyst cavity and will demonstrate a smooth wall. If the fluid is bloody or turbid or the cyst wall is irregular or multiloculated, a complicated cyst (infected) or cystic neoplasm remains a possibility. A further workup is then necessary.

Another common location for a simple cyst is in the renal pelvis. This is referred to as a peripelvic cyst. The renal contour is undisturbed. The IVP shows smooth displacement of the collecting system. The peripelvic cyst may not appear as lucent as a cortical cyst on IVP, since there is overlying renal parenchyma obscuring the lucency. However, the ultrasound, CT, and angiographic criteria remain the same as for the simple parenchymal cyst.

Multiple cysts of the kidney are associated with a number of syndromes, such as tuberous sclerosis and Von Hippel-Lindau syndrome, and with chronic renal dialysis.

DUPLICATED COLLECTING SYSTEM

A common congenital occurrence is the duplicated collecting system, in which the upper group of renal collecting structures are separated from the middle and lower groups of calyces. The upper collecting structure has its own ureter, which may connect with the ureter of the middle and lower calyces either at the level of the kidneys or anywhere before the bladder. The ureters also may never join. When the two ureters do not join, the upper may insert into the bladder at a lower and more medial position than the trigone, or into another ectopic location. This abnormal insertion frequently leads to an obstruction, with a resulting hydronephrotic upper collecting system. This dilated upper system on IVP shows either a delayed nephrogram or no nephrogram if the surrounding renal cortex is so compressed as to be functionless. The later films show an upper-pole "mass" with displacement of the lower calyces inferiorly. This is called the "drooping-lily" sign.

The ultrasound examination may show an anechoic area representing the hydronephrosis with a rind of echoes of renal tissue around it. The separate ureter may also be seen, thus establishing the diagnosis. Ul-

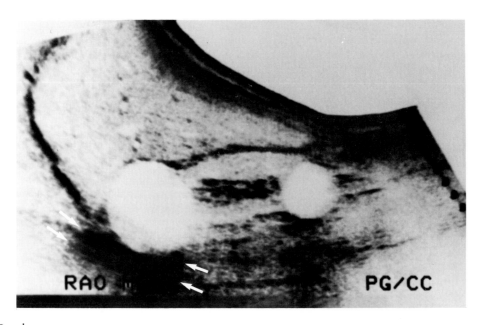

Fig. 3-35 Renal cyst.
History: This 68-year-old male was found to have two masses in his right kidney on an IVP done for microscopic hematuria. The IVP also showed benign prostatic hypertrophy (the reason for his hematuria).
Findings: *US scan:* There are two round, echo-free masses off the upper and lower poles of the right kidney. There is excellent transmission of sound through these masses, as indicated by the strong echoes reaching the tissues behind the masses (arrows). (The gentle echoes seen in the posterior portion of the larger cyst are an artifact of the ultrasound scan.)

trasound will also show separation of the echoes of the pelvis of the two collecting systems by renal tissue of normal appearance.

JUXTARENAL MASS

Often, juxtarenal processes may appear renal in origin on IVP. Careful imaging with ultrasound and CT is then used to delineate the interface between the kidney and the adjacent mass. The adrenal cyst or neoplasm frequently masquerades as a renal lesion. Angiography may be required for a definitive diagnosis if a clear interface cannot be detected by ultrasound and CT. Other lesions that may mimic a renal mass include retroperitoneal tumors and perirenal fluid collections (urinomas, abscesses, and hematomas).

CLINICAL PRESENTATION: PYURIA (ALGORITHM 3-4)

Pyuria is a sequel to chronic or acute infectious process. It may be seen acutely with bacterial infections, such as in acute pyelonephritis, as already dis-

cussed, but is also present in chronic inflammatory processes such as a chronic pyelonephritis, renal abscesses, xanthogranulomatous pyelonephritis, or pyonephrosis. The pyuria may be sterile, with no identifiable organism on routine cultures, such as in tuberculous involvement of the kidney.

RENAL ABSCESS

A renal abscess may be classified as acute or chronic. An acute abscess, also called a carbuncle, is the sequel of severe suppurative pyelonephritis, with many small abscesses coalescing into one or more larger lesions. It is believed to represent the result of a continuum, beginning with acute pyelonephritis and ranging through acute focal bacterial nephritis (or acute lobar nephronia) to frank abscess formation. The abscess may present as a localized mass involving one portion of the kidney, or as a diffuse process involving the entire kidney. The acute abscess does not communicate with the collecting system but is frequently associated with perinephric extension. The most common organism is the gram negative *E. coli,* from an ascending urinary tract infection. *Staphylococcus aureus,*

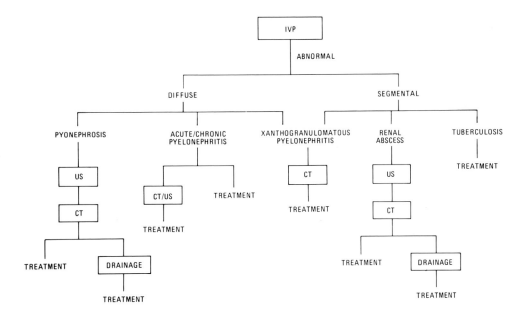

CLINICAL PRESENTATION: PYURIA

Algorithm 3-4

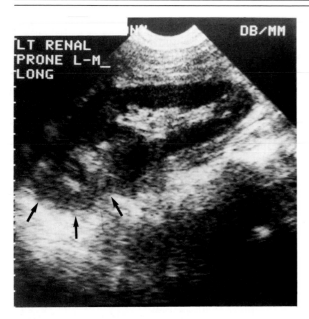

Fig. 3-36 Renal abscess.
History: This 27-year-old male intravenous drug abuser presented with a prolonged fever.
Findings: *US scan:* The longitudinal view of the kidney demonstrates a localized mass involving the upper pole of the left kidney (arrows). The mass is well distinguished from the remainder of the kidney and has hypoechoic, hyperechoic, and anechoic areas. There is no definite perinephric extension.

which reaches the kidney via the blood, is also seen, especially in IV drug abusers.

The localized renal carbuncle presents as an inflammatory mass with displacement and stretching of the surrounding calyces. The calyces about the mass are poorly defined due to their poor function. The diffuse form of renal carbuncle has the same IVP manifestations as acute pyelonephritis.

The ultrasound examination further characterizes the acute mass as a localized hypoechoic area that may contain irregular fluid-density areas (Fig. 3-36). With an accompanying perinephric extension there is loss of the sharp external contour of the kidney and the visualization of an extrarenal mass. Again, the diffuse form demonstrates a large hypoechoic kidney similar to what is obtained in acute pyelonephritis. In fact, it is often impossible to differentiate acute pyelonephritis from a diffuse abscess with IVP and ultrasound.

On the CT scan there is a mass of lower density than the surrounding normal renal parenchyma, with a thick irregular wall as the abscess matures. The wall of the abscess may enhance with contrast medium, but the necrotic core does not. Computed tomography is most beneficial for the evaluation of such complications of an abscess such as perinephric extension. Renal-cell carcinoma may give a similar picture, and its secondary effects are sought on CT to differentiate it from an abscess, as previously discussed.

Interventional procedures, such as the percutaneous drainage of an abscess not responding to therapy, are very helpful. This may be done with the guidance of ultrasound or CT to localize the mass, as with any percutaneous renal biopsy.

Angiographically there is no discrete mass of vessels seen in the acute phase, but a diffuse peripheral blush outlines the abscess, which has an avascular, necrotic core. There is only minimal vascular displacement. Perinephric extension is typically seen as a prominence and displacement of capsular vessels, as well as a loss of the sharp cortical border of the kidney.

An abscess is considered chronic when the surrounding granulation tissue organizes and forms a thick wall. It remains unusual for the abscess to communicate with the collecting system, but perinephric extension is again common.

The plain-film IVP in cases of a chronic abscess may show flocculent or curvilinear calcifications reminiscent of a renal-cell carcinoma. (Fig. 3-24). The thickened wall of the abscess may show a blush on the initial nephrogram phase. The calyces are displaced around the chronic abscess, with poor filling of the most closely surrounding calyces. The ultrasound examination and CT scan will also show a more organized wall than seen with an acute abscess, as well as a complex or inhomogenous center to the abscess.

The angiographic picture of a chronic abscess is even more difficult to differentiate from that of a necrotic renal carcinoma than the image of an acute abscess. The abscess wall often exhibits neovascularity, like a tumor. The vessels are usually evenly tapered, as opposed to the irregular and encased vessels of a renal carcinoma. Early venous opacification during the arterial phase of the angiogram (A-V shunting) is not a typical feature of chronic abscesses.

PYONEPHROSIS

Pyonephrosis is an infected hydronephrotic collecting system. This often results from advanced suppurative destruction of the kidney superimposed on an obstructive hydronephrosis.

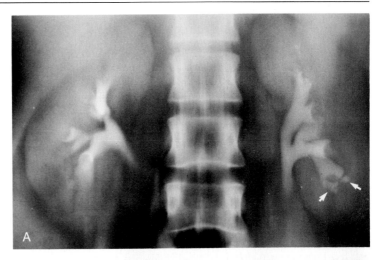

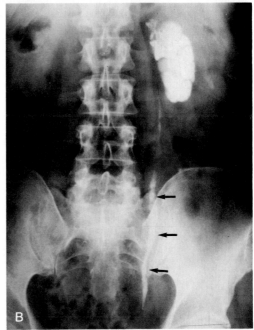

Fig. 3-37 Tuberculosis of the genitourinary system.
History: These pictures illustrate two cases of varying severity of tuberculous involvement of the kidneys.
Findings: (A) *IVP:* Case 1. There is filling of irregular cavities (arrows) by the contrast medium. These cavities connect to the collecting system through narrow, stenotic channels. **(B)** *Plain radiograph:* Case 2. A view of the abdomen before the administration of any contrast material shows a small, diffusely calcified kidney that was found to be without function (autonephrectomy). The left ureter is also diffusely calcified along its entire course (arrows).

The kidney is usually enlarged and not functioning. If the pelvis is opacified it is irregular and has multiple filling defects. With time, as the destruction of the parenchyma continues,[27] the kidneys become small.

Ultrasound suggests the diagnosis by demonstrating, within dilated collecting systems, echoes representing pus and debris-filled calyces. The CT scan demonstrates the renal parenchymal destruction, showing a small, irregular kidney. As in cases of abscess, it is particularly useful for identifying complications such as perinephric extension.

XANTHOGRANULOMATOUS PYELONEPHRITIS

Xanthogranulomatous pyelonephritis is an unusual type of chronic renal abscess. It is associated with a long history of urinary tract infection. *Proteus mirabilis* is the most common pathogen.[24] Eighty-five percent of cases present with a nonfunctioning kidney and 15 percent with a localized mass. Calculi and ureteropelvic junction (UPJ) obstruction are frequently associated with the condition.[25] The calculi may be small, a cast of the collecting system (staghorn calculus), or occur within the parenchyma itself. As with a renal abscess, there is a discrete or tumefactive form and a diffuse form.

The IVP study and CT scan are usually diagnostic, showing a poorly or nonfunctioning kidney along with calculi and hydronephrosis from the ureteropelvic junction obstruction.

TUBERCULOSIS

Tuberculosis of the kidney is a secondary infection from a primary site in the lung or bone. The primary site is often inactive at the time of presentation; only 10 to 15 percent of patients with renal tuberculosis will have concurrent active pulmonary disease. Since the disease is a result of hematogenous dissemination, both kidneys are diffusely exposed to *Mycobacterium tuberculosis.* The subsequent course of the infection is determined by the dose and virulence of the organism and the resistance of the host. Most of the initial renal lesions heal, and only a few progress to clinical or radiographic significance. The renal destruction, when it occurs, can be limited to the papillary tip, or the infection can progress to form masses or eventually destroy the entire kidney. Healing leads to fibrosis, calcium deposition, and nonfunction. Eventually the bladder and genital structures are involved. Coexistent involvement of the liver, spleen, adrenal glands, and lymph nodes is often seen.

The pyelographic findings are multiple and quite varied. The IVP may be completely normal even in patients with symptomatic disease. The earliest urographic abnormality is an irregularity of the papillary surface or calyx. The sharp contour of the calyx is lost, and the calyx is said to "smudge." This may be true for one or more calyces, and leads to an extensive papillary necrosis (Fig. 3-37A). The infundibulum draining the diseased calyx may be narrowed by fibrosis, or the stricture may involve the entire pelvocalyceal system, leading to a localized or total hydronephrosis. Over 70 percent of cases of renal tuberculosis will have radiographic abnormalities limited to only one kidney.

The involvement of the kidney progresses to include the renal parenchyma, giving three basic presentations: a localized mass, an irregular cavity, or a scarred, functionless kidney. The localized mass represents an enlarging granuloma. These masses may be single or multiple, and often contain circumscribed or amorphous calcifications. They may rupture to communicate with the collecting system, yielding an irregular cavity that fills during opacification of the collecting system. Generalized renal parenchymal involvement may lead to tissue atrophy with subsequent healing. There are multiple depressions or scars overlying the irregular calyces. This most severe form of parenchymal involvement produces the calcified, nonfunctioning, end-stage kidney referred to as the "autonephrectomized kidney" (Fig. 3-37B). The calcification is extensive and the kidney is often of near normal size, or may be small. The ureter may be shortened, dilated, or unusually straight, or may demonstrate multiple levels of stricture (Fig. 3-37B). The bladder may also be involved, with a thick wall resulting in a diminished capacity. The epididymis and seminal vesicles calcify.

Ultrasound, CT, and angiography are less specific than IVP and not usually helpful in the differential diagnosis.

CLINICAL PRESENTATION: OLIGURIA (ALGORITHM 3-5)

There are many causes for a decreased urine output, including prerenal etiologies such as dehydration or congestive heart failure, and renal causes, including acute glomerulonephritis and acute tubular necrosis. The most common cause is obstruction in the postrenal portion of the urinary tract, such as a bladder outlet obstruction.

BENIGN PROSTATIC HYPERTROPHY

Benign prostatic hypertrophy is a common disorder that causes a variable degree of bladder-outlet obstruction. This relative obstruction may lead to a secondary obstructive uropathy.

The IVP findings include elevation of the trigone or floor of the bladder, with a posterior and inferior filling defect that represents the prostate. The ureters, just before they enter the bladder, are displaced upward with the elevated trigone. This gives a "fishhook" appearance to the distal ureters. The bladder wall is thickened and irregular or trabeculated from the hypertrophied muscle bundles (Fig. 3-38). The

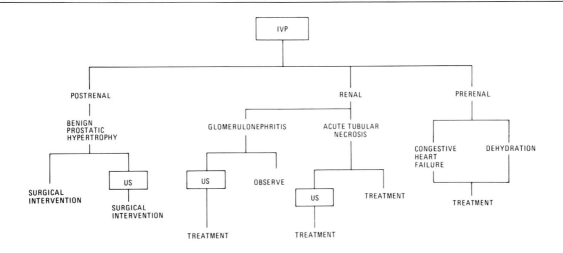

CLINICAL PRESENTATION: OLIGURIA

Algorithm 3-5

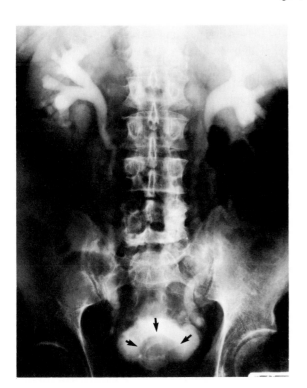

Fig. 3-38 Benign prostatic hypertrophy.
History: This 67-year-old male had increasing hesitancy of the urinary stream and frequency of urination.
Findings: *IVP:* The 15-minute supine view of the abdomen after contrast-medium administration shows blunting of the collecting systems bilaterally, as consistent with a moderate degree of hydronephrosis. Both ureters are dilated and filled with contrast medium along their entire length. The bladder wall is irregular owing to the hypertrophy of its muscular wall as it continually forces urine past the enlarged obstructing prostate. There is a circular defect elevating the floor of the bladder (arrows) which represents an indentation from the enlarged prostate.

post-void bladder is incompletely emptied and there may be vesicoureteral reflux. The outlet obstruction of the bladder leads to ureteral and pelvicalyceal dilatation along with eventual atrophy of the renal parenchyma. This results in worsening renal function.

Recently, ultrasound has been used to estimate the size and volume of the prostate. This helps decide which patients are candidates for surgical intervention, and what type of procedure should be performed.

ACUTE TUBULAR NECROSIS

Acute tubular necrosis or acute renal failure occurs in association with a number of conditions such as hypotension, extensive burns, ischemia during aortic sur-

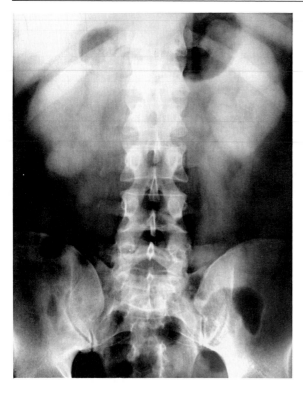

Fig. 3-39 Acute tubular necrosis.
History: This 46-year-old male had a cardiac catheterization 14 hours before the present study. The film shown here was ordered because of 12 hours of anuria.
Findings: *Plain radiograph:* A single view of the abdomen demonstrates a persistent nephrogram without the appearance of the collecting system, ureters, or bladder. The kidneys are mildly enlarged.

gery, sepsis, near drowning, and exposure to renal toxins (e.g., contrast media). It is manifested by several days to weeks of oliguria followed by polyuria and improved renal function in the following days.

The IVP demonstrates a prolonged nephrogram that becomes increasingly dense with time. This blush may last from several hours to several days. There is no or at best poor visualization of the pelvicalyceal system as a result of the poor function (Fig. 3-39). The renal size is variable. The kidneys may be enlarged with interstitial edema from water retention, as seen most obviously with exposure to nephrotoxins. However, in acute renal failure associated with hypotension, such as with blood loss, the kidneys are small.

Ultrasound is used with acute renal failure to rule out an obstructive etiology to the oliguria by demonstrating an absence of hydronephrosis. It is otherwise not helpful in discovering an etiology for the acute renal failure.

The angiogram shows narrowing of the interlobar and arcuate arteries. There is no opacification of the most terminal intrarenal vessels, yielding an irregular renal outline. As on the IVP, the nephrogram is prolonged. There is subsequent poor visualization of the renal vein since blood flow into and through the kidney is decreased and slowed.

CLINICAL PRESENTATION: RENAL TRANSPLANT (ALGORITHM 3-6)

Renal transplants between consanguineous family members are reaching an 80 to 85 percent success rate after 2 years and a 60 percent success rate after 2 years for cadaver kidneys. Radiographic studies have become increasingly important in the postoperative management and long-term follow-up of the transplant patient. Today, nuclear medicine studies lead all others in the postoperative evaluation, giving information about renal size, perfusion, tubular excretion, glomerular filtration, obstruction, and extravasation.

PREOPERATIVE EVALUATION

Preoperatively the donor is studied angiographically or, more recently, with digital subtraction angiography. It is necessary to be aware of any anatomic variations in the donor such as multiple renal arteries. In the past, conventional angiography was the only means of visualizing the renal arteries, but today, DSA offers visualization via a venous injection. This avoids much of the morbidity, mortality, and expense of conventional studies.[28] With more refinement of the resolution of DSA, it may replace angiography for donor evaluation.

POSTOPERATIVE EVALUATION

In the early postoperative period the transplant patient undergoes a baseline renal scan. Two agents are used for this scan, allowing for both qualitative and quantitative evaluation of the graft. The first agent injected is a technetium compound, and most recently one that is bound to dimercaptosuccinic acid

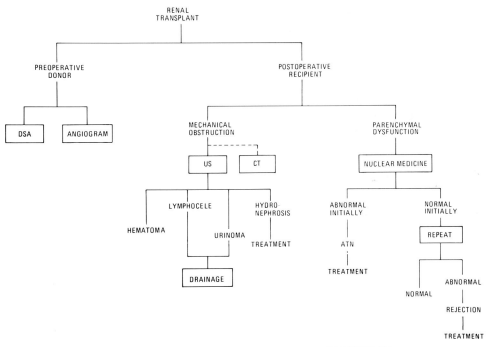

CLINICAL PRESENTATION: RENAL TRANSPLANT

Algorithm 3-6

(DMSA). The resultant technetium labeled-DMSA is injected and followed in a blood-flow study. There is an orderly visualization of the aorta, and in adequately perfused grafts, the transplanted kidney appears directly thereafter within 3 seconds. Views obtained 2 hours later allow anatomic parenchymal evaluation. For example, a segmental or partial infarct may appear as a wedge-shaped defect. After the ^{99m}Tc-DMSA is injected and the flow study completed, the next agent, ^{131}I-hippuran, is administered, also intravenously. Sequential images including the transplant are obtained, and the radioactivity in each scan is compared to the standards for the expected time of appearance of the cortex, collecting system, ureters, and bladder. The amount of activity with respect to time from the moment of injection of the hippuran is also entered into a computer, and the graph called a renogram curve is generated. The hippuran gives information on renal function, as opposed to the anatomic detail given by the technetium portion of the study.

The most common problem the postoperative patient encounters is that of oliguria. The causes of this are divided into parenchymal and mechanical. Acute tubular necrosis and rejection constitute the parenchymal etiologies, while vascular occlusion, ureteral leakage or obstruction, and bladder leakage are the mechanical problems.

ACUTE TUBULAR NECROSIS

Cadaver allografts are usually initially associated with some degree of acute tubular necrosis. For the first 48 hours acute rejection is not a consideration in the differential diagnosis of oliguria. Acute tubular necrosis is characterized by a variably diminished renal blood flow as seen on both the technetium and hippuran studies. The technetium-labeled media fail to show the graft clearly against the background activity (Fig. 3-40). The hippuran renogram show loss of the initial rise of the curve as a result of reduced flow, as well as a slow, progressive increase in parenchymal activity, indicating compromised function. Subsequent activity in the collecting system and bladder may never occur. The abnormalities as seen on a renal

Fig. 3-41 Renal transplant: Acute rejection.

History: A 56-year-old female with improving renal function 4 days after a renal transplant presented with deteriorating renal function 11 days after the transplant.

Findings: (A) *Renal scan:* A hippuran scan done 4 days after transplantation shows a normal renogram and prompt clearing of the radio-pharmaceutical by the kidney by 21 seconds. (B) *Renal scan:* A hippuran study performed 11 days post-transplant reveals, at 21 seconds, the predominant amount of activity within the transplanted kidney, signifying renal functional impairment. (C) *Renogram:* A curve plotted from the second hippuran study above confirms the delay in excretion, with no normal initial peak obtained.

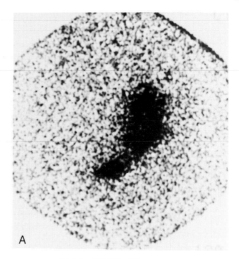

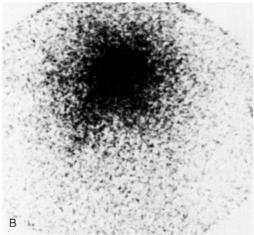

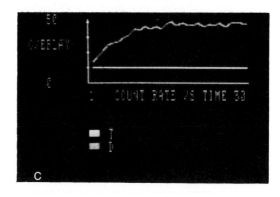

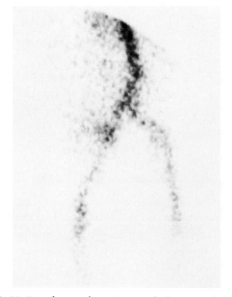

Fig. 3-40 Renal transplant: Acute tubular necrosis.

History: A 59-year-old male who was 2 days past cadaver renal transplantation presented with no improvement in his renal status.

Findings: *Renal scan:* A single view from the technetium flow study shows activity in the aorta for more than 9 seconds, with renal activity not yet apparent. A quantitative measurement of renal activity confirmed a state of impaired perfusion of the cadaver transplant.

scan reach a maximum by 24 to 48 hours, remain constant for a variable period, and then show improvement.[29]

REJECTION

With acute rejection there is a deterioration of perfusion and function after the initial 48 hours after transplantation (Fig. 3-41 A and B). The renographic findings may appear the same as in acute tubular necrosis, but it is the later appearance that is diagnostic of rejection (Fig. 3-41C). The rejection may be superimposed over an initial pattern of acute tubular necrosis. The hippuran examination may anticipate the biochemical changes of rejection by as much as 2 days, allowing the earlier initiation of more intensive medical therapy. For this reason renograms should initially be done several times a week following transplantation. The renogram may also be used to follow the response of renal function and perfusion to subsequent medical therapy.

VASCULAR OCCLUSION

Complete renal artery occlusion and total renal vein obstruction leading to infarction cannot be distinguished in nuclear medicine studies. There is a lack of perfusion with a resulting photon-deficient or lucent zone in the renal area. Angiography is usually done to verify these findings.

URETERAL AND PERIRENAL ABNORMALITIES

Ultrasound is useful in the detection of obstruction and peritransplant fluid collections. Hydronephrosis, abscesses, hematomas, urinomas, and lymphoceles may produce symptoms clinically indistinguishable from those of rejection, and may also compromise renal function. Aspiration of the collected fluid for diagnostic or therapeutic purposes can also be done under ultrasound guidance.

Computed tomography is reserved for cases in which ultrasound fails because of the overlying surgical wound or interposed bowel gas[30] (Fig. 3-42). It is sometimes successful in differentiating between an

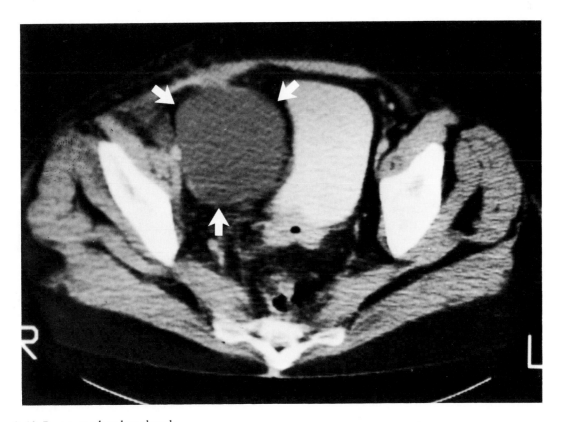

Fig. 3-42 Post-transplant lymphocele.
History: This 39-year-old female who had had a renal transplant 2 months earlier presented with progressively deteriorating renal function.
Findings: *CT scan:* A contrast-assisted CT scan shows the bladder to be filled with contrast medium (white) and compressed by an 8-cm mass (arrows). The CT number of the mass is +10, which is near water density. The mass does not become more dense after contrast medium is administered and so is not contiguous with the urinary tract.

acute hematoma, urinoma, or abscess. The urinoma is a low-density mass with CT numbers close to that of water (0 to 20 HU), while an acute hematoma will have numbers measuring 60 to 80 HU. A chronic hematoma or abscess may be similar in appearance to a urinoma. An abscess may also show gas within it. Computed tomography may also be used for diagnostic and therapeutic biopsy and drainage of the foregoing lesions.

Obstructive uropathy and urinary extravasation are easily detected by radionuclide studies. The technetium scan is superior for demonstrating dilated calyces or rents in the collecting system, but in renal failure hippuran is more useful, since the transit time of technetium through the renal parenchyma is greatly slowed.

REFERENCES

1. Elkin M: Radiology of the Urinary System. Little, Brown & Company, Boston, 1980, pp 341–2
2. Sarti DA, Sample WF: Diagnostic Ultrasound. Text and Cases. GK Hall Medical Publishers, Boston, 1980, p 269
3. Silver TM, Kass EJ, et al: The radiological spectrum of acute pyelonephritis in adults and adolescents. Radiology 118:65–71, 1976
4. Schneider M, Becker JA, Staiano S , Campos E: Sonographic radiographic correlation of renal and perirenal infections. AJR 127:1007–1014, 1976
5. Bosniak MA, Madayag, MA, Ambos MA, LaFleur RS: Renal cell carcinoma detected by chance. In: Abstracts of the 61st Scientific Assembly and Annual Meeting of the RSNA, Chicago, 1975
6. Davidson AJ: Radiologic Diagnosis of Renal Parenchymal Disease. WB Saunders, Philadelphia, 1977, p 218
7. Weyman PJ, McClennan BL, Stanley RJ, et al: Comparison of computed tomography and angiography in the evaluation of renal cell carcinoma. Radiology 137:417–424, 1980
8. Teplick JG, Haskin ME: Roentgenologic Diagnosis WB Saunders, Philadelphia, 1976, p 850
9. Kirchner PT: Nuclear Medicine Review Syllabus. Society of Nuclear Medicine, New York, 1980, pp 350–351
10. Lee JK, Sagel SS, Stanley RJ: Computed Body Tomography. Raven Press, New York, 1983, p 343
11. Elkin M, Becker JA, Fredenberg RM, Lang EK: Genitourinary Tract Disease Syllabus. ACR, 1973, pp 106–109
12. Fedula MP, Cross RA, Jeffery BB, Trunkey DD: Computed tomography in blunt abdominal trauma. Arch Surg 117:650–654, 1982
13. Margulis A: Abdominal trauma: The role and impact of computed tomography. Invest Radiol 16:260–268, 1981
14. Eisenberg RL, Amberg JR: Critical Diagnostic Pathways in Radiology. JB Lippincott, Philadelphia, 1981 p 200
15. Kincaid OW, Davis GD, Hallermann FJ, et al: Fibromuscular dysplasia of the renal arteries: Arteriographic features, classification and observations on natural history of the disease. AJR 104:271–282, 1968
16. Eisenberg RL, Amberg JR: Critical Diagnostic Pathways in Radiology. JB Lippincott, Philadelphia, 1981, p 201
17. Hillman BJ, Ovitt TW, Capp MP, et al: The potential impact of digital video subtraction angiography in screening for renovascular hypertension. Radiology 145:577, 1982
18. Stewart BH, Dustan HP, Kiser WS, et al: Correlation of angiography and natural history in evaluation of patients with renovascular hypertension. J. Urol 104:231–238, 1970
19. Eisenberg RL, Amberg JR: Critical Diagnostic Pathways in Radiology. JB Lippincott, Philadelphia, 1981, p 207
20. Teplick JG, Haskin ME: Roentgenologic Diagnosis. WB Saunders, Philadelphia, 1976, p 779
21. Heiztman ER, Perchek L: Radiologic features of renal infarction. Radiology 76:39, 1961
22. Deming CL, Harward BM: Tumors of the kidney. p 885. In Campbell MF, Harrison JH (eds): Urology. 3rd Ed. WB Saunders Co., Philadelphia, 1970
23. Gammill S, Rabinowitz JG, Peace R: New thoughts concerning xanthogranulomatous pyelonephritis. AJR 125:154–163, 1975
24. Noyes WE, Palubinskas AJ: Xanthogranulomatous pyelonephritis. J Urol 101:132–136, 1969
25. Kirchner PT: Nuclear Medicine Review Syllabus. So-

ciety of Nuclear Medicine, New York, 1980, pp 355–356

26. Elkin M, Becker JA, Friedenberg RM, Lang EK: Genitourinary tract disease syllabus. ACR 1973, pp 63–67

27. Hillman BJ, Zujoski CF, Ovitt TW, et al: Evaluation of potential renal donors and renal allogaft recipients: Digital video subtraction angiography AJR 138:921–925, 1982

28. Kirchner PT: Nuclear Medicine Review Syllabus. Society of Nuclear Medicine, New York, 1980, p 364

29. Lee JK, Sagel SS, Stanley RJ: Computed Body Tomography. Raven Press, New York, 1983, p 375

4

Radiology of the Gastrointestinal Tract

Richard M. Gore

During the past decade, the evaluation of patients with abdominal symptoms has been revolutionized by a number of dramatic and exciting improvements in the ability to image the alimentary tract. In addition to the development and implementation of new technologies such as computed tomography (CT), ultrasound, endoscopic retrograde cholangiopancreatography (ERCP), and percutaneous transhepatic cholangiography (PTC), the old reliable barium upper and lower gastrointestinal tract examinations and small bowel series have been improved by the addition of air-contrast studies. In this chapter, each of these imaging modalities will be presented as they apply to major abdominal problems.

CLINICAL PRESENTATION: GASTROINTESTINAL HEMORRHAGE

The expeditious workup of a patient with gastrointestinal bleeding is essential because it may be the presenting sign for a gastric or colonic neoplasm and because there is an 8 to 14 percent mortality rate for patients who present with acute gastrointestinal hemorrhage.[1] There is an extensive list of common and uncommon causes for upper and lower gastrointestinal hemorrhage, each of which may be evaluated by one or more imaging techniques including barium

133

studies, fiberoptic endoscopy, radionuclide scans, and arteriography. A rational diagnostic approach to this complex problem involves a series of decisions based on the clinically suspected origin of the bleeding as well as on the severity of the hemorrhage. No simple, single scheme can be applied to the gastrointestinal tract as a whole. Patients must be classified as either having acute or chronic blood loss, and then further classified into those with suspected upper and lower gastrointestinal hemorrhage.

A major goal in the diagnosis of these conditions is distinguishing upper from lower gastrointestinal bleeding (proximal or distal to the ligament of Treitz). Hematemesis almost invariably localizes the source of hemorrhage proximal to the ligament of Treitz, where as hematochezia or melena leaves the site of bleeding in doubt. Aspiration of the stomach contents with a nasogastric tube may reveal blood, a finding which is localizing for an upper gastrointestinal hemorrhage. A lack of blood in the stomach contents does not exclude the possibility of an upper gastrointestinal hemorrhage, however, since bleeding may have ceased before passage of the tube or may have occurred distal to a competent pyloric sphincter.

Certain aspects of the patient's history, physical examination, and laboratory tests may also aid in localizing the site of bleeding. For example, a history of peptic ulcer disease, ingestion of aspirin, or alcohol abuse, or a history of severe alcoholic liver disease with portal hypertension, will increase the likelihood that the bleeding is from the upper gastrointestinal tract. On the other hand, a history of inflammatory bowel disease or hematochezia suggests that the bleeding has arisen from a lower gastrointestinal source. If the site of bleeding is still indeterminate but the bleeding is massive, it is probably best to assume that it is from the upper gastrointestinal tract, since the incidence of massive hemorrhage is less common from lesions distal to the ligament of Treitz. In most instances, lower intestinal hemorrhage is an intermittent event that is usually not life-threatening.

CLINICAL PRESENTATION: UPPER GASTROINTESTINAL HEMORRHAGE (ALGORITHM 4-1)

In a single contrast study of the esophagus and stomach, the patient first drinks a cup of thin barium and is then positioned to allow distention of the various components of the stomach by the barium. In an air-contrast study, gas-producing crystals or tablets (which may be likened to Alka-Seltzer), are first ingested, after which a thicker barium is given which provides a thin coating of the walls of the esophagus and stomach (Figs. 4-1 and 4-2).

Additional thin barium medium can then be given to allow filling and evaluation of the subsequent segments of the small bowel in a small bowel series. Films following the barium are obtained as it progesses into the duodenum, jejunum, and finally the ileum and the colon (Fig. 4-3) in the right lower quadrant.

BRISK HEMORRHAGE

About 150 patients per 100,000 population are hospitalized for upper gastrointestinal bleeding each year.

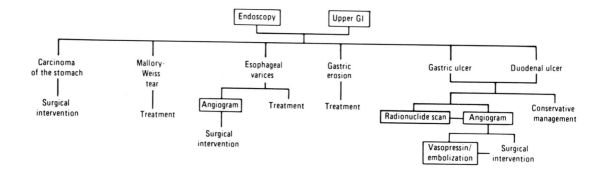

CLINICAL PRESENTATION: UPPER GASTROINTESTINAL HEMORRHAGE

Algorithm 4-1

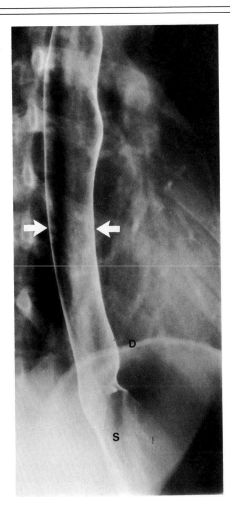

Fig. 4-1 Normal air-contrast esophagram. After the ingestion of gas-producing crystals and thick barium, there is distention of the esophagus, with a thin coating of its wall by the barium (arrows). The esophagus is normally smooth and featureless. S = stomach, D = diaphragm.

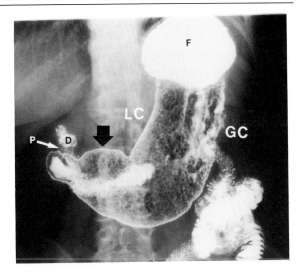

Fig. 4-2 Normal air-contrast view of the stomach. This film was obtained with the patient in the supine position. The barium fills the dependent fundus (F), since it is a posteriorly located part of the stomach. Air fills the anteriorly located body of the stomach, revealing the antrum (arrow). F = fundus, LC = lesser curvature, GC = greater curvature, P = pyloric channel, D = duodenal bulb.

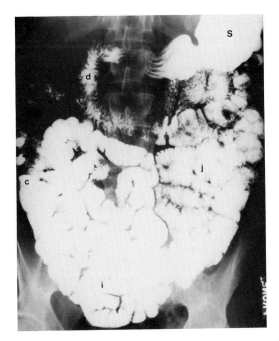

Fig. 4-3 Normal small-bowel examination. Series obtained 1 hour after an upper gastorintestinal examination and the beginning of the small-bowel series. S = stomach, d = duodenum, j = jejunum, i = ileum, c = right side of the colon.

A recent study stated that the major sources of such hemorrhage are duodenal ulcer (24.3 percent), gastric erosions (23.4 percent), gastric ulcer (21.3 percent), varices (10.3 percent), and Mallory-Weiss tears of the esophagus (7.2 percent).[1] These patients should first undergo endoscopy to locate the bleeding site.[2] Barium studies are less successful in this regard, and if they are performed first, residual barium will hinder subsequent endoscopy or angiography.

DUODENAL ULCER

Bleeding duodenal ulcers remain the most frequent cause of massive upper gastrointestinal hemorrhage. Over 90 percent of ulcers occur in the duodenal bulb, and the demonstration of an ulcer crater is the only unequivocal radiographic sign of acute duodenal ulcer disease. The crater appears as a rounded or linear deposit of barium (Fig. 4-4) that is usually surrounded by thickened folds, often in a radiating pattern. In a different projection the ulcer crater may appear as a niche of barium projecting beyond the duodenum (Fig. 4-5).

Secondary signs of duodenal ulcer disease are often more evident than the ulcer crater itself and many, in fact, obscure the crater. The most important secondary sign is deformity and flattening of the bulb due to edema and spasm. The mucosal folds of the bulb may be thickened and edematous due to hypertrophy of Brunner's glands, which are duodenal glands that secrete mucous in an attempt to protect the mucosa from acid.

On occasion, the duodenal ulcer is described as a giant ulcer that involves the entire duodenal bulb and may be difficult to detect. The apparent unchanging appearance of the "duodenal bulb" on multiple views may be the only clue to the diagnosis.

Some ulcers may be found distal to the bulb (postbulbar). They are uncommon and may be difficult to diagnose by clinical, endoscopic, and radiographic methods. They are most commonly found on the inner aspect of the proximal portion of the descending duodenal sweep, above the ampulla of Vater. Localized duodenal narrowing due to spasm and irritability is often associated with these lesions. Healing is commonly followed by fibrosis and stenosis of the proximal descending duodenum. The Zollinger-Ellison syndrome should be considered when a postbulbar ulcer is discovered, because 25 percent of these ulcers occur outside the duodenal bulb (proximal duodenum and jejunum) in patients with the gastrin-producing pancreatic tumors characteristic of the syndrome.

A number of complications accompany both gastric and duodenal ulcers. Free perforation into the peritoneal space may occur, allowing air to leak into the peritoneal cavity. Plain radiographs are conclusive evidence of this complication in the proper clinical setting. Indeed, as little as 1 cc of intraperitoneal air can be detected underneath the diaphragm in patients with a perforated duodenal ulcer. The perforation may also occur into the lesser sac or the pancreas, producing an abscess or pancreatitis.

Fibrosis and scarring develop with chronic ulcers, and may result in relative narrowing of the bulb. The bulb often narrows symmetrically at its midportion, with associated dilated fornices leading to a cloverleaf deformity (Fig. 4-6).

Stenosis is a fairly common complication of peptic

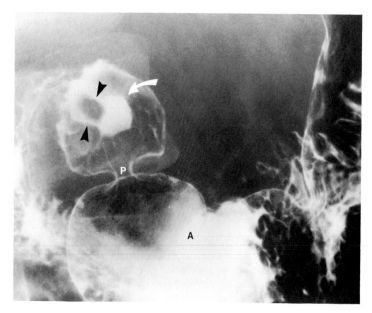

Fig. 4-4 Posterior duodenal bulb ulcer. **History.** A 57-year-old man presented with abdominal pain relieved by eating. **Findings.** *Upper gastrointestinal exam (UGI exam):* The ulcer crater is identified as a barium collection (curved arrow) with radiating folds (arrowheads) on this spot film of the gastric antrum (A). The pyloric channel (P) is well identified. The ulcer is seen en face.

Fig. 4-5 Duodenal bulb ulcer.
History. This 42-year-old man had a coffee-grounds emesis.
Findings. *UGI exam:* There is a persistent collection of barium seen tangentially along the superior aspect of the duodenal bulb (arrow).

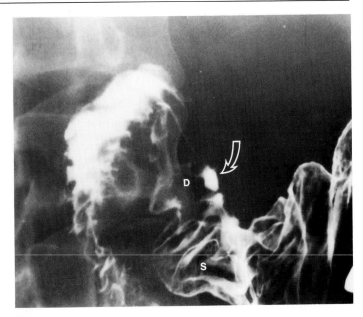

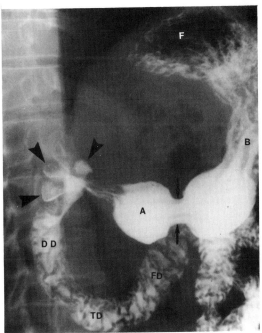

Fig. 4-6 Chronic peptic ulcer disease.
History. This 39-year-old woman had recurrent epigastric pain and a long history of peptic ulcer disease.
Findings. *UGI exam:* There is a cloverleaf deformity of the duodenal bulb. Sacculations (arrowheads) due to scarring are identified; they do not represent ulcers. F = fundus of the stomach, B = body of stomach, A = antrum, DD = descending duodenum, TD = third portion of duodenum, FD = fourth portion of duodenum, arrows = peristaltic wave in stomach.

ulcer disease, with duodenal ulcer being the most common cause of gastric-outlet obstruction. The stenosis is due to marked scarring, inflammatory spasm, or both. The bulb is visualized and appears markedly distorted and narrowed.

GASTRIC EROSIONS

Erosive gastritis is a benign, self-limited disease of the mucosa. It is prone to recurrence and may be incapacitating. The resultant gastric erosions are superficial defects, limited to the mucosal layer, that do not penetrate through the muscularis mucosa. In some series, gastric erosions have been considered the most common source of upper gastrointestinal bleeding. Causative factors in the development of gastroduodenal erosions include alcohol, aspirin, and antiflammatory agents such as aspirin, phenylbutazone, indomethacin, and steroids. Mucosal erosions, particularly in the corpus of the stomach, may also develop within hours of a stressful event, such as major burn injury, multiple injuries, and major operations, especially when these events are complicated by hypotension, sepsis, renal failure, or severe respiratory insufficiency. Bleeding ensues in only 10 percent of patients with such stress related erosions, and usually occurs 6 to 7 days after the stressful event. Gastric erosions may also be seen in patients with Crohn's disease and candidiasis.

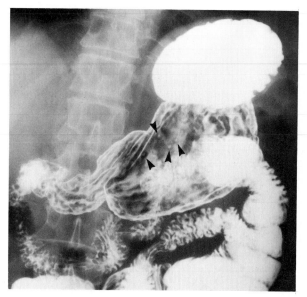

Fig. 4-7 Erosive gastritis.
History. This 27-year-old woman was taking nonsteroidal antiinflammatory medication in a high-dose.
Findings. *UGI exam:* Multiple punctate collections of barium (arrowheads), surrounded by a zone of lucency ("apthous ulcers") are noted in the body of the stomach.

A double-contrast upper GI series is the ideal method of diagnosing gastric erosions radiographically; single-contrast studies are less accurate. The radiographic appearance of an erosion is that of a target lesion with a tiny fleck of barium representing the erosion and a radiolucent halo representing the surrounding edematous mound[3] (Fig. 4-7). Erosions, usually multiple and arranged linearly, like a string of beads, are easiest to detect in the antrum.

GASTRIC ULCER

Gastric ulcers are responsible for acute upper gastrointestinal bleeding in 10 to 20 percent of patients. Emergent operative intervention is accompanied by higher mortality rates for gastric ulcers than for duodenal ulcers. Benign gastric ulcers are more frequently the cause for brisk hemorrhage than are malignant ulcers.

Gastric ulcers are usually located on the lesser curvature of the middle third of the stomach. They may range from several millimeters in diameter to huge excavations 6 to 8 cm in size, with most being 1 to 2 cm in size. The ulcer crater is seen as an abnormal collection or niche of barium. Most gastric ulcers are

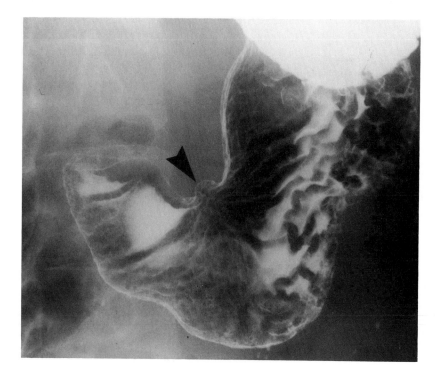

Fig. 4-8 Benign gastric ulcer.
History. This 39-year-old woman had upper abdominal pain and guaiac-positive stools.
Findings. *UGI exam:* There is a 1.3 cm, air-filled ulcer along the lesser curvature of the stomach (arrowhead).

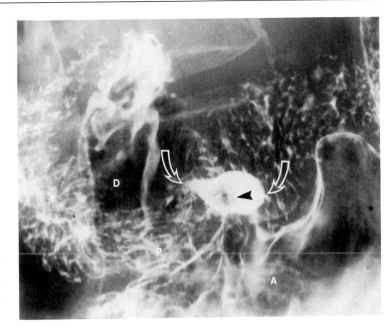

Fig. 4-9 Benign gastric ulcer.
History. This 57-year-old man had a past history of massive upper gastrointestinal bleeding.
Findings. *UGI exam:* This close-up spot film of the lesser curvature of the antrum (A), pylorus (P), and duodenum (D) shows a large ulcer (open arrows) containing a filling defect (arrowhead) which represents a blood clot.

round or slightly oval, running perpendicular to the gastric wall. They have a relatively flat or slightly rounded base (Fig. 4-8).

Once the ulcer is diagnosed, it must then be determined, by careful evaluation of its radiographic features, whether it appears to be benign or malignant or is indeterminate in nature. The size of the ulcer crater is of little value in determining malignancy. The location is also unhelpful unless the ulcer lies in the gastric fundus, in which case it is almost invariably malignant. The following features suggest that an ulcer is benign: (1) an ulcer crater that projects beyond the expected lumen of the stomach (Fig. 4-8); (2) radiation of mucosal folds through the edge and into

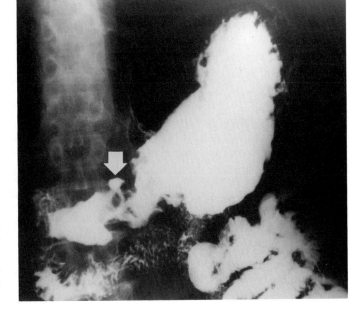

Fig. 4-10 Malignant gastric ulcer.
History. This 72-year-old man had Hemoccult-positive stools and weight loss.
Findings. *UGI exam:* A prone spot film shows an ulcer (arrow) along the lesser curvature of the antrum. This ulcer does not extend beyond the wall of the stomach. Coarse, nodular folds leading to a mass are also seen in the antrum.

the ulcer in a spoke-like fashion (Fig. 4-8); (3) a sharply defined and smooth margin of the ulcer crater (Fig. 4-8); (4) a smooth, symmetric collar of surrounding edema, with the ulcer situated within the center of the mound; (5) a possible symmetric linear defect (Hampton's line) at the orifice of the ulcer crater, due to undermining of the mucosa; (6) a gradual transition of the ulcer to normal mucosal tissue; (7) healing of the ulcer by 8 to 12 weeks; (8) a small, round filling defect (Fig. 4-9) in the center of the crater base, which represents a blood clot (carcinomas ooze blood that usually does not clot, while benign ulcers may bleed rapidly and form a clot in the ulcer base); and (9) an associated duodenal ulcer (this implies the presence of increased gastric acid, whereas most gastric cancers occur in the setting of achlorhydria).

Malignant ulcers typically do not project beyond the lumen of the stomach because they develop within a mass of tumor tissue. Multiple areas of nodularity may be seen about the margin of the ulcer (Fig. 4-10). The ulcer crater is often surrounded by an asymmetric mass, the outer border of which has an abrupt junction with the normal mucosa. There are irregular folds terminating at the tumor mass and not reaching the ulcer crater. Fluoroscopically, the region of the ulcer may be rigid in carcinoma, while there is often a spastic contraction of the stomach opposite a benign gastric ulcer (incisura). More will be discussed on gastric carcinoma in a subsequent section.

Some benign ulcers do not fulfill the radiographic criteria for benignity or malignancy, and are thus called "indeterminate" ulcers. These ulcers and those that fulfill the criteria for malignancy should be examined endoscopically. Some clinicians argue that all gastric ulcers should be endoscoped and biopsied. This is an expensive, time-consuming procedure, with a small return in terms of diagnosing malignancy. About 95 percent of all gastric ulcers are benign, and 0 to 3 percent of seemingly benign ulcers are malignant.

When a benign gastric ulcer is diagnosed radiographically, further studies should be done at 8 weeks and then at 12 weeks. If the ulcer is not significantly reduced (more than 50 percent) in size by 8 weeks and not completely healed by 12 weeks, endoscopy should be performed. If the ulcer is in fact due to a malignant process, this 12-week delay has little impact on the patient's prognosis, since gastric malignancy has a dismal 5-year survival rate.

VARICES

In patients with cirrhosis and portal hypertension, a variety of portosystemic collateral vessels may develop as an attempted means for decompressing the portal circulation. Coronary-esophageal collaterals (varices) are common, and represent the most clinically important shunting pathway of the portal sys-

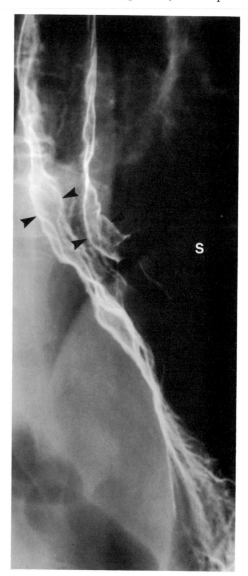

Fig. 4-11 Gastroesophageal varices.
History. This 48-year-old man with chronic alcoholism had massive hematemesis.
Findings. *UGI exam:* There are large, serpiginous filling defects (arrowheads) of the distal esophagus and gastric cardia. At fluoroscopy these folds changed in size. The fundus of the stomach is identified (S).

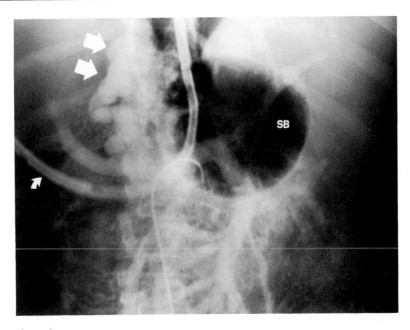

Fig. 4-12 Gastroesophageal varices.
History. This 56-year-old chronic alcoholic male presented with massive hematemesis, hypovolemia, and a history of varices.
Findings. *Angiogram:* A Sangstaken-Blakemore tube (curved arrow) was passed into the stomach and the balloon (SB) was inflated with air in an attempt to tamponade the varices, which were the presumed cause of the patient's hemorrhage. A late venous phase from an angiogram demonstrates multiple, tubular, serpiginous, and dilated coronary veins (arrows), representing varices.

tem. On barium studies of the esophagus, varices usually occur in the lower third of the esophagus, and appear as linear, wormlike filling defects (Fig. 4-11). Changes in size of the varices occur easily, and often disappear during peristalsis or deep inspiration. Not uncommonly, varices of the gastric fundus and cardia are seen in association with esophageal varices. Varices in the region of the fundus and cardia appear as multiple rounded or nodular filling defects. Unlike defects caused by tumors, gastric varices also change size and shape from film to film. Rarely, duodenal varices may be demonstrated. Angiography may confirm the presence of varices (Fig. 4-12). Computed tomography has recently also been used to detect varices.

MALLORY-WEISS SYNDROME

Linear lacerations of the distal esophagus or proximal gastric mucosa near the gastroesophageal junction after an episode of retching are responsible for 2 to 7 percent of acute upper gastrointestinal hemorrhages. About 75 percent of patients with these Mallory-Weiss tears present with a history of vomiting, retching and recent alcohol use. Most of the tears are located at the gastric side of the gastroesophageal junction. Rarely, a linear collection of contrast material can be seen on barium contrast studies. Fiberoptic endoscopy is the preferred method for diagnosis of the syndrome. During active bleeding, celiac angiography demonstrates extravasation of contrast material in the lower esophagus or cardia of the stomach.[3]

SLOW HEMORRHAGE

CARCINOMA OF THE STOMACH

Carcinoma of the stomach is one of the most lethal malignancies in the world, being quite prevalent in Japan. Its incidence is declining in the United States. Because the early symptoms of this malignancy are

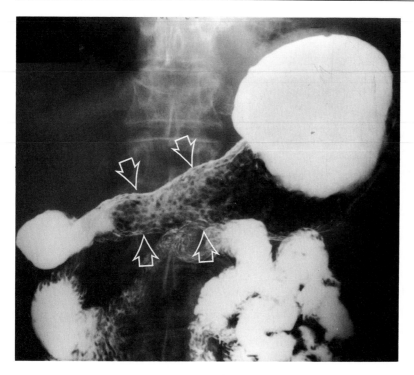

Fig. 4-13 Carcinoma of the gastric antrum.
History. This 78-year-old man presented with weight loss, anorexia, and Hemoccult-positive stools.
Findings. *UGI exam:* A spot film demonstrates a coarse, irregular mucosal pattern of the antrum (arrows). This area was rigid and did not change upon fluoroscopy.

often minimal and nonspecific in the potentially curable phase of the disease, gastric carcinoma is usually discovered when extensive. Indeed, there is a less than 10 percent 5-year survival in patients with this malignancy. Weight loss, ulcer-like symptoms, upper abdominal discomfort of insidious onset, and iron deficiency anemia due to occult bleeding are common presenting findings.

Early gastric cancer presents as a slightly depressed, irregular lesion accompanied by clubbed or irregular converging folds in the gastric mucosa.[4]

Eventually most gastric carcinomas will assume one of the following appearances: (1) infiltrating or scirrhous; (2) polypoid or fungating; or (3) ulcerating.[5] In the scirrhous type, the tumor evokes a pronounced fibrous tissue response in the gastric wall. The gastric wall may become thickened and rigid and does not exhibit peristalsis. Mucosal folds are obliterated and the surface has a fine granular or occasionally a rough, cobblestone appearance. The stomach has a decreased size, and with extension, it has the radiographic appearance of a "leather bottle" or linitus plastica (Fig. 4-13). In fungating or polypoid types of gastric carcinoma the tumor forms a mass that projects into the lumen. The surface of the mass is irregular and nodular. The ulcerating type of gastric cancer has already been discussed (Fig. 4-10).

LYMPHOMA

Lymphoma of the stomach is 5 to 10 times less common than carcinoma. It often occurs in association with systemic non-Hodgkin's lymphoma, but may be isolated to the gastrointestinal tract. Primary lymphoma may radiographically mimic one of the forms of gastric carcinoma. The most common radiographic presentations of this malignancy include considerable nodularity or thickening of all gastric rugae (Fig. 4-14), decreasing gastric peristalsis, or a large, bulky, more localized mass, which is often ulcerated and is quite similar in apperance to an advanced gastric carcinoma.[6]

METASTASIS

Breast carcinoma and malignant melonoma are among the two most common primary malignancies that metastasize to the stomach. Metastatic lesions to

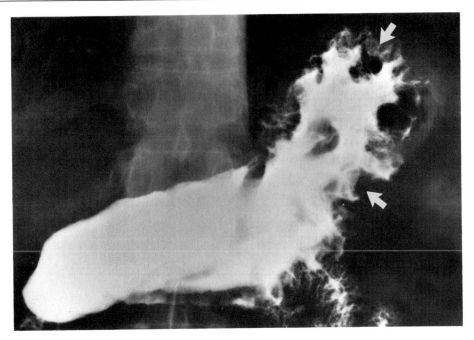

Fig. 4-14 Lymphoma of the stomach.
History. This 74-year-old woman had weight loss and anemia.
Findings. *UGI exam:* There are large polypoid folds throughout the stomach, but most marked in the fundus (arrows).

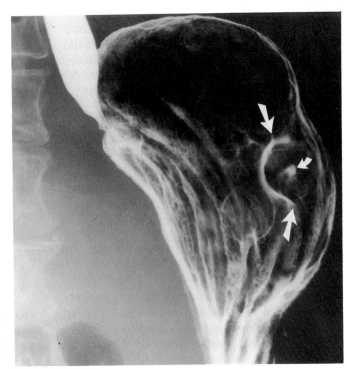

Fig. 4-15 Gastric metastasis.
History. This 61-year-old man with a known malignant melanoma had Hemoccult-positive stools of new onset.
Findings. *UGI exam:* There are round soft-tissue masses noted in the stomach. One lesion has an ulcer that produces a "bull's-eye" appearance (arrows).

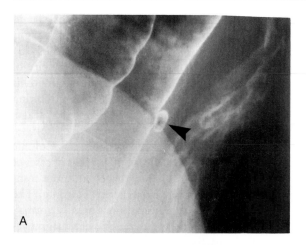

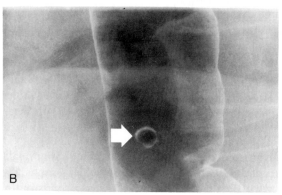

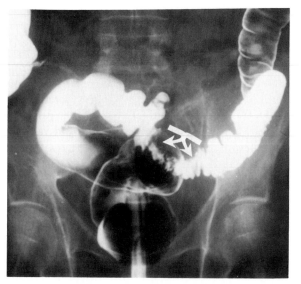

Fig. 4-19 Diverticulitis of the sigmoid colon.
History. This 68-year-old woman presented with fever and left-lower-quadrant pain.
Findings. *Air-contrast exam, LGI:* There is a mass producing a "cushion" defect along the superior aspect of the sigmoid colon, suggesting a small pericolic abscess secondary to diverticulitis (arrows).

Fig. 4-18 Diverticulosis.
History. This 50-year-old man had constipation.
Findings. *Air contrast exam, lower gastrointestinal tract (LGI):* A solitary diverticulum seen in (**A**) profile (arrowhead) and (**B**) en race (white arrow). Diverticulae extend beyond the lumen of the colon and contain barium or air in a double contrast study.

is frequently necessary. Interestingly, diverticular hemorrhage arises from the ascending or transverse colon in 75 percent of cases, despite the predominance of diverticula in the descending and sigmoid colon. The severity of bleeding may range from mild hematochezia to massive hemorrhage.[8]

Diverticulitis is an important complication of colonic diverticular disease and is characterized by perforation of a diverticulum and the formation of a peridiverticular abscess. The clinical findings in this condition include lower abdominal pain, typically associated with fever, a mass, or tenderness, and laboratory evidence of infection. Free intraperitoneal air, as

seen in perforated duodenal ulcers, is rare in diverticulitis because the perforation is sealed off by the surrounding pericolic fat.

Diverticulitis most commonly occurs in the sigmoid colon. Initially the inflammatory changes are limited to the mucosa and there may be no changes seen, or only focal irritability and spasm. If there is extension into the serosa and surrounding tissues, there will be an inflammatory, periocolic soft-tissue mass indenting the neighboring colon (Fig. 4-19). The perforated diverticulum is usually obliterated and not seen during the barium-enema examination. The postevacuation film is occasionally quite helpful in identifying the offending diverticulum. Single-contrast studies are preferred over air-contrast studies.

A frank abscess may become apparent in diverticulitis, and ulceration may lead to internal fistulous tracts, sometimes parallel to the colon or extending into a pericolonic location.[9] Fistulas to adjacent organs such as the bladder, ileum, or female genital organs may also occur.

SLOW HEMORRHAGE

A slow hemorrhage usually results in melena or heme-positive stools. A neoplasm, benign or malignant, is the common etiology.

COLONIC POLYPS

The term polyp is a generic term used to describe any mucosal filling defect, and does not suggest a particular histology. The different histologic types of polyp include hyperplastic and adenomatous polyps. Hyperplastic polyps are usually less than 5 mm in size and are of no clinical significance since they do not bleed, are not true adenomas, and have no malignant potential.

Adenomatous polyps are found in about 10 percent of the population over age 40. They are most common in the distal colon, are multiple in 25 percent of cases, and occur slightly more often in women than in men.[10] All adenomatous polyps are intraluminal as seen with a barium enema. They are usually less than 1.5 cm in diameter, and appear as circular filling defects in single-contrast studies and as "ring shadows"

in air-contrast studies. When larger than 1.5 to 2 cm they are frequently lobulated and occasionally bizarre in appearance. They may be sessile and adherent to the mucosal wall. Adenomatous polyps are often also suspended by stacks or pedicles to the colon wall (Fig. 4-20).

Polyps greater than 1.5 cm and those that are sessile or have a short stalk have an increased probability of harboring malignancy, and should be biopsied and removed colonoscopically. Other clues to malignancy within the polyp include irregularity of the surface of the polyp and an increase in size of the polyp from study to study (Fig. 4-21). There are many recent reports suggesting that all carcinoma of the colon arise from adenomatous polyps.[10]

VILLOUS ADENOMA

Villous adenomas are less common than adenomatous polyps, and are usually seen in the rectosigmoid or cecum. They are soft, roundish masses that are quite friable and bleed easily. On a barium enema villous adenomas exhibit a cauliflower appearance as barium fills the interstices of these polyps (Fig. 4-22). Malig-

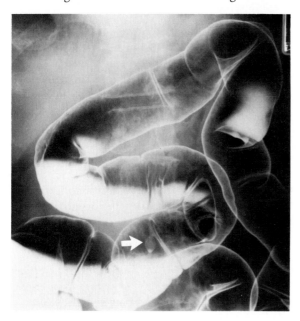

Fig. 4-20 Pedunculated polyp.
History. This 75-year-old man had a previous history of a polyp.
Findings. *Air-contrast exam, LGI:* There is a pedunculated polyp (arrow) in the transverse colon. Note the drop of barium coming off the dependent part of the polyp.

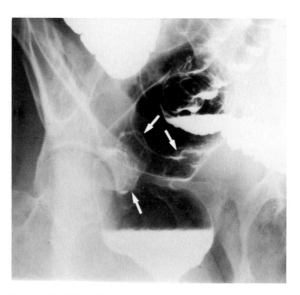

Fig. 4-21 Polypoid carcinoma.
History. This 76-year-old woman had hematochezia.
Findings. *Air-contrast exam, LGI:* In the rectum are two large lobulated polyps (arrows) which proved to harbor malignancy on a proctoscopic biopsy.

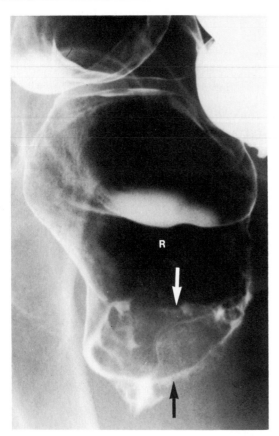

Fig. 4-22 Villous adenoma of the rectum.
History. This 57-year-old man had tenesmus, hematochezia, and a mass on rectal examination.
Findings. *Air-contrast exam, LGI:* A 3-cm lobulated mass (arrows) is demonstrated within the rectum (R).

nant degeneration is seen in 40 to 60 percent of polyps greater than 1 cm in size.[11]

CARCINOMA OF THE COLON

Carcinoma of the colon is the second most lethal cancer in the United States; nearly 60,000 people die annually from this tumor. Approximately 5 percent of the population will develop carcinoma of the colon, and there are 130,000 new cases each year. The symptoms of colon cancer are usually initially vague and nonspecific, with malaise and weight loss quite common. Cancers of the cecum and ascending colon are often silent, with indolent blood loss leading to anemia. Blood in the feces of patients with these malignancies is frequently not recognized because it is thor-

oughly admixed with the liquid fecal matter of the right colon. However, approximately 75 percent of patients will have Hemoccult-positive stools. Noticeable rectal bleeding occurs in 70 percent of cases of cancer of the left colon. These distal neoplasms tend to be obstructive.

Overall, radiographic evaluation for carcinoma of the colon is best done with the air-contrast barium enema. Single-contrast techniques are excellent for demonstrating larger lesions. If carcinoma is to be detected in its ealier and potentially more curable stage, the air-contrast technique is required, in that it

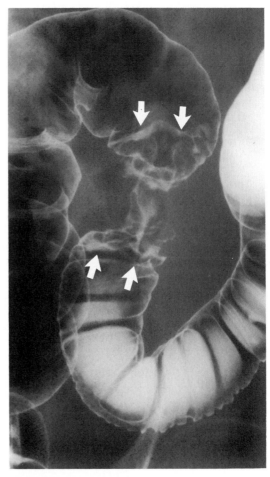

Fig. 4-23 Carcinoma of the sigmoid colon.
History. This 75-year-old man had Hemoccult-positive stools and a change in his bowel habits.
Findings. *Air-contrast exam, LGI:* There is an annular constricting lesion that destroys the mucosa and has abrupt margins (arrows). This is the typical "apple core" or "napkin ring" deformity of carcinoma of the colon.

can better define small polypoid and plaque-like tumors.[12]

Because early colorectal carcinoma usually appears as a polypoid mass, its detection is basically an exercise in the discovery of small polyps, as described in the previous section (Fig. 4-21). Advanced carcinoma encircles the bowel lumen, producing an annular area of narrowing usually less than 6 cm long. The deformity has the appearance of an apple core or napkin ring (Fig. 4-23). The transition from normal mucosa to tumor is usually abrupt, producing an overhanging edge known as a tumor "shelf" or "shoulder" (Fig. 4-23). The mucosal folds in the region of the tumor are destroyed, and there may be associated ulceration.

Carcinomas produce a number of local complications including bleeding, obstruction, perforation, and intussusception. In adults, carcinoma is the most common cause of obstruction of the colon. There is usually dilatation of the colon proximally. There may also be a lesser degree of small-bowel dilatation, depending on the competency of closure of the ileocecal valve. Approximately 5 percent of patients with colorectal cancer have a second, synchronous (coexistent) tumor, and 15 to 20 percent have accompanying adenomatous polyps. Metachronous tumors are those that develop following a primary colon cancer and not at the site of surgery. They are distinguished from recurrent primary lesions, which occur at the surgical anastomotic site. The cumulative risk of a metachronous carcinoma increases with the duration of follow-up, making serial barium studies of the colon necessary for the remainder of the patient's life. A barium study 3 months postoperatively and then annually for 2 years is recommended.

WORKUP OF A BRISK GASTROINTESTINAL HEMORRHAGE

RADIONUCLIDE IMAGING

Recently, nuclear imaging techniques have been used to localize active, occult, or intermittent gastrointestinal bleeding sites at bleeding rates as low as 0.1 cc/min. There are two major methods for doing this, and both depend on the recognition of abnormal radioactivity within the bowel lumen.

One technique involves the bolus injection of ^{99M}Tc-sulfur colloid, to determine whether the patient is actively bleeding. This is the same radiopharmaceutical used for liver and spleen scanning. The reticuloendothelial (RE) system residing predominantly in the liver and spleen rapidly and completely extracts the technetium sulfur colloid from the blood after it passes the splanchnic circulation. No activity is normally seen otherwise within the abdomen (Fig. 4-24). Any activity seen outside the liver or spleen represents extravasated radiopharmaceutical in the bowel lumen that came from a bleeding site before the radiopharmaceutical encountered the liver or spleen. This test has a very high sensitivity for active bleeding, and positive results can be obtained within 10 to 15 minutes. Small amounts of extravasated activity or blood can be detected. The sulfur-colloid bleeding test is often done before an angiogram, and directs the angiographer to a suspicious site. It allows an excellent probability that the bleeding site can be found and the treatment affected. The nuclear medicine study is more sensitive than the angiogram. If it is negative, then angiography should not be performed, since the

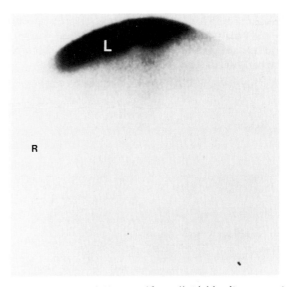

Fig. 4-24 Normal ^{99m}Tc-sulfur-colloid bleeding test. A view of the abdomen shows normal uptake of the labeled sulfur colloid only by the liver (L). No abnormal activity is seen over the abdoman. R = right.

patient is not actively bleeding. A major problem in interpretation of the nuclear medicine study is that areas of bleeding near the liver and spleen may not be diagnosed due to overlying activity in these organs.

ANGIOGRAPHY

Angiography can be used to both localize and treat the source of blood loss in gastrointestinal hemorrhage. The procedure may be performed on severely ill patients and requires very little patient cooperation. This modality is usually reserved for patients who continue to bleed despite conservative management. Following the percutaneous entry of the femoral artery, a catheter is positioned in the celiac, superior mesenteric, or inferior mesenteric artery. After the catheter is properly positioned, contrast medium is injected rapidly and serial films are obtained. Vessels distal to the catheter tip are opacified, and bleeding points are defined by the extravasation or leakage of contrast medium into the bowel lumen (Fig. 4-17). A bleeding rate of at least 0.5 to 1 cc/min at the time of contrast-medium injection is required for the angiographic detection of hemorrhage.

Many reports have documented high success rates in controlling bleeding by the selective infusion of vasopressin and the embolization of bleeding arteries. These methods are very effective when more conservative modes of therapy have failed, and are ideal when the patient is a high-risk surgical candidate. Such interventional angiography can be used as a temporizing measure, buying time for patient stabilization, so that surgery can be performed at a more opportune time rather than on an emergency basis.

Vasopressin is a potent splanchnic vasoconstrictor. The selective infusion of low doses (0.2 U/min) into bleeding arteries at the time of angiography causes sufficient vasoconstriction to stop bleeding without promoting clinically significant ischemia in the various organs and structures of the body. The vasopressin should be infused as close to the bleeding branch vessel as possible. Infusions into the left gastric artery are used for gastric hemorrhages, and infusions into the gastroduodenal artery for bleeding duodenal ulcers. Twenty minutes after the infusion of vasopressin is initiated, a repeat angiogram is performed. If

extravasation is no longer evident and there is good forward flow of blood into the capillary and venous phases, the infusion is considered satisfactory and is continued at the above rate for 24 hours through the indwelling angiographic catheter. The dose of vasopressin is tapered over the next 1 to 2 days. If bleeding recurs during the tapering period, resumption of the initial dose again produces hemostatis. If the repeat angiogram done after the initial 20-minute vasopressin infusion shows continued bleeding, the rate of infusion is doubled, and after an additional 20 minutes another angiogram is performed. If bleeding persists at that time, it is unlikely that any safe dose of vasoconstrictor will be effective, and an alternative means of managing the patient is indicated.

Another useful technique for controlling gastrointestinal bleeding is embolizing the bleeding artery via a catheter, a technique called transcatheter arterial embolization. Several materials are available for injection through the angiographic catheter, including the patient's own clotted (autologous) blood, Gelfoam (gelatin) particles, steel coils, and synthetic glues. The catheter is removed after replacement of the emboli.

Various sites of gastrointestinal bleeding respond better to either vasopressin infusion or embolization. Embolization is more likely to control bleeding from a duodenal ulcer than is a simple vasopressin infusion. Gastric mucosal bleeding, on the other hand, responds readily to vasopressin therapy. Embolization for gastric mucosal bleeding should be limited to those patients in whom the infusion of vasopressin is unsuccessful, or for whom prolonged catheterization is impractical. Vasopressin infusion is usually effective in controlling bleeding from a demonstrated site in most patients with brisk lower intestinal hemorrhage from mucosal ulceration in association with diverticulosis. Embolization is not commonly used in patients with colonic bleeding, since the colon does not have a rich collateral circulation in older patients, and increases the risk of ischemia and infarction of normal portions of the bowel. An emergency or unprepared colectomy in elderly patients with massively bleeding diverticuli carries an operative mortality risk of 30 to 40 percent. Angiographic diagnosis, management (vasopressin), and temporization of these hemorrhages have reduced the subsequent nonemergency surgery mortality rate to 3 percent.[14]

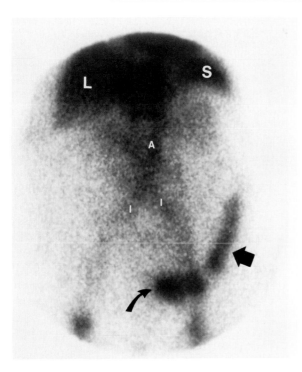

Fig. 4-25 Intermittent hemorrhage from the splenic flexure.
History. This 67-year-old woman had recurrent episodes of hematochezia.
Findings. *Pertechnetate labeled red-blood-cell scan:* This examination shows abnormal activity within the descending and sigmoid colon (arrows). An initial angiogram could not reveal the bleeding site due to the intermittent nature of the bleeding. Normal activity is seen within the liver (L), spleen (S), aorta (A), and iliac arteries (I).

WORKUP OF AN INTERMITTENT OR SLOW GASTROINTESTINAL HEMORRHAGE

RADIONUCLIDE IMAGING

In a technique developed to best detect intermittent sources of gastrointestinal bleeding, the patient's red blood cells (RBC) are withdrawn and labeled with ^{99m}Tc-pertechnetate. This red blood cell-pertechnetate combination circulates through the abdomen normally depositing no activity within the abdomen outside the liver, spleen, and major arterial pathways.

If serial images of the abdomen reveal a focal accumulation of the labeled cells within the abdominal field or within the lumen of a loop of bowel, this represents a pooling of extravasated blood from a slow bleeding point (Fig. 4-25). Serial images can be obtained over a 24-hour period. Intermittent bleeding sites can also be located because the labeled and extravasated blood cells in the bowel lumen are not resorbed. Bleeding that occurs at any time between the time of isotope injection and imaging is identified. This technique differs from both angiography and ^{99m}Tc-sulfur colloid scans in that active bleeding need not be present for detection. Labeled RBC techniques, however, are less sensitive than sulfur colloid scans and require bleeding rates near 0.5 cc/min, resembling those needed in angiography. The sulfur colloid method is superior for active slow bleeding, while the RBC-pertechnetate method is better for intermittent rates of bleeding.

Neither type of nuclear medicine study described above can define individual vessels, as can angiography. However, these tests may suggest which portion of the bowel is bleeding (e.g., activity in the pelvis suggests ileal or sigmoid bleeding, while right-lower-quadrant activity suggests cecal bleeding). If bleeding is found in a portion of the abdomen by the nuclear medicine technique, an angiogram is performed, with special attention given to the suspicious areas.

CLINICAL PRESENTATION: JAUNDICE (ALGORITHM 4-3)

In most patients with jaundice, a careful history and physical examination, combined with routine liver function tests, will suggest the etiology of the causative hyperbilirubinemia. In some patients, however, the clinical distinction between diffuse parenchymal disease, focal liver disease, and extrahepatic biliary obstruction is not possible, and more sophisticated imaging is required. During the past decade, the introduction of computed tomography (CT) and ultrasound has revolutionized the evaluation of the jaundiced patient.

The ultrasound examination of the gallbladder is basically a two-part examination. The first half is the identification of the gallbladder in multiple orientations. The gallbladder is normally oval and gives no

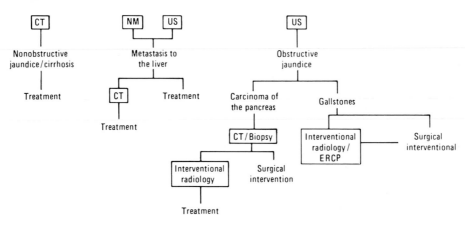

CLINICAL PRESENTATION: JAUNDICE

Algorithm 4-3

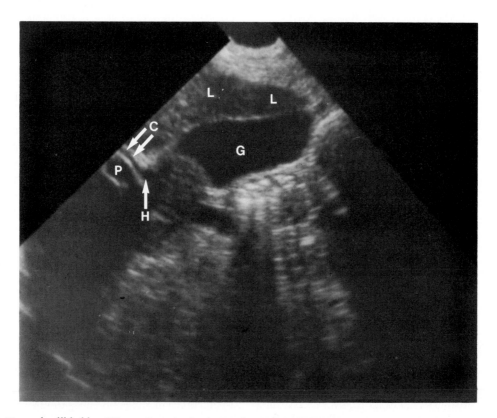

Fig. 4-26 Normal gallbladder, US scan. Longitudinal view through the right upper quadrant. Note the classic relationship of the portal vein (P), common hepatic duct (C), and hepatic artery (H). G = gallbladder, L = liver.

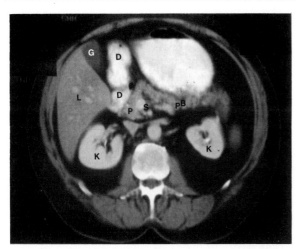

Fig. 4-27 Normal CT scan at the level of the gallbladder; pancreatic head and duodenal sweep. G = gallbladder, D = duodenal sweep, P = pancreatic head, PB = pancreatic body, S = superior mesenteric artery and vein, L = liver, K = kidneys.

echoes from within its lumen (Fig. 4-26). It can be identified by ultrasound in well over 90 percent of normal patients. Imaging of the common hepatic or bile ducts represents the second part of the examination. Here the diameter of the lumen of the bile duct is measured (Fig. 4-26).

A CT scan through the level of the gallbladder images a oval structure of near water density abutting the liver (Fig. 4-27). Anomalies in the position of the gallbladder are not uncommon. The intrahepatic biliary system can be best identified after the injection of intravenous contrast medium as a nonenhancing branching ductal system, again of near water density. The contrast medium is necessary so that the portal veins, now filled with a high-density contrast medium are not confused with the biliary system. The course of the common bile duct can be followed on subsequent levels until its endpoint in the head of the pancreas and ampulla of Vater.

OBSTRUCTIVE JAUNDICE

The early recognition of jaundice caused by extrahepatic biliary obstruction is important because prolonged obstruction may lead to deterioration of liver function, recurrent bouts of cholangitis and sepsis, and occasionally hepatic abscess formation. The relief of a benign obstruction (e.g., from gallstones) often returns the patient to normal. For these reasons, an

ultrasound examination, CT scan, or both are recommended in all patients suspected of having obstructive jaundice. Indeed, these low-risk, high-yield, and noninvasive techniques can reveal early dilatation of the intra- or extrahepatic ducts in patients even before elevated serum bilirubin levels can.

Ultrasound should be the initial screening method in patients with suspected obstructive jaundice because it is rapid, safe, readily available, and has a 97 percent accuracy in detecting obstruction.[15] When the intra- and extrahepatic ducts are well seen sonographically and are normal in caliber, no further radiologic evaluation is needed in most patients. Dilated intrahepatic ducts appear as branching, tubular structures running adjacent to portal venous structures in the ultrasound image. Extrahepatic obstruction is diagnosed when the common hepatic duct is larger than 4 to 5 mm (Fig. 4-28). It is important to visualize both the intra- and extrahepatic ducts because the dilatation of the two may be discordant, and may help localize the abnormality. Ultrasound is quite sensitive in demonstrating cholelithiasis and depicting the gallbladder, as will be discussed. If a mass is demonstrated as the cause of obstruction (a carcinoma of the pancreatic head), a sonographically guided aspiration can then be performed. Unfortunately, bowel gas and body habitus make evaluation of the distal common bile duct difficult in some patients. Additionally, if the ducts are dilated but the etiology or level of obstruction is not apparent, CT or percutaneous transhepatic cholangiography (PTC) are recommended.

The sensitivity of CT (96 percent) in revealing biliary obstruction is comparable to that of ultrasound (97 percent), but it is not recommended as a screening tool because it is much more expensive and time consuming, less available, and uses ionizing radiation. Computed tomography plays a major role for patients in whom sonography indicates ductal dilatation but does not clearly establish the level and cause of obstruction. Furthermore, obese patients and those with prior biliary-enteric anastomoses will often have an unsatisfactory ultrasound study, making CT the preferred procedure. Computed tomography provides unrivaled images of the porta hepatis and pancreas, and has an accuracy of 93 percent in showing the level of biliary obstruction (versus 43 percent for ultrasound), and an 82 percent accuracy in revealing its etiology (versus 30 percent for ultrasound).[16] The CT diagnosis of biliary obstruction is based on the demonstration of

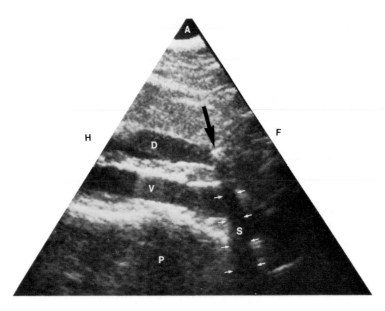

Fig. 4-28 Common duct stone.
History. This 63-year-old woman presented with intermittent jaundice.
Findings. *US scan:* There is dilation of the common hepatic duct (D) proximal to an obstructing stone (black arrow) which casts an acoustic shadow (S). V = portal vein, H = toward head, F = towards foot, A = anterior, P = posterior.

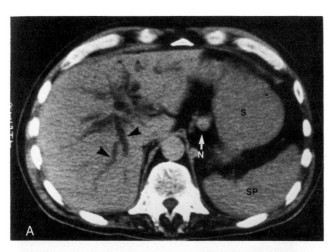

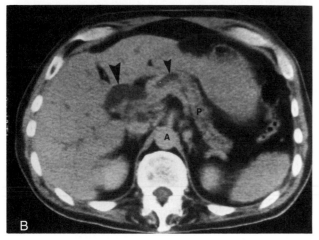

Fig. 4-29 Biliary- and pancreatic-duct dilatation secondary to carcinoma of the pancreas.
History. This 56-year-old woman presented with weight loss, abdominal pain, anorexia, and obstructive jaundice.
Findings. **(A)** *CT scan:* View of the upper abdomen demonstrates multiple, branching, low-density tubular structures within the liver (arrowheads). S = non-opacified stomach, SP = Spleen, and N = enlarged lymph node (arrow) indicating metastasis to surrounding lymph nodes). **(B)** A CT scan obtained 3 cm caudal to the position in (A) shows dilatation of the common hepatic duct (large arrowhead) and pancreatic duct (small arrowhead) within the pancreas (P). Carcinoma of the pancreas often obstructs both the pancreatic and common bile ducts. The aorta (A) is not opacified.

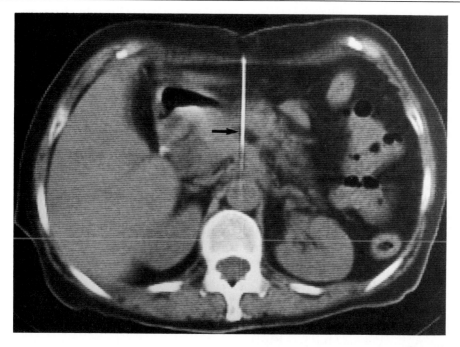

Fig. 4-30 *CT guided needle biopsy.* Localizing scan obtained while performing a CT-guided fine-needle aspiration biopsy of a pancreatic mass. The 22-gauge "skinny needle" (arrow) can be passed through all abdominal structures with impunity.

dilated bile ducts. Dilated intrahepatic ducts appear as linear, branching, or circular structures of near-water density, enlarging as they approach the porta hepatis (Fig. 4-29 A and B).

If a pancreatic mass is identified, it can be staged, since retroperitoneal and mesenteric adenopathy and hepatic and adrenal metastases are readily imaged by CT. The mass may be biopsied under CT guidance as well (Fig. 4-30).

Percutaneous transhepatic cholangiography is performed by putting a needle through the skin and into an intrahepatic bile duct under fluoroscopic control. An iodinated contrast medium is then injected into the ducts for their opacification (Fig. 4-31). It provides a road map of the biliary system for the surgeon or for the interventional radiologist, who may try and snag a stone or pass a tube through an obstructing mass causing the biliary obstruction.

NONOBJECTIVE JAUNDICE

The ability of CT and ultrasound to characterize diffuse parenchymal disease, such as cirrhosis, has not yet

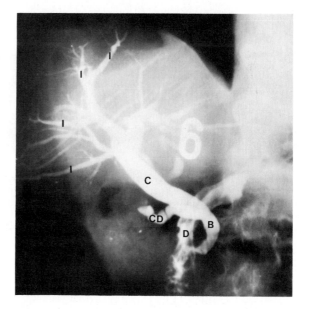

Fig. 4-31 Normal percutaneous transhepatic cholangiogram (PTC). There is excellent visualization of the intrahepatic biliary system (I) and the extrahepatic biliary system, which consists of the common hepatic duct (C), cystic duct (CD) (the gallbladder has been removed), and finally the distal common bile duct (B). Contrast medium flows freely into the duodenum (D).

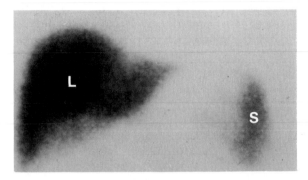

Fig. 4-32 Normal liver and spleen scan. This anterior view is obtained 20 minutes after the intravenous administration of Tc-99mm-sulfur colloid shows intense radioactivity in the liver (L) and less intense uptake by the smaller spleen (S).

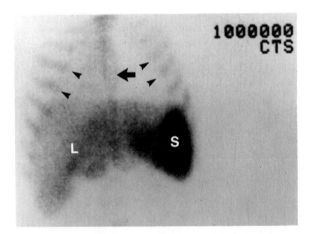

Fig. 4-33 Cirrhosis.
History. This was a 47-year-old alcoholic patient with cirrhosis.
Findings. *Liver and spleen scan:* There is severe parenchymal damage, with less of the colloid taken up by the liver (L). There is secondary increased uptake by the enlarged spleen and reticuloendothelial cells of the spine (arrow) and ribs (arrowheads).

matched the exquisite accuracy of these modalities in revealing obstructive jaundice. Computed tomography can accurately show the liver size, fatty infiltration, (Fig. 1-38), and hemosiderosis, and can strongly suggest the diagnosis of cirrhosis by demonstrating signs of portal hypertension (e.g., ascites, peritoneal and retroperitoneal varices, and changes in liver morphology). Ultrasound is somewhat less accurate in revealing diffuse parenchymal disease, and can only suggest the diagnosis of cirrhosis.[17]

The technetium-99m-labeled sulfur-colloid scan is a quick, low-risk procedure that is less operator-dependent than other radiographic approaches to suspected hepatic disease. This radiopharmaceutical is normally phagocytized by the reticuloendothelial system (RES) of the liver, spleen, and bone marrow. The normal image of the liver and spleen is that of a homogeneous, black structure with that organ's typical shape and location (Fig. 4-32). Bone marrow activity is usually not detected.

Nuclear medicine studies can give the strongest evidence of cirrhosis by demonstrating an intense uptake of radioactive material in an enlarged spleen, and an abnormal uptake in the bone marrow and ribs in a sulfur-colloid liver and spleen scan (Fig. 4-33).

METASTATIC DISEASE

Metastatic tumors are the most common malignancies of the liver. They can be identified either with ultrasound, CT, or nuclear imaging. With this multiplicity of imaging techniques, the problem naturally arises as to which technique should be used as a screening tool and when follow-up scans should be obtained.

In a nuclear medicine liver and spleen scan, any space-occupying process that replaces normal RES cells appears as a hole or cold spot in the usually homogeneous liver image (Fig. 4-34). This nonspecificity is the major drawback of this modality. Cysts, abscesses, and hepatomas may have a similar appearance to metastatic disease. Radionuclide scanning is also relatively insensitive in that it may not reveal lesions smaller than 2 cm when they are deeply situated in the substance of the liver.[18]

Ultrasound is a more sensitive, specific, and accurate modality than nuclear imaging, and does not utilize ionizing radiation. It is exquisitely dependent upon operator expertise, however, and may be limited

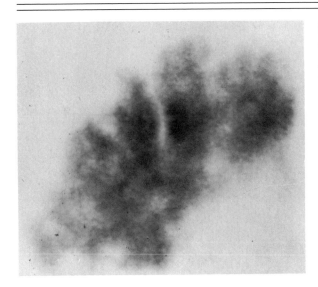

Fig. 4-34 Hepatic metastasis.
History. This 64-year-old woman had adenocarcinoma of the sigmoid colon and presented with elevated liver enzyme readings and an increased carcinoembryonic antigen (CEA) result.
Findings. *Liver and spleen scan:* Note the multiple "holes" or cold areas within the liver. Since metastatic deposits do not contain Kupffer cells, they do not take up the sulfur colloid.

by lack of patient cooperation, gas, obesity, skin wounds, and surgical drains and so is less utilized. Metastases may appear as hyperechoic, hypoechoic, or mixed-echoic lesions that can have a target appearance. These patterns are not histologically specific, although most metastases from colon carcinomas are hyperechoic.

A variety of benign and malignant hepatic mass lesions can be detected with CT. Metastases are the most frequent tumors, and are usually multiple (Fig. 4-35). Primary tumors such as hepatomas, and benign lesions such as adenomas, focal nodular hyperplasia, regenerating nodules, cysts, abscesses, and echinococcal disease can be detected and can be multiple or solitary in their distribution. Unfortunately, CT cannot suggest a histologic diagnosis in most cases; a primary neoplasm cannot be distinguished from a solitary metastasis. However, it can differentiate a neoplasm from a cyst by the near-water density of the cyst and the absence of contrast enhancement. Hemangiomas can usually be confidently differentiated from malignant tumors by their typical CT characteristics. Furthermore, the histologic confirmation needed for

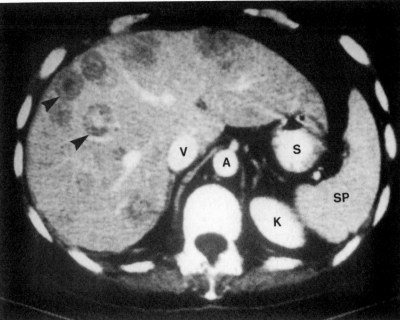

Fig. 4-35 Hepatic metastasis.
History. This 50-year-old woman had breast carcinoma and elevated liver function tests.
Findings. *CT scan:* There are multiple low-density lesions within the liver, some having a "bulls-eye" appearance (arrowheads). A = aorta, V = inferior vena cava, K = left kidney, S = contrast filled stomach, SP = spleen.

the accurate diagnosis of any lesion can be readily facilitated by a CT- or ultrasound-directed needle biopsy.

Metastatic tumors as seen on the CT scan generally have a lower density than normal parenchyma (Fig. 4-35) but have a greater density than cysts. In addition, metastases are less well circumscribed and less uniform in density than cysts. The administration of an intravenous contrast medium usually exaggerates the density difference between normal liver tissue and a metastasis (Fig. 1-43 A and B). The most common CT pattern in metastatic disease is of multiple, low-density masses with contrast-enhancing rims that are brighter than the surrounding normal liver parenchyma. But while such ring enhancement is often encountered, some lesions do not enhance at all and still others become rapidly hyperdense throughout. Calcifications are often seen within metastases from primary mucinous adenocarcinomas (e.g., breast carcinoma).

Computed tomography is somewhat superior to radionuclide imaging and ultrasound for the identification of metastatic tumors.[19] It offers excellent spatial resolution, and can, with bolus contrast enhancement, often differentiate cysts from hemangiomas and other tumors. It also offers the spatial resolution of ultrasound, without the operator dependence and other limiting features of this modality. In short, CT, ultrasound, and nuclear medicine studies are all excellent techniques for the diagnosis of liver metastases. In hospitals where ultrasound has achieved excellence, it should be used as the first modality. Where it has not, nuclear medicine studies should be used. Computed tomography is perhaps the best means for the detection of metastasis, but the least available and most expensive. Unfortunately our society cannot afford a CT scan of every patient with suspected hepatic metastases.

CLINICAL PRESENTATION: RIGHT-UPPER-QUADRANT PAIN (ALGORITHM 4-4)

Right-upper-quadrant pain is a very common presenting complaint in that some of the most frequent disorders of the gastrointestinal tract, such as gallbladder disease and peptic ulcer disease, are responsible for it. Pancreatic disease is also a possible, although less common, etiology.

GALLBLADDER DISEASE

Approximately 20 million people in the United States have gallstones. Indeed, 600,000 cholecystectomies are performed annually, making this the most com-

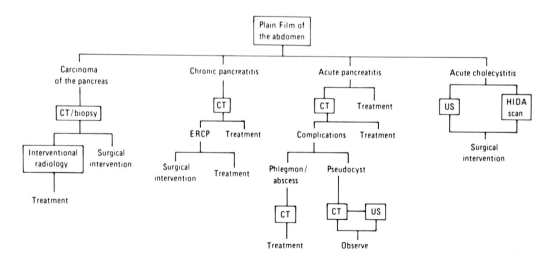

CLINICAL PRESENTATION: RIGHT UPPER QUADRANT PAIN

Algorithm 4-4

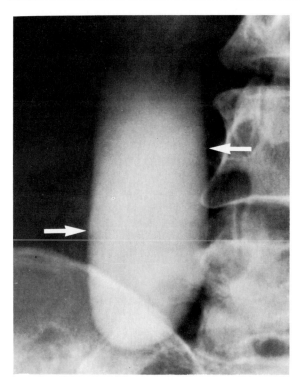

Fig. 4-36 Normal oral cholecystogram (OCG) View of the contrast-filled gallbladder (arrow) obtained 16 hours after the ingestion of Telepaque tablets.

der opacification in from 15 to 25 percent of normal patients, prolonging hospitalization or making a return outpatient visit necessary, both of which are economically expensive and time-consuming. Intestinal absorption and liver function (a bilirubin less than 3 mg/100 ml) must also be adequate for gallbladder visualization.

On a plain film of the abdomen before ingestion of the contrast medium, gallstones are frequently seen to be calcified (Fig. 4-37). On the OCG the stones appear as filling defects within the contrast-filled gallbladder. If composed primarily of cholesterol, the stones float (Fig. 4-38).

The OCG had been the "gold standard" for evaluation of the gallbladder for nearly 50 years, but has been replaced by ultrasound as the imaging modality of choice for the diagnosis of disorders of the gallbladder and biliary tract.[20] The advantages of ultrasound include: (1) establishment of the diagnosis of cholelithiasis in 15 minutes rather than 16 hours; (2) the absence of ionizing radiation, (3) the lack of side effects from contrast medium; and (4) the ability to

mon abdominal surgical procedure in this country. For every patient who eventually undergoes cholecystectomy, it is estimated that 3 to 5 patients have right-upper-quadrant pain that requires gallbladder imaging.

There are currently four modalities available for imaging of the gallbladder: the oral cholecystogram (OCG), CT scanning, cholescintigraphy with ^{99m}Tc-hepatobiliary iminodiacetic acid (HIDA), and ultrasound. In the OCG the patient consumes a 3-gm dose of iodinated contrast medium (Telepaque) that is absorbed in the small bowel, conjugated in the liver, excreted in the bile, and concentrated by the normal gallbladder (Fig. 4-36). Although it has an accuracy near 90 percent, this technique has several important drawbacks. Peak gallbladder opacification occurs within 14 to 19 hours, so that the method is not suitable in patients who present with acute right-upper-quadrant pain. Also, a second-dose examination performed the next day is required for gallblad-

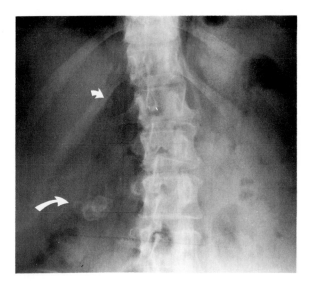

Fig. 4-37 Calcified gallstones.
History. This 58-year-old woman presented with fever and righ-upper-quadrant pain.
Findings. *Plain radiograph of the abdomen:* There are multiple calcified gallstones within the dependent portion of the gallbladder (large arrow). One stone (small arrow) is impacted in the gallbladder neck.

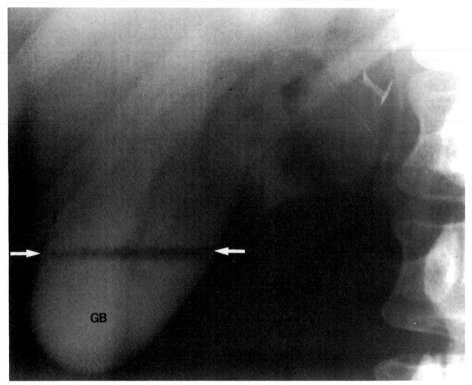

Fig. 4-38 Gallstones.
History. This 43-year-old woman had intermittent right-upper-quadrant pain.
Findings. *OCG:* There is a line of stones floating in the bile within the gallbladder (GB). These are small, light cholesterol stones. No stones were visible on the plain radiograph.

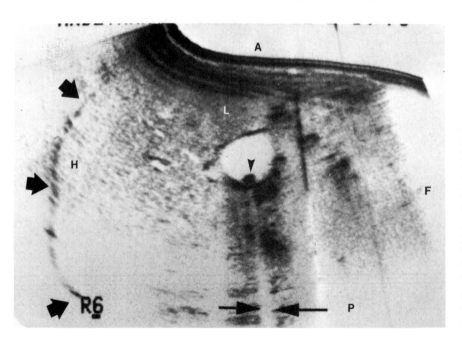

Fig. 4-39 Gallstone.
History. This 49-year-old woman had chronic but worsening right-upper-quadrant pain.
Findings. *US scan:* On this sagittal scan of the right upper quadrant, a gallstone appears as a bright echoic pattern (arrowhead) casting an acoustic shadow (arrows). The stone moved with various gravitational maneuvers. The short arrows demonstrate the right hemidiaphragm. L = liver, H = towards head, F = towards feet, A = anterior, P = posterior.

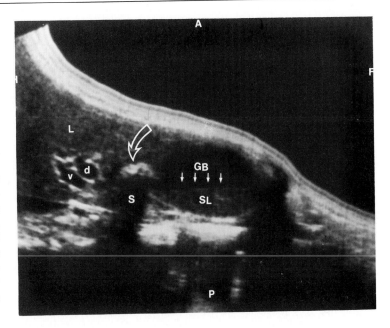

Fig. 4-40 Biliary sludge.
History. This 63-year-old man presented with findings typical of acute cholecystitis.
Findings. *US scan:* Sludge that layers (small arrows) along the dependent, posterior (P) wall of the gallbladder (GB) while the patient is supine produces uniform, low-level echoes (SL). A gallstone lodged in the gallbladder neck (curved arrow), seen from its shadowing (S), is causing obstruction. L = liver, H = toward head, F = toward feet, A = anterior, v = portal vein, d = common hepatic duct.

perform the study in the presence of various disorders, such as liver disease (not dependent on the bilirubin level), jaundice, and malabsorption, and even during pregnancy.

The gallbladder can be identified in 95 percent of fasting patients, and appears as a saccular structure. Optimally, the patient should fast for 8 to 12 hours to allow for maximum filling and distension of the gallbladder, although a scan can be done at any time (Fig. 4-26). Failure to identify the gallbladder in an ultrasound examination of the fasting patient usually indicates a shrunken or calculus-packed gallbladder.

Sonographically, gallstones characteristically produce echogenic foci within the gallbladder, show movement with a change in position of the patient, and produce a posterior acoustic shadow (Fig. 4-39). This shadow is produced because gallstones absorb most of the sound beam, leaving none available to produce echoes from deeper structures. All three of these conditions must be fulfilled for a confident diagnosis of gallstones. When meticulously done real-time sonography can reveal calculi as small as 1 mm, and has a reported sensitivity as high as 98 percent.[21]

Tiny stones or biliary sludge may give a fine echogenic pattern in the gallbladder without producing shadows (Fig. 4-40). Sludge or echogenic bile is caused by calcium bilirubinate granules and cholesterol crystals in the bile. This occurs when there is biliary stasis, as in patients who are fasting, postoperative, or on total parenteral nutrition. This echogenic material layers out in the dependent portion of the gallbladder. Gallbladder polyps may be confused with gallstones since they also appear as a bright focus of echoes, but they cast no shadow and are adherent to the gallbladder wall and so do not change with position (Fig. 4-41). In questionable cases, the presence of polyps should be documented by an OCG.

Besides the detection of gallstones, the ultrasound examination can give information on the intra- and extrahepatic biliary system as well as the gallbladder wall thickness. The common hepatic duct can be seen lying anterior to the portal vein (Fig. 4-26). In normal patients, this duct measures 4 to 5 mm in diameter or less. If the patient has had a cholecystectomy, the duct usually remains normal in caliber. The gallbladder wall thickness can also be assessed, and is found to be thickened in a variety of conditions including acute and chronic cholecystitis, ascites, total parenteral nutrition, portal hypertension, leukemia, lymphoma, and hypoproteinemia.

Because of its expense, limited availability and relatively poor efficacy when compared with ultrasound in detecting gallbladder stones, CT is of limited value

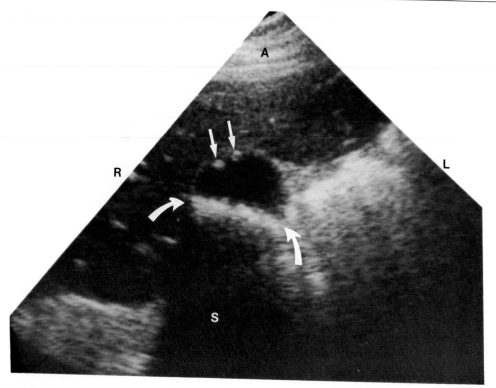

Fig. 4-41 Gallbladder polyps.
History. This 56-year-old man had chronic right-upper-quadrant pain.
Findings. *US scan:* Two gallbladder polyps (straight arrows) are seen along the anterior (non-dependent) wall of the gallbladder on this transverse scan of the upper abdomen. Multiple gallstones are seen layering posteriorly (curved arrows) on the dependent wall of the gallbladder. These are stones since they cast an acoustic shadow (s), whereas the polyps do not. A = anterior, R = right, L = left.

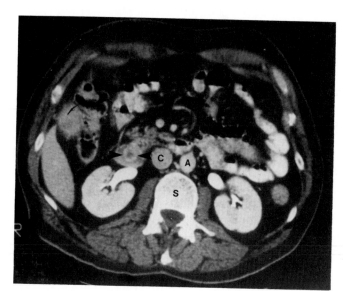

Fig. 4-42 Common-duct gallstone.
History. This 56-year-old man presented with jaundice and biliary sepsis. A CT scan was performed after an ultrasound examination showed biliary dilation but not its etiology.
Findings. *CT scan:* There is a large, partially calcified stone (arrowheads) within the pancreatic segment of the common bile duct. C = inferior vena cava, A = aorta, S = spine.

in the diagnosis of gallbladder disease. However, it is quite sensitive (85 versus 25 percent, respectively)[22] as compared to ultrasound (Fig. 4-42) in the diagnosis of stones in the common bile duct or common hepatic duct.

ACUTE CHOLECYSTITIS

Biliary colic and ultimately acute cholecystitis occur if a calculus becomes impacted in the neck of the gallbladder or cystic duct. Two modalities are of great value in evaluating the acutely ill patients with these conditions: nuclear medicine cholescintigraphy (HIDA scan) and ultrasound. There is currently great controversy about which study should be performed first.

Ultrasound, as previously discussed, is an ideal modality for the identification of gallstones. In the vast majority of cases, however, it cannot demonstrate cystic-duct obstruction by a stone, which is the sine qua non of acute cholecystitis. In some patients, additional clues may be present and may help establish this diagnosis. There may, for example, be a thickening of the gallbladder wall with a surrounding or pericholecystic fluid collection. Also, a stone may be visualized in the gallbladder neck, with a dilated gallbladder full of sludge (Fig. 4-40). Additionally, there is a sonographic "Murphy's sign" in which the gallbladder is exquisitely tender when the transducer of the ultrasound scanner is passed over it. About 90 percent of patients with acute cholecystitis demonstrate such a "Murphy's sign". The absence of this sign is especially useful if there is tenderness in an adjacent structure such as the right kidney or gastric antrum. Even lacking these specific features, one need not prove that the cystic duct is obstructed to justify cholecystectomy in patients with the typical pain and sonographic proof of gallstones.[23]

The HIDA gallbladder scan is another excellent modality for the diagnosis of acute cholecystitis. It is done after the intravenous administration of isotopically labeled compounds that are cleared and rapidly excreted by hepatocytes of the liver into the biliary tree. These compounds fill the gallbladder by retrograde passage through the cystic duct and later enter the duodenum via the common duct. Normally the gallbladder and duodenum exhibit radioactivity within 1 hour or less (Fig. 4-43). If the gallbladder is visualized, cystic-duct patency is assured and the like-

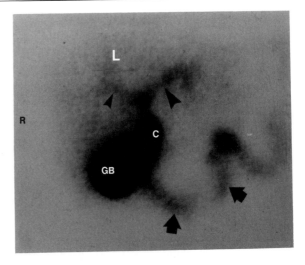

Fig. 4-43 Normal hepatobiliary iminodiacetic acid (HIDA) scan. A view of the right upper quadrant obtained 45 minutes after the injection of radioactive HIDA. There is activity within the gallbladder (GB) lumen. Note that activity is also present in the intrahepatic ducts (arrowheads) and duodenum (arrows). R = right, L = liver, C = common bile duct, GB = gallbladder.

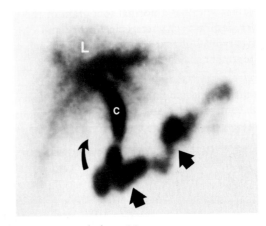

Fig. 4-44 Acute cholecystitis.
History. This 53-year-old woman presented with classic symptoms of acute cholecystitis.
Findings. *HIDA scan:* On this 90-minute scan, the isotope is seen within the common bile duct (c) and duodenum (arrows), but no activity was seen in the region of the gallbladder fossa (curved arrow). This strongly suggests cystic duct obstruction. L = liver.

lihood of acute cholecystitis is minute. If the gallbladder does not fill by 4 hours, the diagnosis of acute cholecystitis with cystic duct obstruction should be suspected (Fig. 4-44).[24]

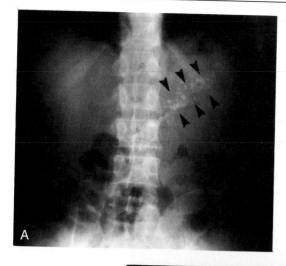

Fig. 4-47 Chronic calcific pancreatitis.
History. This patient was a 42-year-old chronic alcoholic.
Findings. (A) *Plain abdominal radiograph:* There are multiple left-upper-quadrant calcifications (arrowheads). **(B)** *CT scan:* At the level of the gallbladder (GB) one sees enlargement of the pancreas (arrowheads), which contains many high-density calcifications.

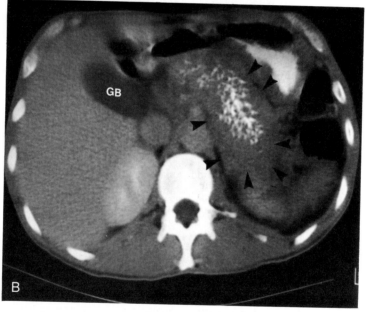

graphic evaluation of the upper abdomen. The pancreas may be enlarged and have a low attenuation on CT (Fig. 4-47 B and 4-48). The CT scan is probably the best single imaging means for evaluating pancreatic disorders.[26] Besides this, CT is superior to ultrasound in easily and consistently revealing the tail of the pancreas, lesser sac, and various retroperitoneal compartments, and is preferred for the detection of various complications of acute pancreatitis. Ultrasound, however, is better able to image the gallbladder for gallstones, which are a major cause of acute pancreatitis.

COMPLICATIONS OF ACUTE PANCREATITIS

One of the most important roles of the various modalities for imaging the pancreas is in the diagnosis, evaluation, and even treatment of the complications of pancreatitis. These complications include pseudocysts, phlegmon and abscess formation, and chronic pancreatitis.

Intra- or extrapancreatic fluid collections, called pseudocysts, occur in up to 50 percent of patients with inflammatory diseases of the pancreas. These fluid collections are composed of cellular debris, fluid,

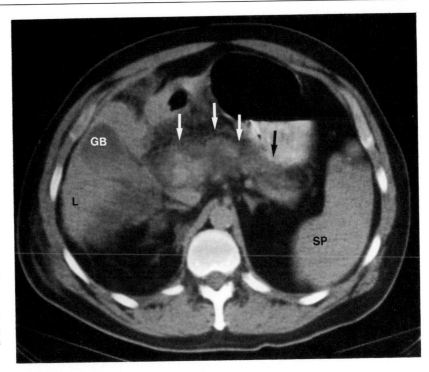

Fig. 4-48 Acute pancreatitis. **History.** This 38-year-old man had fever, chills, and intense right-upper-quadrant pain. **Findings.** *CT scan:* The pancreas is diffusely enlarged, with loss of its normally sharp borders (arrows). L = liver, GB = gallbladder, SP = spleen.

blood, and pancreatic enzymes; they are rich in proteolytic enzymes and most frequently found in the lesser sac, but can extend along retroperitoneal tissue planes in any direction. Rarely these pseudocysts may dissect up into the mediastinum and reach the neck, or course down the retroperitoneum as far as the groin. The wall of the pseudocyst is initially formed by whatever tissue structure first limits its spread. As the pseudocyst matures, the evoked inflammatory reaction encapsulates the contents of the pseudocyst with granulation tissue and ultimately forms a fibrous wall. Pseudocysts often resolve spontaneously.

On ultrasound examination, pseudocysts are typically round, smooth, cystic collections that can be detected with an accuracy ranging from 50 to 100 percent (Fig. 4-49 A and B). On a CT scan pseudocysts are usually homogeneous and have attenuation numbers close to that of water, (+6 H and 20 H; Fig. 49C). Computed tomography is probably the preferred imaging modality for the initial detection of a pseudocyst because it can reveal both intra- and extrapancreatic locations and is not hindered by bowel gas. If a pseudocyst is demonstrated on the CT scan, an

ultrasound examination may be done to correlate its location with that in the CT image. If the cyst is well seen on the ultrasound scan, then ultrasound may be used to monitor the patient. Pseudocysts should be followed until their resolution is demonstrated or surgery planned.[27]

Pseudocysts are dynamic lesions and can increase or decrease in size over several days or remain stable for months. In the first 3 weeks of their development, 20 percent resolve spontaneously, (Fig. 4-44C), but as chronicity sets in, their spontaneous resolution becomes much less likely, and the rate of complication increases to 75 percent by 13 to 18 weeks. The complications of pseudocysts include infection, intraperitoneal rupture with pancreatic ascites, and erosion into adjacent arteries, with gastrointestinal hemorrhage, aneurysm formation, or occlusion of the splenic vein. If a pseudocyst suddenly increases in size or exhibits a change in echogenicity or CT attenuation, hemorrhage or infection should be suspected.

Pancreatic phlegmon occurs in approximately 10 percent of patients with pancreatitis. It represents an amorphous collection of necrotic tissue and inflam-

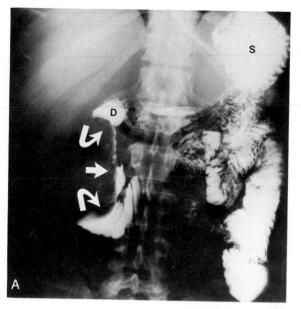

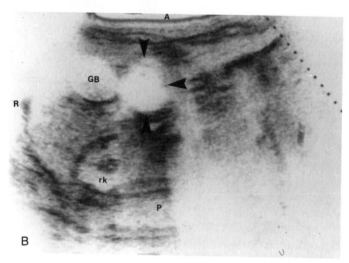

Fig. 4-49 Pancreatic pseudocyst.
History. This 48-year-old man had recurrent pancreatitis.
Findings. (A) *Small-bowel series:* A large mass is causing extrinsic compression along the lateral wall (arrows) of the duodenum (D). S = stomach. **(B)** *US scan:* In the upper abdomen the mass demonstrated to be a 5-cm pseudocyst (arrowheads) with no internal echoes and acoustic enhancement posteriorly (P). GB = gallbladder, A = anterior, R = right, rk = right kidney. **(C)** *CT scan:* The low-attenuation pseudocyst (arrowheads) is identified next to the gallbladder (GB). c = inferior vena cava, a = aorta, v = left renal vein, s = superior mesenteric artery, d = crus of right hemidiaphragm, rk = right kidney, lk = left kidney.

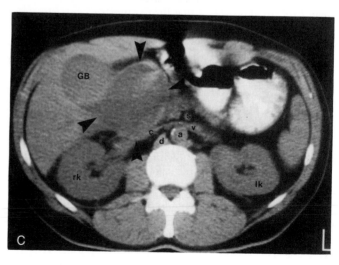

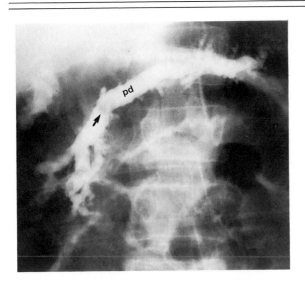

Fig. 4-50 Chronic pancreatitis.
History. This 57-year-old alcoholic man presented with symptoms of pancreatic insufficiency, chronic pain, and recurring bouts of acute pancreatitis.
Findings. *ERCP:* The pancreatic duct is markedly enlarged (1.4 cm) and there is dilatation of primary and secondary pancreatic radicles (white arrows). A pancreatic stone (black arrow) also lies within the pancreatic duct.

matory debris. This disorder is usually seen in patients with acute hemorrhagic pancreatitis. The pancreas is massively enlarged by interstitial edema and tissue necrosis. In an ultrasound examination the pancreas appears enlarged, with an inhomogeneous echogenicity. On the CT scan there is diffuse pancreatic enlargement with inhomogeneous attenuation of the parenchyma and loss of tissue planes around the pancreas. Most phlegmons resolve in 3 to 4 weeks. If they do not resolve, a secondary abscess should be suspected.

Pancreatic abscess is a very serious complication of acute pancreatitis, occurring in up to 40 percent of patients with hemorrhagic or necrotizing pancreatitis and 26 percent of all patients with pancreatitis. If untreated, the mortality from this complication reaches 100 percent. Computed tomography is the preferred modality for imaging this complication, but unfortunately many abscesses do not yield specific CT findings. On CT, an abscess may present as an irregular mass or as extraluminal air in the region of the pancreatic bed.

The diagnosis of chronic pancreatitis is suggested by previous attacks of pancreatitis with recurrent right upper quadrant pain, steatorrhea, malabsorp-

tion, diarrhea, weight loss, and abdominal pain. In this setting, the use of several imaging modalities may be of benefit. Pancreatic calcifications are easily detected on plain radiographs (Fig. 4-47A). On ultrasound this disorder may have a variety of presentations, but often the gland is small and of increased echogenicity. The pancreatic calcifications may cast an acoustic shadow, as seen with gallstones. Computed tomography is again the preferred modality in this situation because it may be better able to define small, subtle calcifications (Fig. 4-47B) and even an abnormal ductal configuration. More importantly, CT can help differentiate between pancreatic malignancy and chronic pancreatitis. Endoscopic retrograde cholangiopancreatography may also be useful because of its high degree of accuracy in revealing the changes of pancreatitis (Fig. 4-50), such as an irregular or beaded ductal configuration. Defining of the ductal anatomy by ERCP is also necessary in the event that surgical drainage of the pancreatic duct or partial pancreatectomy is to be undertaken.

CARCINOMA OF THE PANCREAS

Carcinoma of the pancreas remains an elusive tumor because of its nonspecific symptoms including abdominal pain, weight loss, jaundice, early satiety, nausea and vomiting, anemia, and gastrointestinal hemorrhage. The disease is the fifth most lethal cancer in the United States. The 5-year survival rate is a dismal 1 percent. Cures are rare because the tumor is rarely diagnosed prior to extensive local growth or metastatic spread.

Because of the nonspecificity of the symptoms of pancreatic carcinoma, the final diagnosis is usually made radiographically. There are a variety of diagnostic techniques available for evaluating patients with suspected pancreatic carcinoma including CT, ultrasound, ERCP, angiography, PTC, and selective venography.

Computed tomography has proven the most reliable method for evaluating for pancreatic carcinoma and should be the initial examination performed for this disease.[28] The diagnosis of pancreatic carcinoma with CT is based on alterations in the size and shape of the gland. Two-thirds of cases of pancreatic carcinoma occur in the pancreatic head, and are characterized by an abrupt alteration in the contour of the head that renders it disproportionate to the thickness of the body and tail (Fig. 4-51A). There is often secondary

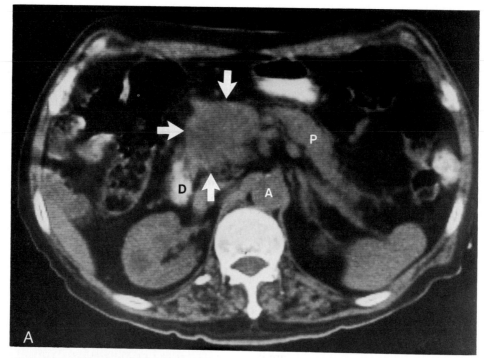

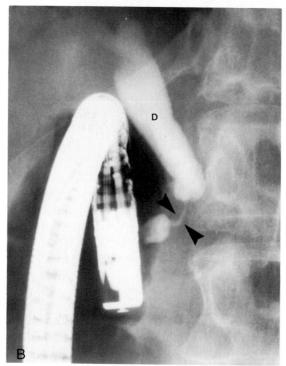

Fig. 4-51 Carcinoma of the pancreas.
History. This 71-year-old man had prolonged right-upper-quadrant pain and worsening jaundice.
Findings. (A) *CT scan:* There is obvious replacement of the pancreatic head by a large irregular mass (arrows). P = pancreas, D = duodenum, A = aorta. **(B)** *ERCP:* There is tight narrowing of the intrapancreatic portion of the distal common bile duct from "encasement" by the pancreatic carcinoma. This is the etiology of the jaundice. D = distal common bile duct.

dilatation of the common bile duct and pancreatic duct. Tumors of the body and tail of the pancreas are often larger than those in the head at the time of initial evaluation because they fail to produce symptoms for a longer period. The tissue density of a pancreatic carcinoma on CT is similar to that of the normal pancreatic parenchyma, with the result that if a focal mass is not present, the tumor is usually not diagnosed. Areas of low density, representing regions of necrosis or cystic degeneration, may occasionally be seen within the tumor, but in these instances an advanced and obvious mass is usually present.

Computed tomography is also helpful in the staging of pancreatic carcinoma. By the time the diagnosis is made, the tumor is often unresectable, having spread to surrounding celiac lymph nodes or invaded the neighboring splenic vein. There is ready invasion of surrounding structures by the tumor, since the pancreas does not have a surrounding capsule. Also, the lymphatic and vascular supply to the pancreatic head provides ready access for metastasis to the lymph nodes and liver.

Computed tomography can be further used in directed fine-needle aspiration biopsy. It is an effective means of establishing the histologic diagnosis of carcinoma of the pancreas, and may therefore reduce the need for exploratory laparotomy by providing both diagnosis and staging of the tumor. There is considerable savings of patient discomfort and money in a disease with a 1 percent 5-year survival rate.

On ultrasound examination, carcinoma of the pancreas usually presents as a mass with low-intensity echoes (hypoechoic) (see Fig. 1-30), although it may have the same echogenicity as the remainder of gland. In these cases, abnormalities of the pancreas are detected only by a localized bulge in the contour of the gland.

Endoscopic retrograde cholangiopancreatography continues to play an important but diminished role in the diagnosis of pancreatic carcinoma. It is useful when the CT findings are normal or equivocal in a patient with a high index of suspicion for carcinoma. Indeed, ERCP is probably the most accurate and sen-

sitive means of detecting small pancreatic lesions. Also when CT is equivocally abnormal, with only ancillary findings of tumor (adenopathy), ERCP may assist in confirming the diagnosis. Besides this, ERCP can reveal secondary invasion of the intrapancreatic portion of the distal common bile duct (Fig. 4-51B).

CLINICAL PRESENTATION: DYSPHAGIA (ALGORITHM 4-5)

Dysphagia, or difficulty in swallowing, is a symptom that usually indicates an anatomic lesion or neuromuscular dysfunction of the esophagus. Patients with this condition most commonly describe a sensation of food "sticking" somewhere during its passage to the stomach. This usually occurs at the level of obstruction, but the sensation is sometimes referred to the suprasternal notch. There are a variety of imaging modalities available for evaluating the patient with dysphagia. The single-contrast and air-contrast barium esophagram with videotaping is probably the best initial modality for studying this problem (Fig. 4-1). Spot films reveal the mucosal abnormalities while disorders of esophageal motility can be recorded and replayed by the videotape.

ACHALASIA

Unlike the more distal segments of the alimentary tube, the esophagus is predisposed to a wide variety of well-defined functional disorders. Achalasia is a dis-

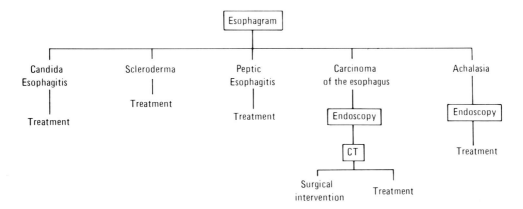

CLINICAL PRESENTATION: DYSPHAGIA

Algorithm 4-5

order characterized by failure of relaxation of the lower esophageal sphincter, which produces progressive esophageal dilatation. The condition is caused by generalized degeneration of the myenteric plexus of the esophagus, which leads to further esophageal dilatation that varies with the duration and severity of the disease. The onset of achalasia is usually noted in the young adult years; affected patients present with dysphagia and aspiration of retained esophageal contents. Patient nutrition is often adversely affected by this disease.

Radiographically, the diagnosis can often be suggested by a routine plain radiograph of the chest obtained for other reasons. An air-fluid level may be visible in the region of the upper esophagus as fluid and retained food are trapped in that organ. A gastric air bubble is typically not seen.

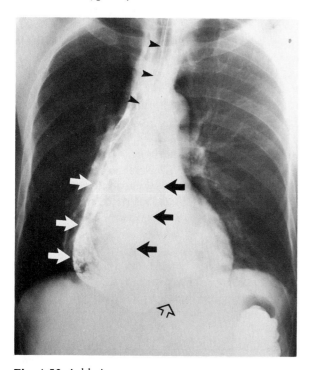

Fig. 4-52 Achlasia.
History. This 24-year-old patient had a long history of dysphagia. A chest radiograph suggested an extra soft tissue density to the right of the right heart border.
Findings. *Esophagram:* After barium is instilled through a nasogastric tube (arrowheads), the extra-soft-tissue density proves to be a markedly dilated esophagus whose margins are outlined by the arrows. Note that the gastroesophageal junction (open arrows) does not relax, preventing passage of barium and the nasogastric tube.

In a barium esophagram the esophagus is usually dilated, tortuous, and elongated, often in a sigmoid fashion (Fig. 4-52). Retained secretions and food are often encountered. Normal peristaltic waves do not occur, and only weak, irregular, and ineffectual contractions of the esophagus are seen. At the gastroesophageal junction a long, narrow, 1- to 4-cm segment is seen, having an appearance resembling a "rattail."[29] With the patient in the recumbent position, very little barium enters the stomach.

Although the tapered narrowing of the distal esophagus in achalasia is characteristic of the condition, the differential diagnosis must include carcinoma of the esophagus. A tumor originating in the distal esophagus or stomach may invade the more proximal esophageal submucosa, destroy the myenteric plexus, and mimic achalasia. In these cases the distal esophagus is extremely rigid and the mucosa may have a polypoid appearance. Thus, endoscopy should be performed in all newly discovered cases of achalasia, especially if the patient is over 30 years of age. Unfortunately, since the bulk of the tumor is often submucosal, an endoscopic biopsy may initially not reveal it.

CARCINOMA OF THE ESOPHAGUS

Most patients presenting with esophageal symptoms caused by a tumor usually have an advanced carcinoma. No alimentary-tract cancer, with the possible exception of carcinoma of the pancreas, has a worse prognosis. Difficulty in swallowing solids is the patient's first and usually only complaint as the tumor encroaches upon the esophageal lumen. Although initially intermittent, the dysphagia progresses. The disease occurs in middle-aged and older persons, and is four times more prevalent in men than in women. It is associated with heavy smoking and drinking, celiac disease (sprue), primary squamous carcinoma of the head and neck, achalasia, and Barrett's esophagus. About 25 percent of squamous-cell esophageal cancers occur in the upper third, 50 percent in the middle third, and 25 percent in the lower third of the esophagus. Nearly half of all neoplasms in the distal esophagus prove to be adenocarcinomas probably arising from the stomach.[30]

In its early stages, carcinoma of the esophagus appears as a small plaque on barium studies. Unfortunately, the tumor is only rarely discovered in this

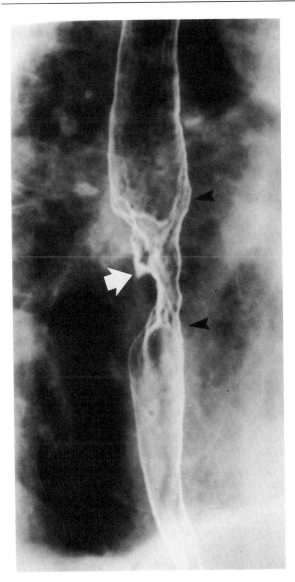

Fig. 4-53 Carcinoma of the esophagus.
History. This 58-year-old man, who had an extensive smoking and drinking history, presented with progressive dysphagia.
Findings. *Esophagram:* There is an annular constricting neoplasm (arrowheads) and a large ulcer (arrow) of the mid-portion of the esophagus.

form. More commonly, it is first diagnosed when it has become more extensive, usually involving several centimeters of the esophageal wall. The radiographic features of esophageal cancer can be classified into four patterns: annular constricting, polypoid, infiltrative or stenosing, and ulcerative.

The annular constricting pattern of carcinoma is the most frequent, and has a radiographic configuration similar to that of the annular type of colon cancer. Abrupt overhanging margins are often seen, and there may be modest dilatation of the esophagus proximal to the stricture. The narrowed area of lumen is characteristically irregular and ulcerated, without a recognizable mucosal pattern (Fig. 4-53). The polypoid pattern is the next most common. At first it may asymmetrically involve the wall of the esophagus, but with further growth the neoplasm may encircle the esophagus, creating an annular configuration. Occasionally the tumor may infiltrate the esophageal wall, simulating varices.

When the diagnosis of esophageal carcinoma is suggested by the esophagram, endoscopy and biopsy should be undertaken. Since this neoplasm has such a dismal prognosis, all cases should be staged with CT prior to any exploratory or curative surgery. The CT scan may demonstrate tumor extension to the adjacent mediastinum, enlarged lymph nodes in the mediastinum or gastrohepatic ligament, or metastasis to the liver.

PEPTIC ESOPHAGITIS

With advent of double-contrast barium techniques it has become possible to detect even minor morphologic changes of the mucosa associated with reflux esophagitis from the continued reflux of gastric contents. Peptic esophagitis is at least as common as peptic ulcer disease and is often associated with a hiatal hernia. However, the hernia plays a passive role in that the reflux is actually due to an incompetent lower esophageal sphincter. Patients with hiatal hernia do not clear their refluxed gastric material as well as those who do not have hernias leading to prolonged irritation.

Patients with low-grade esophagitis frequently exhibit a normal double-contrast esophagram, or show minor degrees of esophageal dysmotility. As the inflammation progresses, erosions and superficial ulcerations may be seen extending up from the gastroesophageal junction (Fig. 4-54). The superficial ulcerations may have a linear configuration with fine, radiating folds. There may also be minimal retraction and contour deformity of the esophageal wall. With more severe esophagitis, a coarse granular appearance of the mucosa may develop in association with deep

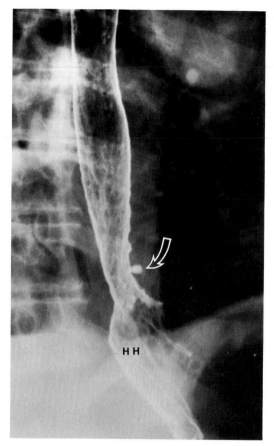

Fig. 4-54 Reflux esophagitis.
History. This 68-year-old woman had a history of heartburn and a brackish taste in her mouth postprandially.
Findings. *Esophagram:* There is demonstrated a sliding hiatal hernia (HH), narrowing, and ulceration (arrow) at the gastroesophageal junction.

ulcers. Strictures ultimately result from persistent, severe esophagitis.

SCLERODERMA

While achalasia results from neural dysfunction, scleroderma of the esophagus causes degeneration and fibrous replacement of the smooth-muscle components of the esophageal wall. Patients with this condition have symptoms of dysphagia associated with systemic manifestations such as sclerodactyly or Raynaud phenomenon. The disease is limited to the lower two-thirds of the esophagus because the proximal esophagus is lined by skeletal muscle, which is spared.

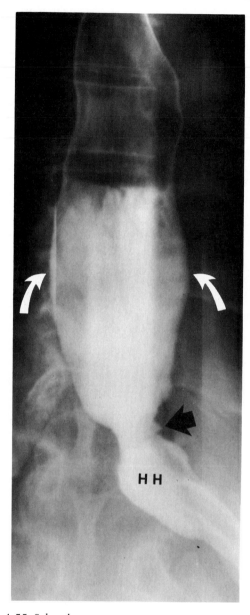

Fig. 4-55 Scleroderma.
History. This 34-year-old woman with scleroderma presented with a 1-year history of increasing dysphagia.
Findings. *Esophagram:* Single views show a dilated esophagus (curved arrows) proximal to a stricture, and an ulcer (black arrow) associated with a hiatal hernia (HH). The gastroesophageal junction is patulous in these patients, and allows free gastroesophageal reflux.

On plain radiographs, and especially on the lateral view, air may be seen filling the esophagus. On bar-

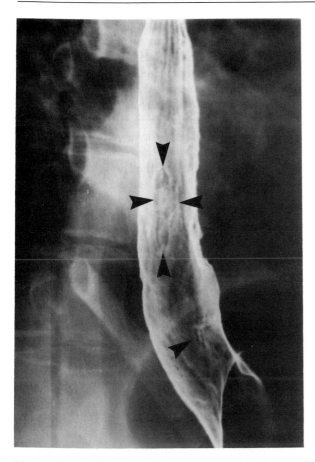

Fig. 4-56 Monilia esophagitis.
History. This 65-year-old immunocompromised woman, undergoing chemotherapy for carcinoma of the breast, presented with odynophagia.
Findings. *Esophagram:* There are multiple, plaque-like lesions (arrowheads) of the distal esophagus.

ium studies the most common presentation of scleroderma is that of a dilated distal esophagus lacking normal peristalsis. Initially, the gastroesophageal junction is wide open or patulous, and the esophagus empties freely by gravity when the patient is in the erect position, in contrast to the case in achalasia. Hiatal hernia is a common finding. Patients with scleroderma are predisposed to gastroesophageal reflux, which can be quite painful, inducing spasm and eventually leading to stricture formation (Fig. 4-55).[31] Advanced scleroderma may thus present as a dilated, atonic esophagus with hiatal hernia associated with esophagitis and a stricture of the most distal portion of the esophagus.

MISCELLANEOUS CAUSES OF STRICTURE

The esophagus is a frequent site of metastatic disease, either as a result of direct extension or less commonly by hematogeneous metastasis in patients with carcinoma of the lung and breast. Thus, when a stricture of the esophagus is encountered in an older individual with these primary neoplasms, the possibility of metastatic disease rather than a primary neoplasm should be considered.

Other disorders leading to esophageal stricture include scarring following the lodgement of a pill (e.g., iron or quinine tablet) in the esophagus. Patients with severe infectious esophagitis may also eventually develop a stricture.

CANDIDA ESOPHAGITIS

Most patients with esophageal candidiasis present with acute dysphagia and retrosternal pain. In some cases gastrointestinal hemorrhage occurs. Most of these patients are immunosuppressed either by neoplasms, chronic antibiotic or steroid use, cancer-chemotherapeutic agents, or acquired immune deficiency syndrome (AIDS). Candidiasis also occurs with increased frequency in patients with diabetes.

The radiographic findings in cases of candida esophagitis vary considerably and depend on the degree of mucosal involvement. The earliest radiographic signs of candidiasis on the barium esophagram are isolated mucosal plaques (Fig. 4-56) or a granular mucosal surface. This is often associated with disturbed esophageal motility. As the disease becomes more severe, a cobblestone appearance becomes apparent as shallow ulcerations and pseudomembranes form (Fig. 4-56). Endoscopy usually reveals an edematous mucosa covered by whitish pseudomembranes. The esophagus of immunosuppressed patients with herpes or cytomegalovirus infection may have a similar radiographic appearance.

CLINICAL PRESENTATION: DIARRHEA (ALGORITHM 4-6)

Diarrhea can be defined as an abnormal increase in stool liquidity and in daily stool weight (greater than 200 g). It is usually associated with an increased stool

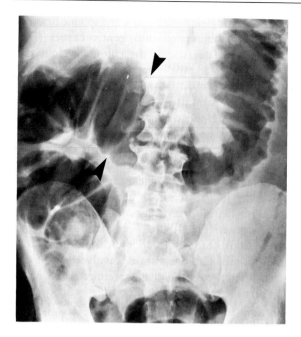

Fig. 4-59 Toxic megacolon.
History. This 64-year-old man who had an 8-year history of ulcerative colitis, presented with 10 hours of abdominal pain and bloody diarrhea. His vital signs showed tachycardia and hypotension.
Findings. *Abdominal Radiograph:* Note the marked dilation of the transverse colon (arrowheads) typical of toxic megacolon.

present as a subtle, persistent irregularity in the contour of a segment of bowel, that appears to be out of proportion to the inflammatory disease elsewhere in the colon. Carcinomas in association with longstanding ulcerative colitis may also be multifocal.[34]

One of the most ominous complications of ulcerative colitis is the rapid development of a striking colonic dilatation called toxic megacolon. This may occur in either the acute or chronic phase of the disease and is associated with a high fever, tachycardia, and pronounced diarrhea. It results from a paralysis of motor function of the colon. The dilated colon wall is very thin and prone to perforation, for which reason a barium enema examination is contraindicated.

A plain radiograph shows colonic dilatation (greater than 6 cm), especially of the transverse colon (Fig. 4-59). Air collects in this segment because it is the highest portion of the colon when the patient is both supine and upright. The haustra are obliterated and there may be broad-based nodular pseudopolyps

projecting into the lumen of the colon, representing the superimposed inflammatory process.

CROHN'S DISEASE

Crohn's disease (regional enteritis) or granulomatous ileocolitis, is a chronic, idiopathic, cicatrizing inflammatory disorder of the colon. The disease most commonly occurs in the terminal ileum but has been reported in all portions of the alimentary tract.[33] About 60 percent of the affected patients have small-bowel and colon involvement, 20 percent have disease restricted to the small bowel, and 20 percent have disease limited to the colon. Regional enteritis is characterized by recurrent inflammatory involvement of segments of the small bowel, with diverse clinical manifestations and a chronic, unpredictable course of exacerbation and remission. The disease usually occurs in the second through fourth decades of life, and two to three times more frequently in patients of Jewish origin. The diverse pathologic features and variable intestinal involvement by regional enteritis account for the protean manifestations of this disorder. The clinical features are a direct reflection of the location of the inflammatory lesions, and their extent, activity, and relationship to contiguous structures. Typically the disease presents in a young adult with a history of fatigue, weight loss, right-lower-quadrant discomfort, pain, and diarrhea. A low-grade fever, anorexia, nausea, and vomiting may be present as well. The diarrhea is often moderate, usually without gross blood. It is usually due to a combination of factors, including bile-salt deficiency resulting from the impaired ileal absorption of bile salts. This latter fact also accounts for a 30 percent incidence of cholelithiasis in patients with extensive ileal involvement.

The earliest radiographic manifestation of Crohn's disease of the small bowel and colon is an enlargement and inflammation of submucosal lymphoid follicles, accompanied by an inflammatory submucosal and mucosal thickening. Although lymphoid follicles can normally be seen, they are typically less than 2 to 3 mm in size. In early Crohn's disease the follicles are enlarged. As they grow, the overlying mucosa tends to ulcerate at the apices of the enlarged follicles, producing small, discrete mucosal ulcerations (Fig. 4-60) known as aphthae (aphthous ulcers), which may occur against a background of normal or smoothly edematous mucosa.[36]

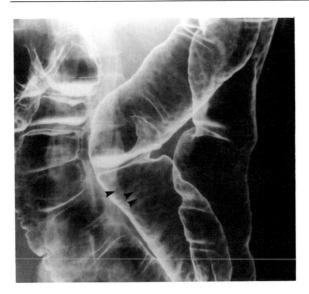

manifested by the tendency of the lesions to appear asymmetrically on the mesenteric wall (medial) of the intestine and sparing the antimesenteric wall (lateral), resulting in sacculations or puckering of the bowel.

Fistulae frequently develop in Crohn's disease. While air-contrast studies are ideal for demonstrating mucosal abnormalities, the single-contrast barium enemas are the best way to demonstrate such fistulae.[37] The fistulae may occur between the small bowel and colon, or between contiguous segments of small bowel (Fig. 4-62). There are also fistulas frequently between the bowel and skin, bladder, vagina, or even thecal space. In a significant number of patients, the first indication of Crohn's disease may be the presence of a persistent rectal fissure, a perirectal abscess, or a mesenteric or retroperitoneal abscess.

Fig. 4-60 Crohn's disease.
History. This 17-year-old woman presented with a 3-week history of abdominal pain and diarrhea.
Findings. *Air-contrast exam, LGI:* There are punctate collections of barium surrounded by a zone of lucency, indicating aphthous lesions (arrowheads).

As the disease progresses, these aphthae enlarge in depth and diameter, and may become confluent. The resulting ulcers may then deepen and penetrate the bowel wall, producing fistulae and sinus tracts. The ulcers may also extend along the bowel wall longitudinally and transversely, producing a crisscross pattern of ulceration that has a "cobblestone" appearance.

As Crohn's disease becomes more chronic there is marked inflammatory induration of the bowel wall and adjacent mesentery. Involved segments of the bowel have a fixed and rigid appearance and are separated from adjacent loops. This separation is due to thickening of the bowel wall and mesentery, the enlargement of regional lymph nodes, and occasionally interloop abscess formation. The diameter of the lumen may be narrowed down to a few millimeters. The lumen appears irregular, and when the terminal ileum is involved, as is typical, it has the appearance of a "string" ("string-sign") (Fig. 4-61).

There are two fundamental characteristics of Crohn's disease that are decisive factors in its diagnosis. First there may be intervening areas of normal mucosa between involved segments of the bowel: the so called "skip lesions." The second characteristic is

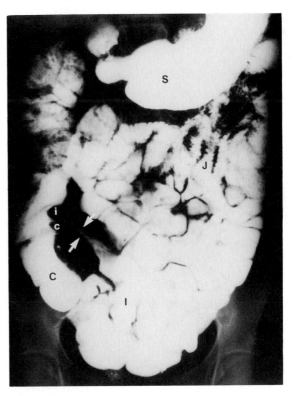

Fig. 4-61 Crohn's disease of the terminal ileum.
History. This 27-year-old woman had a 7-month history of abdominal pain and diarrhea.
Findings. *Small-bowel series:* There is marked narrowing of the terminal ileum (arrows) and separation of this segment from more normal appearing small-bowel loops. S = stomach, J = jejunum, I = ileum, C = cecum, ic = ileocecal valve.

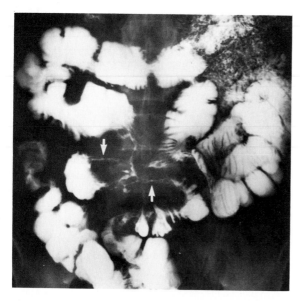

Fig. 4-62 Entero-entero fistula in Crohn's disease.
History. This 25-year-old man had a 7-year history of Crohn's disease.
Findings. *Small-bowel series:* Multiple fistulae (arrows) are demonstrated between various small bowel loops.

GRANULOMATOUS COLITIS VERSUS ULCERATIVE COLITIS

Crohn's disease of the colon typically does not present with the massive rectal bleeding as seen in ulcerative colitis unless the rectosigmoid colon is involved. The rectum is almost always involved in ulcerative colitis, while sigmoidoscopy shows a normal rectum in 50 percent of patients with granulomatous colitis. Skip lesions, asymmetric wall involvement, and cobblestoning are not seen in ulcerative colitis.

Discontinuous lesions are seen in 90 percent of cases of Crohn's disease. There may be aphthous lesions present on one side of the colon while the opposite wall is involved. In advanced granulomatous colitis, fibrosis may shrink one wall of the colon while leaving the other wall normal, producing sacculations. Ulcerative colitis diffusely, symmetrically, and contiguously involves the colon. Fistulae and abscesses are common in granulomatous colitis but are rare in ulcerative colitis. Strictures are often found in Crohn's disease, but the risk of neoplasm is much smaller than in ulcerative colitis, albeit greater than in the general population.

REFERENCES

1. Larson DE, Farnell MB: Upper gastrointestinal hemorrhage. Mayo Clin Proc 371–387, 1983
2. Gore RM, Goldberg HI: Current indications for radiology and endoscopy in the evaluation of upper gastrointestinal tract disease. IMJ 3:77–85, 1982
3. Catalano D, Pagliari U: Gastroduodenal erosions: Radiological findings. Gastrointest Radiol 7:235–240, 1982
4. Gold RP, Green PHR, O'Toole KM, et al: Early gastric cancer: Radiographic experience. Radiology 152:283–290, 1984
5. Thompson G, Sommers S, Stevenson GW: Benign gastric ulcer: A reliable radiologic diagnosis. AJR 141:331–333, 1983
6. Brady LW: Malignant lymphoma of the gastrointestinal tract. Radiology 137:291–298, 1984
7. Smith GF, Ellyson JH, Parks SN, et al: Angiodysplasia of the colon. Arch Surg 119:532–536, 1984
8. Fleischner FG: Diverticular disease of the colon. New observations and refined concepts. Gastroenterology 66:316–324, 1971
9. Gore RM, Calenoff L: Roentgenographic manifestations of diverticulitis. Ill Med J 159:293–297, 1981
10. Spencer RJ, Melton LF, Ready RL, et al: Treatment of small colorectal polyps: A population-based study of the risk of subsequent carcinoma. Mayo Clin Proc 59:305–310, 1984
11. Ott DG, Gelfand DW: Colorectal tumors: Pathology and detection. AJR 131:691–695, 1978
12. Skukas J, Spataro RF, Cannucciari DP, et al: The radiographic features of small colon cancers. Radiology 143:335–340, 1982
13. Bunker SR, Brown JM, McAuley RJ, et al: Detection of gastrointestinal bleeding sites. JAMA 247:789–792, 1982
14. Athanasoulis CA, Waltman AC, Novelline RA, et al: Angiography: Its contribution to the emergency management of gastrointestinal hemorrhage. Radiol Clin North Am 14:265–280, 1976
15. Honickman SP, Mueller RP, Wittenberg J, et al: Ultrasound in obstructive jaundice: Prospective evaluation of site and cause. Radiology 147:511–515, 1983
16. Baron RL, Stanley RJ, Lee JKT, et al: A prospective comparison of the evaluation of biliary obstruction using computed tomography and ultrasonography. Radiology 145:91–98, 1982
17. Gosink BB, Lemon SK, Scheible W, et al: Accuracy of ultrasonography in diagnosis of hepatocellular disease. AJR 133:19–23, 1979
18. Bernardino ME, Lewis E: Imaging hepatic neoplasms. Cancer 50:2666–2671, 1982

19. Alderson PO, Adams DF, McNeil BJ, et al: Computed tomography, ultrasound, and scintigraphy of the liver in patients with colon and breast carcinoma: A prospective comparison. Radiology 149:225–230, 1983

20. Cooperberg P, Golding RH: Advances in ultrasonography of the gallbladder and biliary tract. Radiol Clin North Am 20:611–633, 1982

21. Cooperberg PL, Burhenne JH: Real-time ultrasonography: A diagnostic technique of choice in calculous gallbladder disease. N Engl J Med 302:277–279, 1980

22. Mitchell SE, Clark RE: A comparison of computed tomography and sonography in choledocholithiasis. AJR 142:729–733, 1984

23. Laing FC, Federle MP, Jeffrey RB, et al: Ultrasonic evaluation of patients with acute right upper quadrant pain. Radiology 140:449–455, 1981

24. Weissman HS, Badia J, Sugerman LA, et al: Spectrum of 99m-Tc-1DA cholescintigraphic patterns in acute cholecystitis. Radiology 138:167–175, 1981

25. Shuman WP, Mack LA, Rudd TG, et al: Evaluation of acute right upper quadrant pain: Sonography and 99M Tc-PIPIDA cholescintigraphy. AJR 139:61–65, 1982

26. Hessel SJ, Siegelman SS, McNeil BJ, et al: A prospective evaluation of computed tomography and ultrasound of the pancreas. Radiology 143:129–133, 1982

27. Segal I, Epstein B, Lawson HH, et al: The syndromes of pancreatic pseudocysts and fluid collections. Gastrointest Radiol 9:115–122, 1984

28. Martinex A, Velasco M, Caceres J: Fine-needle biopsy of the pancreas using real-time ultrasonography. Gastrointest Radiol 9:231–234, 1984

29. Seaman WB: Pathophysiology of the esophagus. Semin Roentgenol 16:214–227, 1981

30. Wiot JW, Felson B: Current concepts in cancer. I. Esophagus: Radiographic differential diagnosis. JAMA 226:1548–1552, 1973

31. Donner MW, Saba GP, Martinez CR: Diffused diseases of the esophagus: A practical approach. Semin Roentgenol 16:198–213, 1981

32. Margulis AR, Goldberg HI, Lawson TL, et al: The overlapping spectrum of ulcerative and granulomatous colitis: A roentgenographic pathologic study. AJR 113:325–334, 1971

33. Sommers SC: Ulcerative and granulomatous colitis. AJR 130:817–823, 1978

34. Laufer I: The radiographic demonstration of early changes in ulcerative colitis by double contrast technique. J Can Assoc Radiol 26:116–121, 1975

35. Kelvin FM, Woodward BH, McLoed ME, et al: Prospective diagnosis of dysplasia (precancer) in chronic ulcerative colitis. AJR 138:347–349, 1982

36. Goldberg HI, Caruthers SB, Nelson JA, et al: Radiographic findings of the National Cooperative Crohn's Disease Study. Gastroenterology 77:925–937, 1979

37. Laufer I, Mullens EJ, Hamilton J: Correlation of endoscopy and double-contrast radiography in the early stages of ulcerative and granulomatous colitis. Radiology 118:1–5, 1976

5

Radiology of the Bones and Joints

Ronald W. Hendrix

Unlike other chapters in this book, this chapter will not be oriented around patient symptoms since the characteristic symptoms or clinical findings produced by bone pathology, if there are any at all, consist of pain, a soft-tissue mass, or swelling. Furthermore, the presentation of bone pathology provides scant information for a differential diagnosis. Therefore the chapter will deal with the clinical questions that most commonly prompt a radiographic examination of the bones and joints.

Almost all bone pathology is of traumatic, infectious, neoplastic, arthritic, vascular, congenital, metabolic, dysplastic, or degenerative etiology. Since bone has a relatively limited number of responses to pathologic processes, several abnormalities may cause the same or similar changes in it. The radiographic differential diagnostic findings will be considered for each of the categories of bone abnormality considered.

Through much experience it has been demonstrated that to identify most pathologic processes in any given area requires a group of standard radiographic views for the examination of each area of the skeleton. A barely minimal radiographic study should include two radiographs obtained at right angles to one another. Occasionally additional views in different projections, or special studies such as tomography or radionuclide bone scans, are needed to supplement routine studies in order to identify subtle fractures, such as some fractures of the femoral neck or scaphoid bone, stress fractures (Fig. 5-1A) or other pathologic processes.

A nuclide bone scan involves injecting into a vein a radioisotope-tagged (polyphosphate, diphosphonate, etc.) compound that will be taken up by bone (Fig. 5-1B). Areas of increased or decreased bone turnover or remodeling can be identified by this method for the entire skeleton. The technique is exquisitely sensitive to very small differences in bone turnover caused by

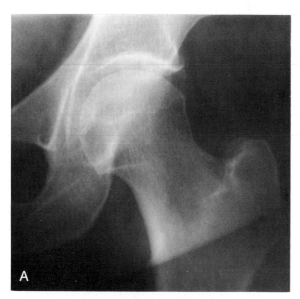

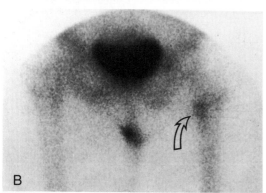

Fig. 5-1 Subtle fracture.
History. This patient was unable to bear weight after a fall.
Findings. (A) *Plain radiograph:* The routine plain radiograph does not demonstrate a fracture. No fracture was demonstrated on conventional tomography. **(B)** *Bone scan:* Linear, abnormally increased activity across the intertrochanteric area (arrow) indicates a fracture, which accounts for the patient's inability to bear weight.

disease processes of all kinds, and allows the detection of abnormal areas long before they are visible on plain radiographs.

A tomographic examination provides views of any selected plane within the body by blurring out the tissues above and below that plane. Tomography is useful when there are dense superimposed structures, such as surrounding bone, which obscure an area of interest.

CT has become useful recently in diagnosing fractures in certain bones, bony destruction from tumor and soft tissue masses.

IS THE BONE FRACTURED?

During any given day, the most frequent question asked of radiologists about bone pathology is whether a bone is fractured, particularly if the radiology department is servicing an active emergency department. A fracture consists of an interruption in the continuity of a bone. Many fractures are easily identified and cause little or no diagnostic difficulty (Fig. 5-2 A, B, and C). Adequate treatment depends on an accurate diagnosis, which in turn depends on an adequate and accurately interpreted radiographic examination.

Fractures are caused by direct forces applied to a bone (e.g., a gunshot, kick, etc.) or by forces applied to the body at a site remote from the fracture and indirectly transmitted to the bone. Most fractures are caused by the latter mechanism. Usually a combination of simultaneous forces is responsible for a given fracture. Different types of force will produce fractures with characteristic radiographic features, and the fracture line will reflect the combination of forces applied. These forces include bending, rotation, compression, tension, shearing, and combinations of all of these. Bending forces are usually operative in the shaft of a long bone, causing tension of the cortex on the side convex to and compression on the side concave to the applied force, which results in a transverse fracture (Fig. 5-2A). Rotation or torsion forces cause a spiral fracture and are commonly seen in a long bone (Fig. 5-2B,C). Compression forces cause fractures with telescoping of the bone trabeculae (Fig. 5-3); these include fractures of the tibial plateau or surgical neck of the humerus. Tension forces cause transverse fractures as well and are commonly seen in ankle injuries.

Fractures may produce one or more direct or indirect radiographic features that allows their diagnostic identification. The most common such feature is a radiolucent line (Fig. 5-2A). The width of the line depends on the amount of displacement of the bone fragments; the wider the line the more easily it is seen. A fracture is most easily seen on a radiograph obtained

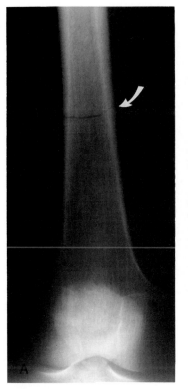

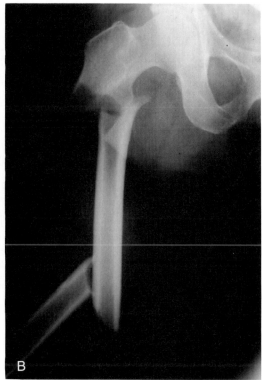

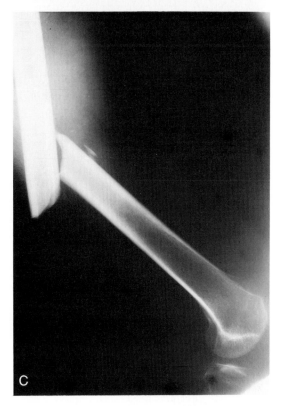

Fig. 5-2 Fracture.

History. Two patients with obvious fractures after a car accident.

Findings. *Plain radiograph:* **(A)** Nondisplaced femoral fracture consisting of a radiolucent line with interruption of the cortex. **(B, C)** Transverse subtrochanteric and midshaft fractures provide no diagnostic difficulty. A lateral angulation of the midshaft fracture is seen only on the anterior-posterior view, while the anterior angulation is visible only on the lateral view. A minimum of two views obtained at 90 degrees to one another, as seen here, is needed to reconstruct a three-dimensional image of the fractured bone from the two-dimensional radiographic images.

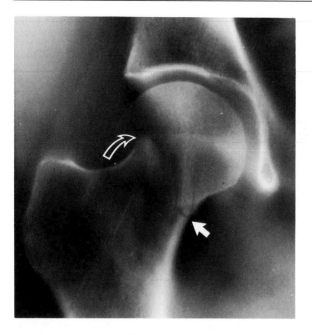

with the x-ray beam parallel to the fracture line (Fig. 5-4A), and is virtually impossible to see if the beam is perpendicular to the plane of the fracture. Radiographs obtained at angles between these extremes vary in the difficulty they present for identifying a fracture (Fig. 5-4B).

Suture lines and vascular grooves in the skull are frequently mistaken for fractures (Fig. 5-5). How-

Fig. 5-3 Compression fracture.
History. This patient had hip pain after a fall.
Findings. *Tomogram:* There is a fracture of the femoral neck with compression of the bone trabeculae on the lateral side of the neck forming a radiodense line (open arrow) and a slight distraction of the medial cortex (closed arrow).

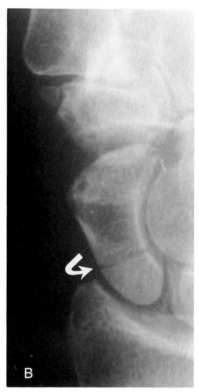

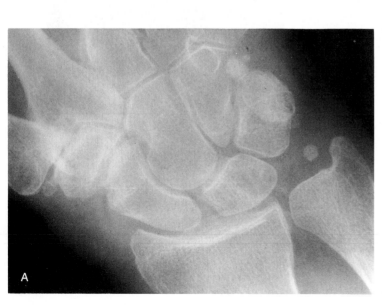

Fig. 5-4 Fracture.
History. The patient had point tenderness in the anatomic snuff box after a fall onto an outstretched hand.
Findings. (A) *Navicular view:* Done with ulnar deviation of the wrist, this view aligns the x-ray beam parallel with the fracture line and clearly demonstrates the navicular waist fracture. **(B)** *Plain radiograph:* The routine wrist radiograph does not demonstrate a visible fracture as the beam is oblique to the fracture line.

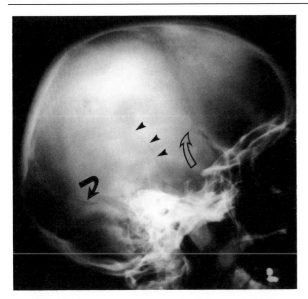

Fig. 5-5 Skull fracture.
History. This patient lost consciousness following a car accident.
Findings. *Skull radiograph:* A linear skull fracture (arrowheads) is more lucent than adjacent vascular grooves (open arrow) and is more regular than suture lines (solid arrow).

ever, a fracture is more radiolucent than a vascular groove because it extends through both tables of the skull, whereas the latter indents only one table. The vascular groove also has a fine, dense margin and frequently branches; whereas branching is unusual for linear skull fractures. Suture lines are serpiginous and have dense margins. They occupy a similar position in all patients, which is helpful in differentiating these normal, lucent lines from a fracture.

Interruption of the bone cortex is the second most useful finding for diagnosing a fracture. The cortex may be discontinuous, with or without distraction of the fragments, either telescoped on itself or with a step deformity (Figs. 5-3 and 5-4).

A radiodense line occurs when there is impaction or telescoping of the fractured bone ends on one another. The dense line occurs because the telescoped bone trabeculae fill up much of the space previously occupied by the marrow (Fig. 5-3). This finding is usually accompanied by interruption of the bone cortex and

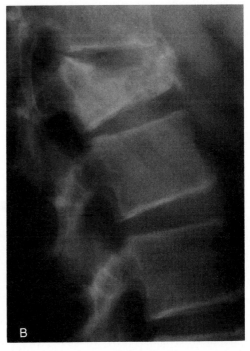

Fig. 5-6 Vertebral-body fracture.
History. This patient had back pain following a fall from a ladder.
Findings. *Spine radiographs:* Anterior-posterior (**A**) and lateral (**B**) views show that the deformed vertebral body is denser than other vertebra because it contains approximately the same amount of bone mineral but within a much smaller volume.

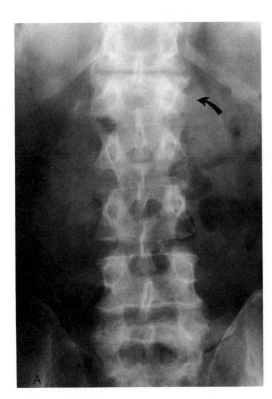

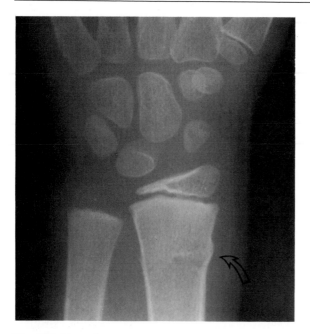

Fig. 5-7 Torus fracture.
History. This child had arm pain and swelling after a school "recess."
Findings. *Plain radiograph:* A typical torus or greenstick fracture is seen in the radius, its most common site of occurrence (arrow).

interruption of multiple bone trabeculae within the radiodense line. Fractures of the femoral neck and surgical neck of the humerus are the most common examples of those that present as radiodense lines. The same type of fracture is seen in vertebral bodies but is called a compression fracture rather than an impacted fracture (Fig. 5-6 A and B).

Buckling of the cortex with or without an associated transverse line of wavy bone trabeculae is seen in infants and children and is called a torus or greenstick fracture (Fig. 5-7). Part of the bone structure remains intact, as does a green twig which snaps but does not separate into two pieces, and hence the name. Torus fractures are not seen in adults because with age the bones become more brittle and normally fracture through. The distal radius is the most frequent site of a torus fracture (Fig. 5-7).

In children, a fracture can occur through an epiphyseal growth plate and displace it. Most often a small metaphyseal fragment is chipped off with the epiphysis (Fig. 5-8). An epiphyseal fracture must be reduced to put the fragments in their normal anatomic position so as to prevent growth disturbances and deformities. These fractures are frequently subtle, and comparison with the normal contralateral bone is often helpful. The Salter-Harris classification of epiphyseal fractures shown in Figure 5-9 is widely used in describing these fractures.

A fracture through bone that is abnormal as the result of another disease entity is known as a pathologic fracture. The fracture may occur through a solitary destructive bone lesion (e.g., metastasis, cyst, primary bone tumor, etc.) or through a bone which has a generalized abnormality (e.g., Paget's disease, infection, etc.). The fracture through generally abnormal bone usually causes no diagnostic problem, although

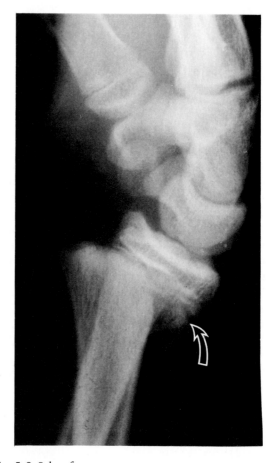

Fig. 5-8 Salter fracture.
History. This patient suffered a fall.
Findings. *Plain radiograph:* A Salter type 2 fracture through the radial epiphysis includes a small metaphyseal fragment (arrow).

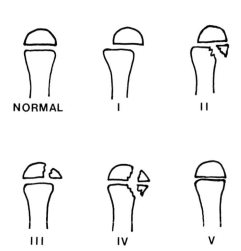

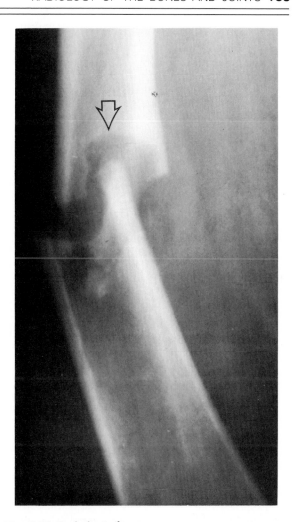

Fig. 5-9 Salter-Harris Classification of Epiphyseal Fractures. Type I to V fractures occur with a frequency of 6%, 75%, 8%, 10%, and 1% respectively. Type V fractures represent crushing of the epiphysis.

the pathologic fracture through a solitary lesion may be easily identified while the lesion itself is overlooked (Fig. 5-10). The tipoff is that the bone ends appear smooth and minimally irregular, and the fracture is transverse across a long bone. In identifying the destructive lesion, it may be helpful to mentally visualize what the bone would look like if the fracture fragments were returned to their normal anatomic positions.

Clinicians treating fractures wish to know about alignment, apposition, and rotation of the bone fragments. They want to know the amount of deviation of the distal fragment from the normal axis of the bone in degrees, as seen with the anterior-posterior (AP) and lateral projections. In common practice the distal fragment is said to be angulated medially, laterally, anteriorly, or posteriorly by a certain number of degrees with respect to the proximal fragment. Apposition is described in terms of the number of centimeters the fracture end of the distal fragment is displaced with respect to the fracture end of the proximal fragment. If the distal bone fragment is rotated from its normal axis the rotation must be estimated and noted, since a rotational deformity is the one least corrected by the healing process. If it is not corrected it will lead

Fig. 5-10 Pathologic fracture.
History. This was a patient with known multiple myeloma who suffered a fall.
Findings. *Plain radiograph:* There is a pathologic fracture of the femur through a lesion of multiple myeloma. Notice the smooth contour (arrow) of the proximal femoral fragment produced by the destructive lesion, and the transverse orientation of the fracture.

after healing to abnormal loads on adjacent joints and to the rapid development of degenerative arthritis.

IS THE FRACTURE HEALED?

The decision of when to remove a cast or when to allow weight bearing is that of the orthopedic surgeon, not the radiologist. Radiographs are periodically obtained to follow the stages of healing of a

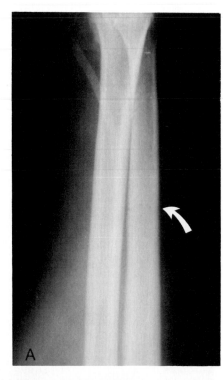

Fig. 5-11 Healing fracture.
History. This patient had an acute fracture of an ulna.
Findings. (A) *Plain radiograph:* This shows the healing sequence of an ulnar fracture. The transverse fracture is undisplaced. **(B)** Two weeks after the fracture, a radiograph taken through a plaster cast shows that the fracture line is wider than in **(A)** from normal resorption of the bone ends. **(C)** Twelve weeks after the fracture, following cast removal, a significant amount of calcified callus has accumulated with bridging of the fracture margins. This amount of callus will safely stabilize a fracture in a non-weight-bearing bone. In a weight-bearing bone, more mature callus than this is needed before unaided weight-bearing is safe. **(D)** Six months after the fracture, there is solid fusion of mature callus with the bone on both sides of the fracture. The fracture line has been virtually obliterated by endosteal callus. Bone remodeling is in progress.

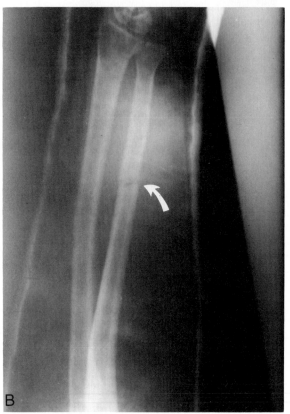

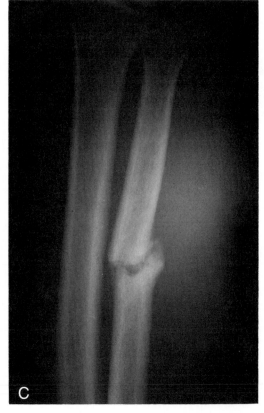

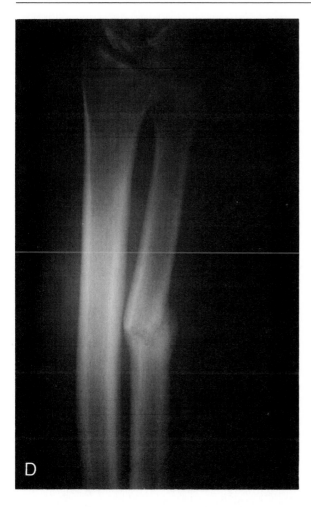

The reparative phase ensues, with invasion of the hematoma by capillaries and fibroblasts and the formation of granulation tissue. Dead bone at the fracture ends is resorbed, causing indistinctness of the fracture margins and widening of the fracture line by approximately 10 to 14 days after the injury. Cells from the granulation tissue, endosteum, and periosteum all participate in the healing process. The clotted blood is replaced by collagen fibers and matrix for the immature woven bone known as callus that will initially hold the fracture fragments together. Callus surrounds the bone ends and stabilizes the fracture. It then calcifies and is first seen radiographically as a hazy density at the margins of the fracture, after which it progressively becomes denser. Eventually the callus becomes as dense as the adjacent cortex and fuses with it on both sides of the fracture line, forming a bridge of bone (Fig. 5-11C). The fracture margins then become hazy and the fracture line becomes progressively less distinct and finally disappears as calcified callus forms between the ends of the fracture fragments and in the medullary canal (Fig. 5-11D). The woven bone which makes up the callus is homogeneously dense and is slowly replaced by trabecular bone and a marrow cavity. The latter is part of the final stage of fracture healing, which also includes remodeling of the bone at the fracture site if the healing has occurred with any deformity. The degree of remodeling is greatest in an infant and least in an adult.

Fracture union is best determined by clinical evidence of stability. This includes lack of pain, lack of motion with stress at the fracture site, and ability to use the body part that has sustained the fracture without external support. The radiographic appearance of the injured bone is taken into consideration as well. Calcified callus completely bridging a fracture line will provide stability even when a fracture line is still visible (Fig. 5-11C). However, in a weight-bearing bone the callus must be thick and well developed, with a distinct peripheral margin, before weight bearing is safe. In a non-weight-bearing bone the fracture may be stable and allow some use of the part when the callus bridges the fracture line but before it becomes dense with a well-defined outer margin.

Small irregular bones (carpal and tarsal bones) and flat bones heal with little or no peripheral callus formation. Callus formation is also minimized by impaction (telescoping of the bone ends on one another, as

fracture. Within 1 to 2 weeks there is bone demineralization along the fracture margins (Fig. 5-11 A and B). This causes the fracture line to appear more prominent than at the time of occurrence of the fracture. A subtle fracture (e.g., in a rib, or a stress fracture) not initially detected may first be seen at this time.

Fracture healing is frequently divided into inflammatory, reparative, and remodeling phases for conceptualization. Immediately after a fracture there is hemorrhage from the fractured bone ends and from the laceration of adjacent soft tissues. A hematoma forms around the fracture. Tissue may be destroyed either by the force of the injury or by devascularization due to vessel disruption. The resulting necrotic debris produces an acute inflammatory response with vasodilatation and the exudation of plasma and leukocytes.

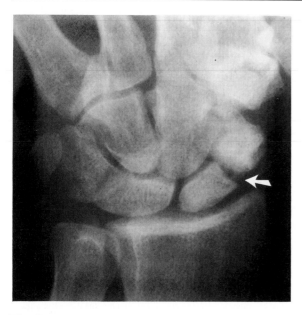

Fig. 5-12 Fracture nonunion.
History. This patient had a fractured wrist 2 years earlier, but had continued pain.
Findings. *Plain radiograph:* There is nonunion osteonecrosis of the distal fracture fragment of the navicular (scaphoid) bone from loss of its blood supply.

in the femoral or humeral necks), and is less prominent when a fracture occurs through a thin cortex. No periosteal callus is seen in fractures of the skull or femoral neck. The periosteum of the skull lacks osteogenic capacity, and the intracapsular part of the femoral neck is not covered by periosteum. A greater than normally anticipated amount of peripheral callus forms with comminution (multiple fracture fragments), with increased separation of the fracture fragments, in areas with a thick cortex and large overlying muscles, in the presence of infection, and with insufficient immobilization.

Delayed union is the term applied to a fracture that heals more slowly than usual. Nonunion is the term used for a fracture which fails to heal with bony union. Delayed union, nonunion, or both are most frequently seen in fractures of the carpal scaphoid, middle third of the humerus, junction of the middle and distal thirds of the tibia, distal end of the clavicle, and middle third of the radial shaft (Fig. 5-12). Infection, damage to the blood supply of one fragment of a fracture, inadequate immobilization, excessive separation of the fracture fragments or interposition of

soft tissue between the fracture ends all predispose to nonunion. Radiographically, the opposing fracture margins become sclerotic and the fracture line persists. Calcified callus may heap up at the periphery of the fracture fragments and extend medially and laterally into the soft tissues on both sides of the fracture line.

IS THE JOINT DISLOCATED OR SUBLUXED?

Dislocation and subluxation, which are different entities, are terms often confused and carelessly used interchangeably. A joint is dislocated when the opposing articular surfaces are displaced and are no longer in contact with one another. Subluxation occurs when the articular surfaces are no longer normally opposed but are instead displaced, so that only a portion of each surface remains in contact with the other. A subluxation is therefore not as severe a displacement as a dislocation. Because it is not always clinically possible to distinguish a fracture from a dislocation, the radiographic examination is important. Fractures often accompany dislocations (Fig. 5-13A), and may not be visible until after reduction of the latter—thus emphasizing the importance of the postreduction x-ray examination. A postreduction radiograph is also necessary to evaluate the results of manipulation of a fracture or dislocation (Fig. 5-13B). The interphalangeal joints of the hands are those most commonly dislocated, and the shoulder is the most frequently dislocated large joint in the body.

IS OSTEOMYELITIS PRESENT?

This question is frequently asked by orthopedists, internists, emergency care physicians, surgeons in most of the subspecialities, and an assortment of other physicians with regard to a bone. Osteomyelitis may be caused by organisms including mycobacteria, fungi, viruses, protozoans, rickettsiae, and worms. The present discussion will be limited to pyogenic osteomyelitis. The routes of microbial inoculation leading to osteomyelitis are hematogenous, penetrating (including surgical), and contiguous, from adjacent infected soft tissue. Since radiographic changes in the bone lag behind the clinical course of osteomye-

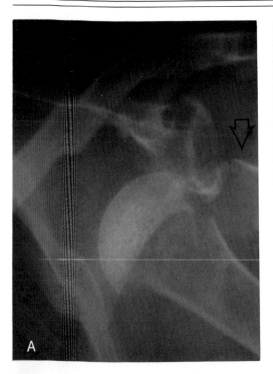
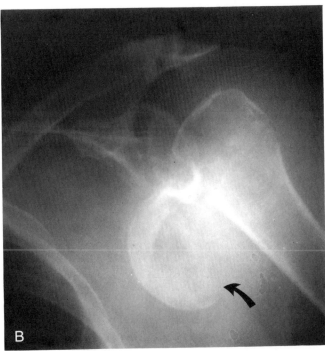

Fig. 5-13   Dislocation and fracture.
History. Shoulder pain and loss of motion following a football game.
Findings.   **(A)** *Plain radiograph:* Anterior dislocation with avulsion of the greater tuberosity (arrow) is a common combination. **(B)** *Post-reduction radiograph:* Although the humeral shaft was returned to its normal position by manipulation in order to reduce the dislocation, the surgical-neck fracture, seen only indistinctly as a sclerotic line in **A**, has been distracted, with the humeral head now grossly displaced and dislocated (arrow). A post-reduction radiograph is needed after manipulation of a fracture or dislocation in order to evaluate the result.

litis by at least 10 to 14 days, appropriate antibiotic therapy must be instituted before identifying specific radiographic changes if there is a reasonable suspicion of this disease. Staphylococci are responsible for most cases of acute osteomyelitis, and are found primarily in children following skin infections, in adults after orthopedic procedures, in diabetic patients' foot infections, and after penetrating trauma.

Hematogenous osteomyelitis characteristically begins in the medullary canal of the metaphysis of a long bone. The infection may extend through to the cortex, in which case the pus collects beneath the periosteum. The periosteum is very poorly attached to the underlying bone cortex in infants and children, but becomes quite tightly attached by adulthood. In infants and children, therefore, the pus strips the periosteum from the cortex. This causes an extensive periosteal reaction, which may extend a considerable distance away from the cortex (Fig. 5-14). The reaction may completely surround the bone and is called an involucrum. When the cortex is stripped away, periosteal vessels may be interrupted with resulting osteonecrosis of the outer one-third to one-half of the cortex. Fragments of dead bone called sequestra, which are more dense than adjacent viable bone and result from early loss of their blood supply and lack of participation in the ensuing hyperemia and osteoporosis, are the result of this necrosis (Fig. 5-15). As described, the infection in an adult, rather than elevate the periosteum, will more likely penetrate both the cortex and adherent periosteum, causing relatively little periosteal reaction but extending into adjacent soft tissue and even to the skin as a sinus track.

In children aged 1 to 16, the epiphyseal plate com-

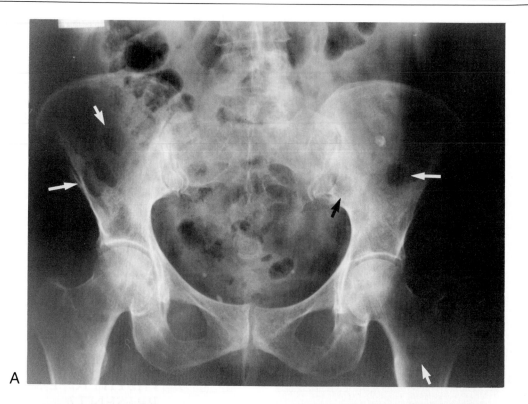

A

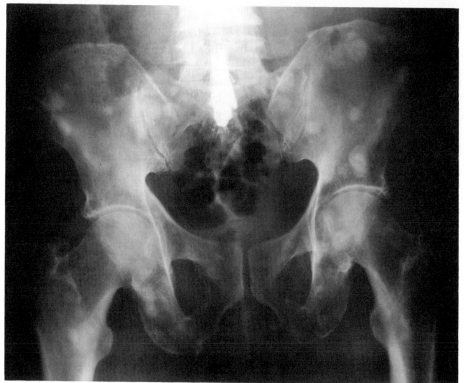

B

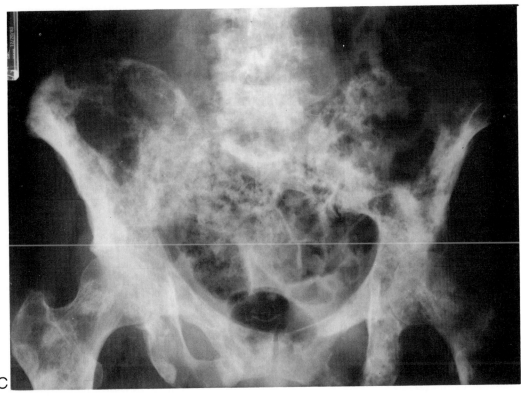

C

Fig. 5-19 Bone metastasis.
History. These were three patients with known primary tumors and bone pain.
Findings. *Plain radiograph:* **(A)** There are extensive lytic metastases (arrows) in the pelvis and proximal femur from breast carcinoma. **(B)** Dense sclerotic metastases from prostate carcinoma involve all of the visualized bones. **(C)** There is extensive metastatic disease with both lytic and sclerotic lesions from treated breast carcinoma.

is due to changes caused by healing in the bone rather than to bone made by the tumor (Fig. 5-19B). This type of lesion is most often seen with metastases from prostate tumors, and occasionally in lymphomas. Mixed lesions are of an aggressiveness intermediate between that of purely lytic and purely blastic lesions. They are usually seen with osteolytic metastases after treatment with radiation or with breast metastases after treatment with radiation, hormones, or chemotherapeutic agents, or after sterilization (Fig. 5-19C).

Lytic metastases are detected radiographically when bone trabeculae or cortex are destroyed. Any lesion is more difficult to detect in areas rich in trabecular bone such as the spine, ribs, or pelvis, than in long bones, where dense cortical bone predominates. Fifty percent or more of the bone-mineral content may

have be destroyed in the spine, ribs, or pelvis before a metastasis or any lesion becomes visible in a routine radiograph. By comparison, conventional tomographs of an involved area may reveal a lytic metastasis when only 20 to 30 percent of the bone mineral is destroyed, and computed tomography may be even more sensitive for identifying metastases, although its primary use is to determine the extent of the lesion. Nuclear medicine bone scans are used as the most sensitive way of detecting individual sites of metastatic disease. In patients with possible or suspected metastatic disease, all areas with positive activity demonstrated on a bone scan should be radiographed. The bone scan is exquisitely sensitive to abnormal areas of bone turnover, but is also extremely nonspecific. Radiographs, on the other hand, are specific but insensi-

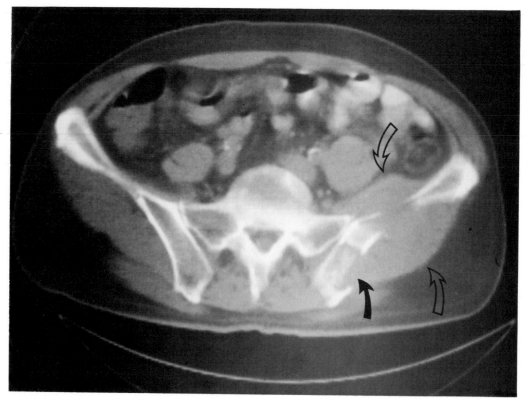

Fig. 5-20 Bone metastasis.
History. This patient with lung carcinoma had pelvic pain. The pelvis film was reported as normal.
Findings. *CT scan:* Further studies were obtained because of continued pelvic pain. A large destructive lesion in the iliac bone, with an associated soft-tissue mass (open arrows), is clearly demonstrated. A second destructive lesion in the innominate bone is also seen (closed arrow).

tive. In cases of metastastic disease it is typical for the patient to complain of pain in one or more areas of the body. If a bone scan of the area is abnormal but a radiograph of the same area is negative, either conventional or computed tomography may be able to demonstrate a bone lesion (Fig. 5-20).

IS A SOLITARY BONE LESION A MALIGNANT BONE TUMOR?

Bone metastases occurs much more frequently than primary bone tumors. Therefore, when a solitary bone lesion is found, a diligent search, such as by bone scanning, is needed to exclude other, similar lesions. If more than one lesion is found, it is remotely likely that the lesions are due to a primary bone tumor, and some other disease entity, such as metastases from a

tumor, osteomyelitis, fibrous dysplasia, the brown tumors of hyperparathyroidism, Paget's disease, and so forth should be sought as the diagnosis.

Although most primary bone tumors or tumor-like lesions of bone cause bone destruction, a few cause increased bone density (Fig. 5-21). Included in tumor-like lesions are fibrous dysplasia, bone cysts, the brown tumors of hyperparathyroidism, and eosinophilic granuloma, because all of them can be sufficiently aggressive to simulate a primary bone tumor.

Tumors will occasionally cause a lesion more dense than the surrounding bone. This is seen in only one type of tumor—osteosarcoma—in which actual tumor bone is made and ossified (Fig. 5-22). Dense bone is also seen with lesions in which the host bone reacts to the tumor and lays down normal bone to heal itself either spontaneously (only in the case of very slow-growing tumors) or after treatment. Ossifying

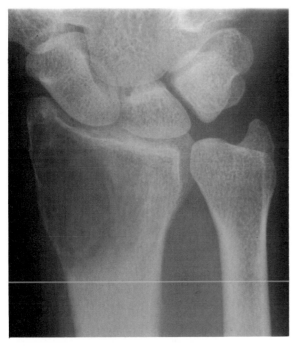

Fig. 5-21 Giant-cell tumor.
History. This patient had a mass with pain in the forearm.
Findings. *Plain radiograph:* A tumor is present and is causing destruction and expansion of the radius. The tumor margin is well defined, but no reaction of the adjacent normal bone has been stimulated.

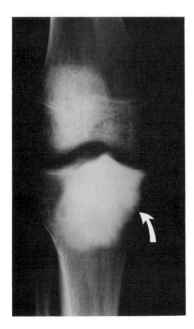

Fig. 5-22 Osteosarcoma.
History. This young man had a short history of bone pain.
Findings. *Plain radiograph:* There is extraordinarily dense tumor bone (arrow).

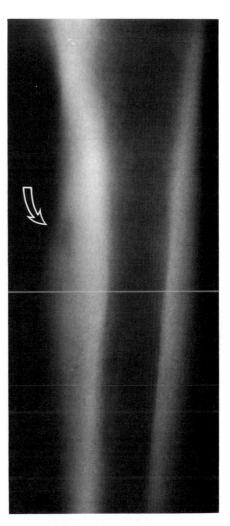

Fig. 5-23 Osteoid osteoma.
History. This patient had mild pain, especially at night.
Findings. *Tomogram:* There is visualization of the eccentric, lucent tumor nidus (arrow), which has stimulated enormous cortical thickening.

fibromas, osteoid osteomas (Fig. 5-23), and bone cysts are common examples of the former, while brown tumors after treatment of the underlying hyperparathyroidism, or most primary tumors after radiation therapy (although this may not be the best mode of therapy), are examples of the latter.

The age of the patient, pattern of bone destruction, appearance of the margins of the lesion, type of periosteal reaction, interruption of the bone cortex by tumor, calcification of the tumor matrix, and growth rate all provide useful diagnostic information about a solitary bone lesion. The patient's age is the most useful piece of historical information, since many

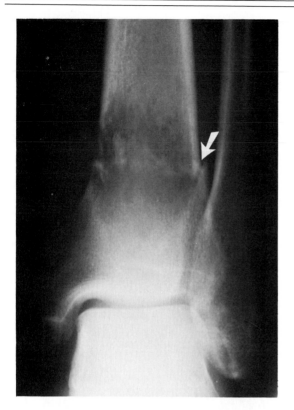

Fig. 5-24 Malignant fibrous histiocytoma.
History. This patient had a "fracture" after a fall.
Findings. *Plain radiograph:* An anterior-posterior view demonstrates a tumor with ill-defined margins proximally and distally, moth-eaten destruction of the posterior cortex, and a pathologic fracture (arrow).

malignant lesions are more aggressive and grow faster than benign lesions. A lucent lesion (Fig. 5-21) is less aggressive and slower growing than one composed of multiple small holes that have coalesced to create an ill-defined larger lesion (Fig. 5-24), although this intermediate lesion is slower growing than a permeative lesion composed of a multitude of tiny holes in the cortex but which does not have a discernible margin (Fig. 5-25). This latter type of lesion grows so rapidly that it leaves behind a large amount of adjacent normal bone. A dense, well-defined margin indicates slow growth with reactive bone forming at the margins (Fig. 5-26). In fact, the thicker the sclerotic mar-

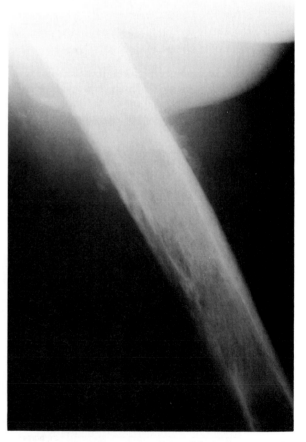

Fig. 5-25 Leukemia of the bone.
History. This middle-aged man had leukemia.
Findings. *Plain radiograph:* There is permeative destruction of the proximal femur which has penetrated the cortex and produced an extensive periosteal reaction. This is a rapidly growing lesion without clearly definable margins.

tumors are age dependent. Metastases and multiple myeloma are the most frequent causes of destructive lesions after age 40. Osteomyelitis frequently mimics malignancy but most frequently occurs before skeletal maturity. Ewing's sarcoma, osteosarcoma, aneurysmal bone cysts, chondroblastoma, and nonossifying fibromas occur most frequently in the second decade and are mainly seen in patients under age 15. Metastatic neuroblastoma is the most frequent malignant tumor seen in bone in patients under the age of 1 year. Fibrosarcoma, chondrosarcoma, and lymphoma are most common in the 30-to-70 age range. Giant-cell tumors are seen in the 20-to-40 age range.

The radiographic appearance of the interior and margin of the lesion provides information about the growth rate of a bone tumor. With a few exceptions,

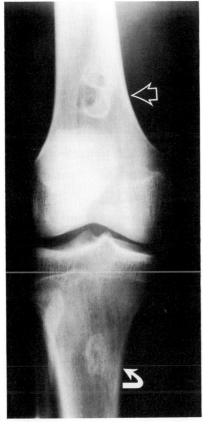

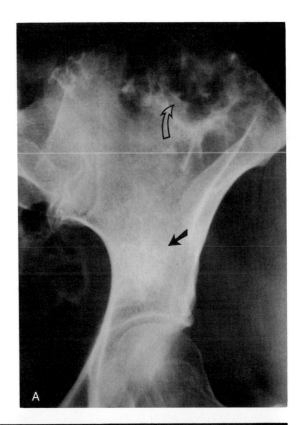

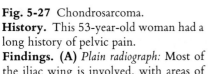

Fig. 5-26 Non-ossifying fibroma.
History. This young man had prolonged bone pain.
Findings. *Plain radiograph:* Non-ossifying fibromas with dense margins (arrows) that indicate their slow growth rate are seen in the tibia and femur. The greater internal density of the tibial lesion is due to healing; eventually this cortical lesion will heal and be uniformly dense.

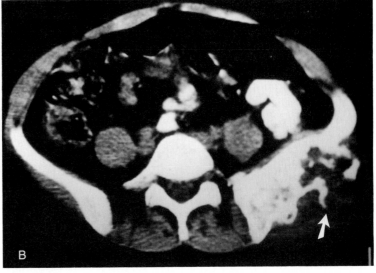

Fig. 5-27 Chondrosarcoma.
History. This 53-year-old woman had a long history of pelvic pain.
Findings. (A) *Plain radiograph:* Most of the iliac wing is involved, with areas of destruction (open arrow) and areas of calcified cartilage matrix (solid arrow). **(B)** *CT scan:* The same findings as in **(A)** are demonstrated, plus extension of the tumor mass through the bone cortex with formation of a large, soft-tissue mass (arrow).

gin of a lesion the slower is the growth rate. A sharp, nonsclerotic margin indicates more rapid growth (Fig. 5-21) and an ill-defined margin indicates the fastest growth of all (Fig. 5-25). Extension of the tumor through the bone, with the formation of a soft-tissue mass is more likely due to a malignant than a benign tumor (Fig. 5-20 A and B) as well.

Primary bone tumors are classified according to the matrix they produce, which is determined by the cytology of the tumor. Tumors include hematopoietic tumors (multiple myeloma, lymphoma, leukemia), chondrogenic tumors (enchondroma, chondroblastoma, osteochondroma, chondromyxoid fibroma, chondrosacroma), osteogenic tumors (osteoid osteoma, osteoblastoma, osteosarcoma), fibrogenic tumors (nonossifying and ossifying fibromas, fibrosarcomas), and tumors of unknown origin (giant-cell tumor, Ewing's sarcoma, adamantinoma, etc.). Calcification occurs frequently within cartilage-matrix tumors, while mineralized, dense tumor bone occurs only within osteosarcomas. Calcification within a cartilage matrix produces punctate or amorphous densities, as opposed to ossification in the osteoid matrix of an osteosarcoma, where bone trabeculae, even though they may be randomly directed, can be identified (Figs. 5-22 and 5-27 A and B).

DOES THE PATIENT HAVE HYPERPARATHYROIDISM?

The parathyroid glands recognize the amount of ionized calcium in the blood and alter the rate of parathyroid hormone release to maintain the serum calcium level within relatively narrow limits. Parathormone is manufactured by the chief cells and acts upon bone by stimulating osteoclastic bone resorption. The calcium from the resorbed bone is released into the blood and elevates the serum calcium level. By affecting vitamin D metabolism, increased parathormone levels also cause an increased absorption of calcium from the gut and an increased renal tubular reabsorption of calcium.

Hyperparathyroidism may be divided into primary and secondary types. Primary hyperparathyroidism results from the secretion of more parathormone than is necessary for maintaining a normal serum calcium concentration. It is caused by an adenoma in approximately 90 percent of cases and by glandular hyperpla-

sia in the remainder. Patients with hyperparathyroidism often complain of bone or joint pain or both, abdominal pain due to pancreatitis, a duodenal ulcer, or renal stones, and may manifest personality disturbances.

Secondary hyperparathyroidism occurs when the serum calcium level is depressed and abnormal amounts of parathormone must be secreted to restore and maintain a normal calcium level. Most causes of secondary hyperparathyroidism result from calcium deficiency associated with vitamin D abnormalities. In the United States, renal failure is by far the most frequent and important cause of secondary hyperparathyroidism. In this condition phosphorus absorption by the gut is normal while renal phosphorus excretion is reduced. The resulting high serum phosphorus

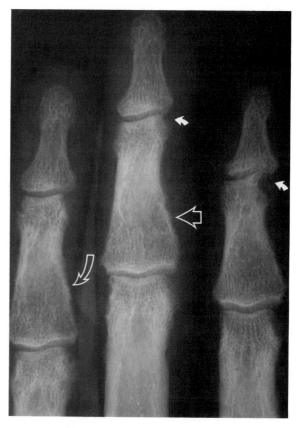

Fig. 5-28 Secondary hyperparathyroidism.
History. This patient had a long history of renal failure.
Findings. *Plain radiograph:* There is subperiosteal bone resorption along the radial aspect of the middle phalanges (open arrows), and marginal erosions (closed arrows).

level reduces the ionized serum calcium level, which in turn stimulates parathormone secretion. The elevated serum phosphorus level also decreases the hydroxylation of 25-OH-vitamin D to the dihydroxyform, which is essential for absorption of calcium from the gut. This mechanism is protective since it prevents the absorption of calcium from the gut and an increase in the serum calcium concentration leading to an abnormally high calcium-phosphorus product. The latter, if high enough, will allow extraskeletal mineralization, which may occur in the kidneys and vessels, with further renal damage. However, the abnormally high parathormone level stimulates osteoclastic bone resorption and causes generalized osteopenia or radiolucent bones.

The mineralization of cartilage and bone requires adequate concentrations of both phosphorus and calcium. Low serum values for calcium or phosphorus may lead to the failure of bone mineralization and cause an accumulation of large amounts of unmineralized osteoid in some patients with secondary hyperparathyroidism due to renal failure. Increasingly, the parathyroid glands become less able to maintain normal serum calcium levels, and the levels of parathormone may become astronomical, far exceeding those seen in the primary form of the disease. For this reason

the bone findings in secondary hyperparathyroidism are more exaggerated than in the primary form. Bone resorption, osteopenia, and fractures are the common radiographic manifestations of the disease (Fig. 5-28).

Parathormone stimulates bone resorption in almost every conceivable site within a bone, such as beneath the periosteum (subperiosteal), within the cortex (intercortical), on the inner cortical surface (endosteal), adjacent to the articular surfaces (subchondral), and on the surfaces of the medullary trabeculae (trabecular). Subperiosteal resorption is essentially diagnostic of hyperparathyroidism, and is most frequently seen involving the radial margin of the phalanges of the hands, especially the middle phalanx of the second and third digits (Fig. 5-28). Other involved areas include the phalangeal tufts and rib margins, and the proximal medial cortex of the femur, tibia, and humerus. This subperiosteal resorption may involve joint margins in the hands, wrists, and feet, and the sacroiliac, acromioclavicular, and sternoclavicular joints (Fig. 5-28). The resorption of medullary bone trabeculae results in a loss of trabecular detail and gives a granular appearance to the medullary canal. In the skull this causes a characteristic appearance called a "salt and pepper" skull (Fig. 5-29).

Brown tumors are primarily accumulations of fi-

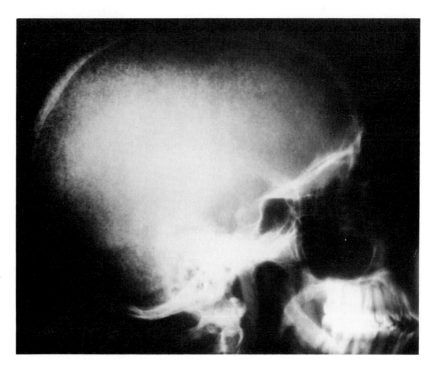

Fig. 5-29 Secondary hyperparathyroidism.
History. Renal failure.
Findings. *Skull radiograph:* Typical mottled appearance of the "salt and pepper" skull.

brous tissue which may undergo necrosis and lique-
faction to form a cyst. They occur in both primary and
secondary hyperparathyroidism but are more frequent
in the primary form (Fig. 5-30). They may occur as
single or multiple destructive lesions with well-defined, lucent margins indicating an intermediate aggressiveness. They occur in the medullary canal or in
the cortex, may be eccentric, and may attain a large
size. Removal of the parathyroid adenoma underlying
these lesions may lead to the healing of brown tumors
with the formation of a dense sclerotic margin and
later with progressive filling in of the tumor area by
sclerotic bone.

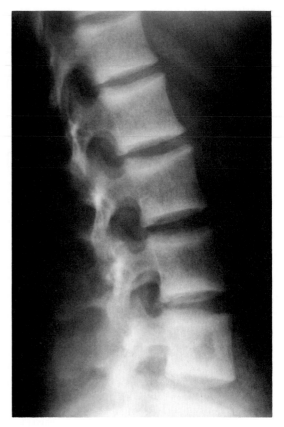

Fig. 5-31 Secondary hyperparathyroidism.
History. Chronic renal failure.
Findings. *Plain radiograph:* There is increased density adjacent to the end plates of the vertebral body, producing a
"rugger jersey" spine along with osteomalacia.

Occasionally, patchy or even generalized bone
sclerosis may be seen in patients with hyperparathyroidism. The mechanism of this abnormality is not
understood, but is often attributed to the effect of
thyrocalcitonin.

Chondrocalcinosis—the deposition of calcium
within cartilage—is a frequent finding in primary
hyperparathyroidism but is rare in the secondary form
of the disease.

In addition to showing the changes produced by
hyperparathyroidism, patients with renal osteodystrophy may also demonstrate features of osteomalacia.
Several nonspecific radiographic findings are seen.
There is a decrease in the number of bone trabeculae,
while those that remain are thickened, causing a

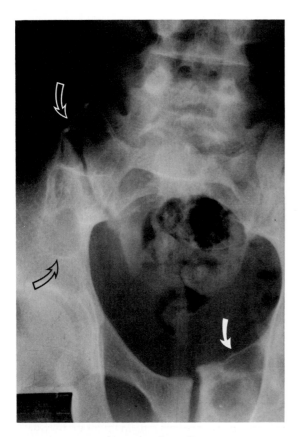

Fig. 5-30 Primary hyperparathyroidism.
History. Swelling of the left groin with pain.
Findings. *Plain radiograph:* Large brown tumors involve
the right iliac bone (open arrows) and left pubic bone
(closed arrow).

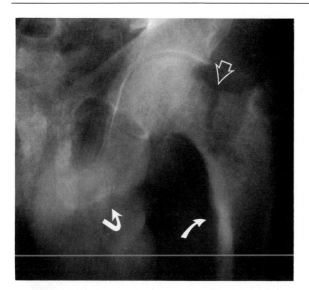

Fig. 5-32 Osteomalacia.
History. Unknown.
Findings. *Plain radiograph:* There is a Looser's zone or pseudofracture in the left femoral neck (arrow), along with subperiosteal bone resorption inferior to the lesser trochanter and at the ischiopubic junction (closed arrows), and resorption of the margins of the symphysis pubis. The bone trabeculae are ill-defined, causing a washed out appearance of all of the bones due to osteomalacia.

prominent, dense and coarse trabecular appearance in the presence of osteopenia. The spine, long bones, and pelvis are the most common examples. In the spine there is an increased density near the vertebral endplates while the center of the vertebral body remains relatively lucent. The resultant alternating, striped appearance is reminiscent of British football jerseys (Fig. 5-31) and is known as a "rugger jersey" spine. In a long bone, the subperiosteal deposition of osteoid may thicken the cortex and cause a fuzzy cortical margin. Additionally, the pseudofractures known as Looser's zones are common (Fig. 5-32). These are lucent areas within and oriented perpendicular to the cortex, which extend only partway across an involved bone and tend to occur symmetrically. They may involve the superior or inferior pubic rami or both, the medial margins of the proximal femurs, the ribs, and the medial margins of the scapulae.

DOES THIS PATIENT HAVE OSTEOPOROSIS?

Osteoporosis, the most frequent metabolic bone disease, results from a generalized decrease in bone mass. This is most evident in the spine, pelvis, and proximal humeri and femora (Fig. 5-33 A and B). The bone that is present is qualitatively normal, but there is quantitatively less of it than normal. The diagnosis is usually made coincidentally from routine radiographs obtained for some other reason and only after the disorder is well established. The bones are more radiolucent than normal (Fig. 5-33 A and B). Caution must therefore be taken to ensure that an overpenetrated film is not misinterpreted as demonstrating radiolucent bone when the radiographic technique used is at fault.

The early diagnosis of osteoporosis can be made only by bone biopsy or sophisticated imaging modalities such as computed tomography or photon absorptiometry, since plain radiographs may not reveal trabecular bone loss until more than 50 percent of the bone mineral content is gone. The common etiologies of general osteoporosis include postmenopausal or senile age, exogenous steroid therapy, alcoholism, chronic liver disease, idiopathic sources, endocrine states (e.g., hyperparathyroidism, Cushing's disease, or hyperthyroidism), and anemic states. Regional osteoporosis can also occur and is most frequently seen secondary to disuse or immobilization of a limb. Local osteoporosis is most often seen in association with arthritis, infection, and tumor (especially metastases).

In osteoporosis, radiographs demonstrate an increased lucency of bone that is best described as osteopenia or a poverty of bone. Since the causes of increased radiolucency of bone — including senile and postmenopausal osteoporosis, tumor, hyperparathyroidism, and osteomalacia — may not be distinguishable from one another with plain radiographs, osteopenia is a more accurate generic term than osteoporosis in cases of such radiolucency because it applies whenever the amount of bone destruction exceeds that of bone production. Looser's zones in osteomalacia, brown tumors or subperiosteal bone re-

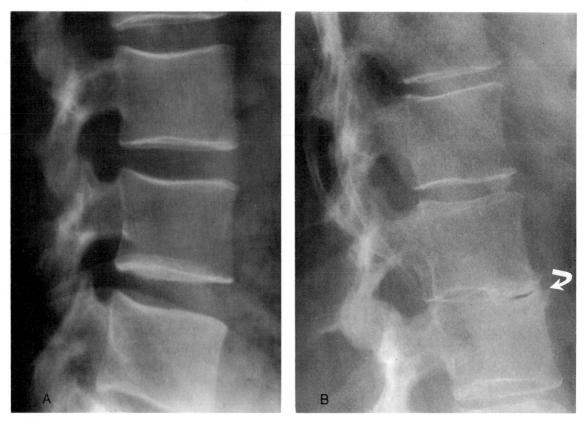

Fig. 5-33 Osteoporosis.
History. This patient had used steroids chronically for asthma.
Findings. **(A)** *Plain radiograph:* A lateral view of the lubar spine in a normal, skeletally mature adult demonstrates normal cortical and trabecular bone. **(B)** *Plain radiograph:* A lateral view of the spine in a patient with osteoporosis. The cortex of the vertebral bodies is as thin as a pencil line, and the interior of the bodies has a ground-glass appearance. Disc space narrowing is seen at one level (arrow).

sorption in hyperparathyroidism, and small, destructive bone lesions in metastatic disease or multiple myeloma are useful for identifying the etiology of the osteopenia. Besides these specific findings, which identify the etiology in a specific case of osteopenia, nonspecific findings are also seen radiographically. These include a decreased number of trabeculae, with thickening of the remaining trabeculae due to reinforcement in response to stress. The loss of trabeculae can be severe enough to give the interiors of the bones an empty appearance (Fig. 5-34 A and B), which is best appreciated in the vertebral bodies. The cortex becomes thin and in the vertebral bodies may be reduced to a thin white line. Fractures are frequently seen in the vertebral bodies, with compression of the end-plates and anterior wedging. The former gives the vertebral bodies a biconcave configuration sometimes referred to as "fish vertebrae" (Fig. 5-35). The latter causes a loss of height and increased thoracic kyphosis which, if severe enough, may reduce the lung volume. Spontaneous fractures of the femoral neck and distal fractures of the radius and ulna are also encountered as frequent complications, particularly of postmenopausal osteoporosis.

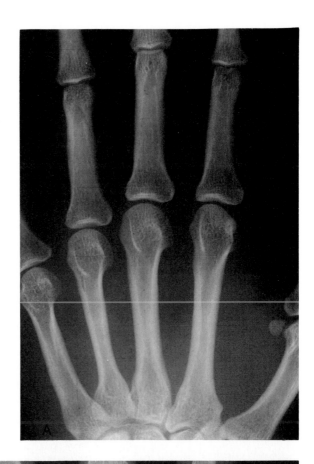

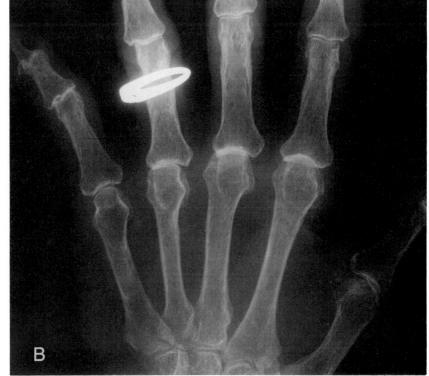

Fig. 5-34 Osteoporosis.
History. This patient was a 70-year-old woman.
Findings. (A) *Plain radiograph:* Normal cortical and trabecular bone is shown in a 34-year-old woman for comparison. **(B)** *Plain radiograph:* This patient has severe thinning of the cortex and a decrease in the number of bone trabeculae at the ends of the bones.

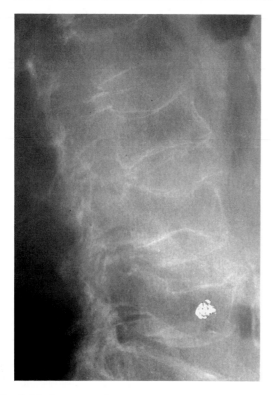

Fig. 5-35 Osteoporosis.
History. This patient had ingested steroids for asthma.
Findings. *Plain radiograph:* Compression fractures of the end-plates of all of the lumbar vertebral bodies has produced the appearance known as "fish vertebrae."

DOES THIS PATIENT HAVE RHEUMATOID ARTHRITIS OR SOME OTHER TYPE OF ARTHRITIS?

Arthritis is a general term used when joints are affected by a host of different disease processes. The patient characteristically experiences stiffness, swelling, and pain in the affected joint(s). Arthritis can conveniently be divided into three categories: degenerative joint disease, inflammatory arthritis, and metabolically induced arthritis. Degenerative joint disease arises from the destruction of cartilage due to trauma, infection, other forms of arthritis, and several miscellaneous causes. Almost all inflammatory arthritis is due to rheumatoid arthritis, rheumatoid variants, infection, and connective-tissue disorders.

Metabolic arthritis is most often due to gout, calcium pyrophosphate dihydrate (CPPD) arthropathy, and hemochromatosis. It results from an abnormal substance deposited in and around the joints, causing localized cartilage and bone erosion. Because the pathologic process is not a primary disease of cartilage and synovium, as contrasted to inflammatory and degenerative arthritis, the joint space remains normal until late in the disease.

An easily remembered and helpful way to approach any joint for determining an arthritic change in it is to evaluate the joint according to the ABCs of arthritis.[3] The ABCs here is mnemonic for alignment, bone mineral, cartilage space, and soft tissue, all of which should be checked when evaluating a joint for potential change due to any type of arthritis. Such an evaluation requires that the observer have a visual image of

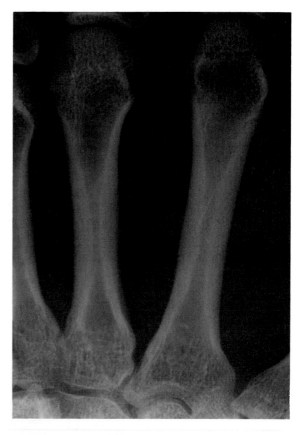

Fig. 5-36 Normal hand. Normal tubular bones of the hand serve as a standard for comparison with the examples of arthritis shown in Figures 5-36 through 5-39.

what a given joint appears like normally. Unfortunately this comes only with time and the repetitive study of many patients. A very detailed and precise image of a normal joint may allow the detection of quite subtle abnormalities, although many arthritic changes are so gross that they are difficult to miss.

Deviations from normal alignment tend to be more easily detected than the other parts of the ABCs mnemonic, probably because even untrained observers have a good idea of what a normal alignment for most joints look like. In long and short tubular bones the outer cortical margin of the bone is smooth and regular (Fig. 5-36). The cortex is thickest at the midpoint of the bone and becomes progressively thinner toward the bone ends until it is only a thin white line covering the metaphyseal and epiphyseal areas. In the latter two areas, individual bone trabeculae, appearing as thin white lines, fill the medullary cavity. In the middle two-thirds or diaphysis, the cortical bone is thickest, the medullary cavity is narrow and has a ground glass density, and individual trabeculae may not be detectable. The bone appears whitest in this area and progressively becomes grayer toward the bone ends. Joint spaces are characteristically of the same width at all points along the articular surface. Comparison with the contralateral normal joint or with an adjacent joint, especially in the hands and feet, can help in detecting subtle differences and reminding

one what a normal joint looks like. Care must be exercised when doing this, since arthritic abnormalities may be symmetrically distributed and involve multiple joints. Normally, the soft tissues around a bone generally follow the contour of the underlying bony prominences. Adjacent to most joints, except small joints in the hands and feet, fat planes can be seen separating individual muscles. Joint effusions may displace these fat planes, and soft-tissue edema will obliterate them.

INFLAMMATORY ARTHRITIS

RHEUMATOID ARTHRITIS

Early rheumatoid arthritis (RA) may present a puzzling diagnostic problem for the clinician and the wish for help from a radiographic examination. The most prominent changes are seen in the hands, wrists, feet, knees, atlantoaxial joint of the cervical spine, acromioclavicular joints, elbows, and glenohumeral joints. One of the most useful diagnostic features of RA is its symmetric distribution between the two sides of the body (Fig. 5-37). If the right third metacarpophalangeal joint is involved, the left third metacarpophalangeal joint is usually also involved. The radiographic changes in RA include fusiform soft-tissue swellings around the affected joints, periarticular (ad-

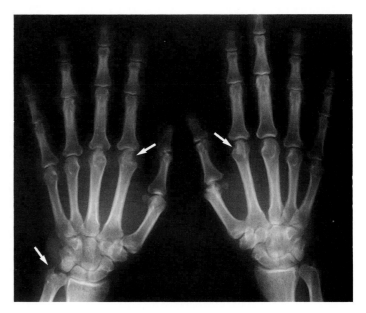

Fig. 5-37 Rheumatoid arthritis.
History. This 35-year-old woman had known RA.
Findings. *Plain radiograph:* There is arthritis of symmetric distribution. There is also soft-tissue swelling of the extensor carpi ulnaris tendon sheath over each ulnar styloid, and fusiform swelling around the proximal interphalangeal joints of the fourth digits. Marginal erosions, without reaction of the adjacent bone, involve several metacarpophalangeal and proximal interphalangeal joints, multiple carpal bones, and each ulnar styloid (arrows).

jacent to the articular surface) osteoporosis, bone ero-sions at joint margins early in the disease and at the central articular surface late in the disease, a uniform loss of the joint space, and either fibrous or bony an-kylosis with joints that are severely involved (Fig. 5-38).

The synovium that lines the joints, bursae, and ten-don sheaths becomes involved by an inflammatory process in RA. The synovial inflammation precipi-tates a surrounding soft-tissue edema and also causes an exudation of fluid into the joint, which manifests itself as a soft-tissue swelling and sometimes as a tran-sient widening of the joint space. These are the earli-est radiographic changes in RA. Hyperemia occurs because of the synovial inflammation. This increased blood flow also involves the bone, causing a more

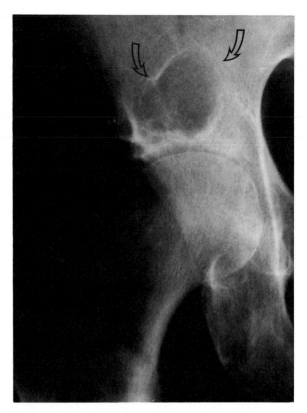

Fig. 5-39 Rheumatoid arthritis.
History. This 64-year-old woman had RA.
Findings. *Plain radiograph:* A large subchondral cyst (arrows) is present. A similar cyst was symmetrically present in the opposite acetabular roof. There is uniform narrowing of the joint space in the superior, axial, and medial direc-tions, with a minimum of reactive bone.

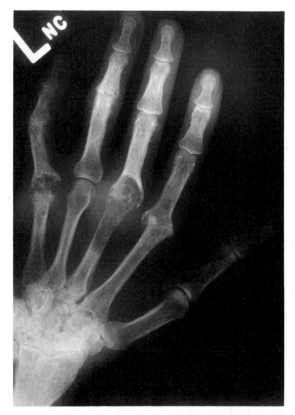

Fig. 5-38 Rheumatoid arthritis.
History. This 57-year-old man had longstanding RA.
Findings. *Plain radiograph:* Severe changes of rheumatoid arthritis are demonstrated, with extensive erosions and ad-jacent soft-tissue swelling in the metacarpophalangeal joints. There is also fusion of most of the carpal bones and loss of the radiocarpal and midcarpal joints. Osteopenia, with thinning of the cortex of most of the bones, is also present.

rapid loss of bone mineral which is seen as periarticu-lar osteoporosis (Figs. 5-37 and 38). This is the second radiographic finding. The inflamed, hypertrophied synovium soon extends from the joint recesses and lining of the joint capsule to the articular cartilage, and eventually covers it. This covering is a hyperemic connective tissue called pannus which interferes with cartilage nutrition provided by the synovial fluid and also releases proteolytic enzymes that destroy the car-tilage. A relatively early radiographic manifestation of the cartilage destruction is a uniform narrowing of the entire joint space. At the margin of the articular cartilage, areas of bare bone are present in many joints. Pannus covers these bare areas in the same way as it does the articular cartilage, and invades it even more readily than the cartilage. The radiographic findings at this stage consist of bone erosions at the margins of the articular cartilage involving the proximal and distal bones of the joint (Fig. 5-37). The erosions usually do not have sclerotic margins unless the disease process has been arrested or slowed by drug therapy. Pannus may also erode through the cartilage and destroy the subchondral bone, forming a cystic area. The resultant cystic structures may be multiple and form clusters, or in large joints such as the hip and knee may become quite large (Fig. 5-39). Radiographically they are located in the subchondral bone and usually do not have sclerotic margins.

Advanced rheumatoid arthritis is characterized by extensive bone erosion and joint deformities including subluxation and dislocation (Fig. 5-40). The osteoarthritic changes occur after cessation of the synovial inflammation but with the continued use of a joint that has damaged cartilage. Friction of the damaged bone ends against one another causes a further destruction of cartilage, subchondral cyst formation,

osteophytes at the joint margins, and thickening and sclerosis of trabeculae in the subchondral bone. Bony ankylosis will occur in some joints, especially the interphalangeal joints of the hands and carpal joints of the wrists, before osteoarthritic changes have a chance to occur (Fig. 5-38). Other joints may develop fibrous ankylosis rather than bony ankylosis.

Tendon sheaths and bursae may also become involved by the synovitis of RA, since they have a synovial lining. They typically fill with exudate from the synovitis and appear radiographically as soft-tissue swellings or masses (Fig. 5-37). A tendon may become involved and be weakened or rupture. Bone resorption contiguous to an inflamed bursa or tendon sheath is commonly seen in the posterior calcaneus and ulnar styloid, respectively.

Many other changes may be seen in rheumatoid arthritis, but those described above are the most com-

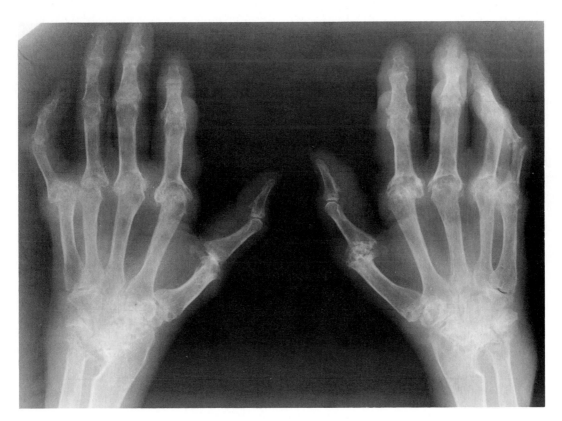

Fig. 5-40 Rheumatoid arthritis.
History. Longstanding RA.
Findings. *Plain radiograph:* There is severe generalized osteoporosis and fusion of most of the carpal bones, extensive erosions in the wrists, metacarpophalangeal joints, and proximal interphalangeal joints, soft-tissue swelling, and protrusion of the metacarpal head into the base of the proximal phalanges (a "mortor and pestal deformity"). Notice the characteristic symmetry of the abnormalities.

mon abnormalities. An understanding of the radiographic findings discussed for RA will form a basis for understanding the structural changes seen in any inflammatory arthritis, which, like RA, will have synovitis as a significant feature.

RHEUMATOID VARIANTS

The three rheumatoid variants or seronegative (rheumatoid-factor-negative) spondyloarthropathies are psoriatic arthritis, Reiter's syndrome, and ankylosing spondylitis. All three share soft-tissue swelling, joint-space narrowing, marginal erosion, and bony ankylosis due to synovial inflammation as common features. The three diseases also demonstrate more severe changes in cartilagenous joints (e.g., sacroiliac and discovertebral joints) than is seen in rheumatoid arthritis, and bone resorption at the site of attachment of tendons or ligaments to bone. With the involvement of synovial joints, the seronegative spondyloarthropathies usually demonstrate a lack of osteoporosis, frequent ankylosis, and bone proliferation adjacent to erosions, which is not seen in rheumatoid arthritis. Ankylosing spondylitis causes conspicuous ankylosis of the sacroiliac joints and parts or all of the spine, producing a characteristic bamboo appearance of the spine (Fig. 5-41 A and B). Reiter's syndrome primarily affects the joints of the lower extremity in an asym-

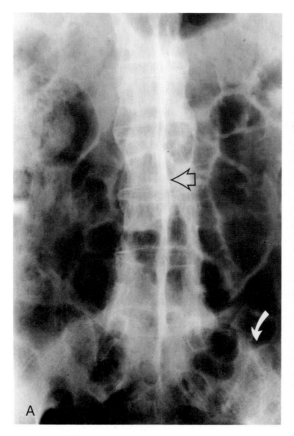
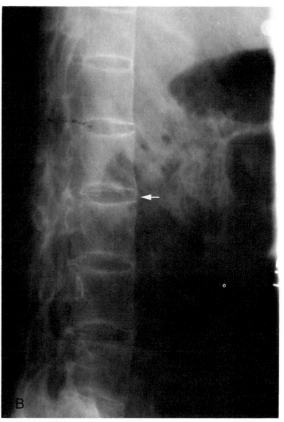

Fig. 5-41 Ankylosing spondylitis.
History. This elderly man had a long history of pelvic and back pain.
Findings. **(A)** *Plain radiograph:* A frontal view shows fusion of the interspinous ligaments (open arrow) and fusion of the sacroiliac joints (closed arrow). **(B)** A lateral view shows squaring of the anterior margins of the vertebral bodies, with fusion of the vertebral bodies by thin vertical bone struts (arrow) called syndesmophytes. The resulting spine is called a bamboo spine because of its appearance.

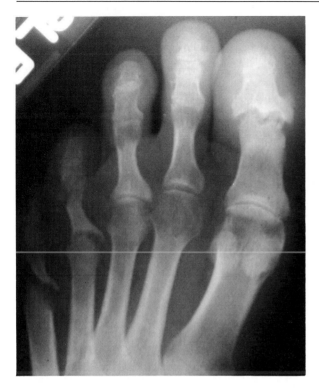

Fig. 5-42 Reiter's arthritis.
History. This young woman had foot and ankle pain.
Findings. Erosions are present on the margins of the interphangeal joints of the great toe and the metatarsophalangeal joints of the fourth and fifth digits. The abnormalites were asymmetrically distributed in the feet.

metric fashion, and may be accompanied by sacroiliitis and spondylitis (Fig. 5-42). Psoriatic arthritis involves the hands, wrists, and feet in a distribution similar to that in rheumatoid arthritis but with less symmetry and with frequent involvement of the distal interphalangeal joints of the hands, which is unusual in RA (Fig. 5-43).

DEGENERATIVE JOINT DISEASE

Degenerative joint disease is the most commonly encountered type of arthritis and is most commonly referred to as osteoarthritis. The factors that predispose to osteoarthritis include chronic and repetitive joint abuse (associated with many athletic enterprises and numerous occupations), single traumatic episodes, chronic abnormal stresses across any joint, underlying

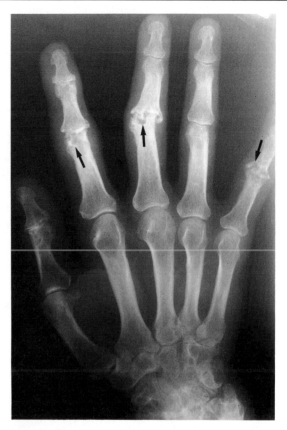

Fig. 5-43 Psoriatic arthritis.
History. This 56-year-old man had joint pain and a long-standing skin rash.
Findings. *Plain radiograph:* Erosions are present in most of the carpal bones, several proximal interphalangeal joints, and in the distal interphalangeal joint of the second digit. Sclerotic margins, from healing reaction of the host bone, are seen around many of the erosions (arrows).

articular abnormalities or incongruities, and prior inflammatory joint disease. In simplest terms, one of the above disease processes produces an area of cartilage destruction. The radiograph demonstrates nonuniform joint-space narrowing at the site of the cartilage loss (see Fig. 5-45). Because the joint cartilage normally acts as a shock absorber for the underlying bone, its loss leads to increased stress on the bone, which responds to the extra stress by laying down new bone on existing trabeculae immediately beneath the cortical surface. This increased bone mass is known as subchondral sclerosis. Next, bony spurs or osteophytes, another form of new bone which are a major feature of osteoarthritis, form at the joint margins

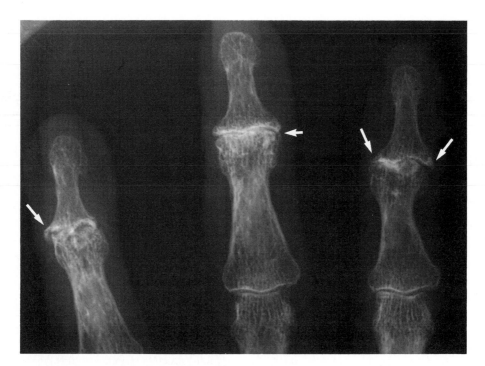

Fig. 5-44 Osteoarthritis.
History. The patient was a 75-year-old woman.
Findings. *Plain radiograph:* The distal interphalangeal joint is one of the most common sites affected by osteoarthritis. Irregular joint-space narrowing, osteophyte formation (arrows), and subchondral-cyst formation are all visible.

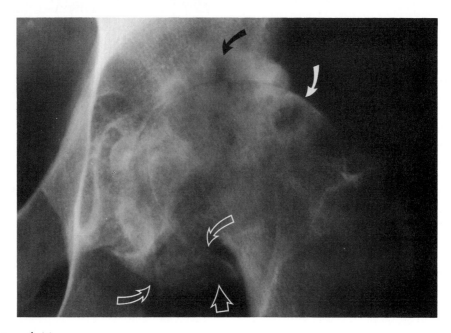

Fig. 5-45 Osteoarthritis.
History. This 59-year-old man had hip pain and stiffness.
Findings. *Plain radiograph:* The joint space is destroyed, with subchondral sclerosis and subchondral cyst formation (closed arrows). There is migration of the femoral head in a superior-lateral direction and the formation of a huge medial osteophyte which is partially intra-articular (open arrows).

(Figs. 5-44, 5-45). Cystic areas called subchondral cysts, which develop immediately beneath the articular surface, are frequently seen (Fig. 5-45), but may also be seen in inflammatory and metabolic arthritis.

METABOLIC ARTHRITIS

GOUT

Gout occurs when the body produces sodium urate faster than it can excrete this salt. The joints most often involved include the interphalangeal joint of the great toe, multiple joints of the feet, ankles, knees, hands, wrists, and elbows. The sodium urate is deposited within the joints and in adjacent soft tissues, producing two characteristic types of soft-tissue change. Effusion and synovitis occur when urate crystals are precipitated into a joint, and a radiographically symmetric, fusiform soft-tissue swelling is seen about joints affected in this way. When the acute arthritic attack resolves, the soft-tissue changes usually also disappear. After many years of recurrent arthritic attacks, accumulations of urates called tophi may collect in soft tissues near the joints, causing the second typical change in gout: eccentric soft-tissue swelling. Such eccentric swelling may be seen adjacent to or at a distance from a joint, and is to be differentiated from the effusion or synovitis that cause symmetric swelling around a joint.

Even in extremely severe cases, bone mineralization and joint alignment remain normal in most patients with gout until late in the disease process. Extensive cartilage and underlying bone erosion can occur in articular surfaces with the adjacent cartilage remaining relatively normal. This accounts for preservation of the normal joint space until the late stages of articular disease even in the presence of extensive erosion. In gout, as opposed to rheumatoid arthritis, a dense bone reaction is stimulated around bone erosions (Fig. 5-46). A lip or shell of bone that acts as a covering for a tophus may extend into the soft tissues from erosions at the margin of a joint or at some distance from the joint. This is seen in approximately 40 percent of patients with gouty erosions and is called an overhanging margin (Fig. 5-46). When present, it strongly suggests gouty arthritis. If the tophus is deposited into a bone, a cystic area with a sclerotic margin is produced. Uniform joint-space narrowing may occur late in the disease and is most often seen in the hands, wrists, feet, and knees. Anky-

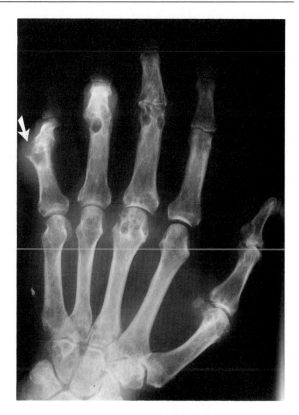

Fig. 5-46 Gout.
History. This patient had uncontrollable gout for many years.
Findings. *Plain radiograph:* There are extensive erosions, with an overhanging margin in the fifth digit (arrow). There are also flexion deformities in the fourth and fifth digits. Joint space narrowing is not a prominent feature of gout, which helps to differentiate it radiographically from rheumatoid arthritis.

losis may occur but is rare except in the intercarpal joints and interphalangeal joints of the hands and feet. A mutilating arthritis, indistinguishable from that produced by extremely severe RA or psoriatic arthritis, is occasionally seen in the hands and feet.

DOES THIS PATIENT HAVE EVIDENCE OF AVASCULAR NECROSIS?

The question of possible avascular necrosis usually arises because the patient has pain in or around the hip, shoulder, ankle, or wrist. The terms aseptic necrosis, avascular necrosis, and ischemic necrosis all refer to

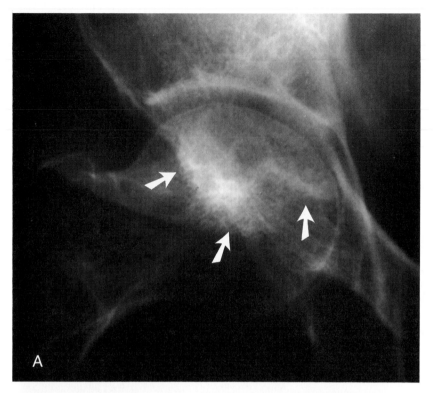

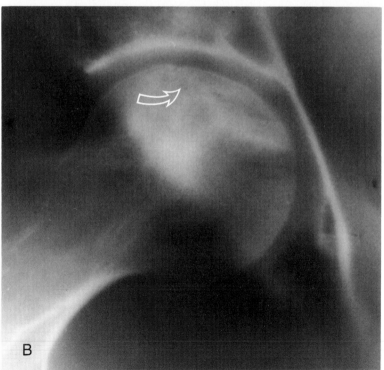

Fig. 5-47 Avascular necrosis. **History.** This patient had sickle cell anemia. **Findings. (A)** *Plain radiograph:* The healing changes of osteonecrosis or avascular necrosis of the femoral head have produced a wedge-shaped area of sclerosis (arrows) with a central lucency. This is a frog-leg lateral view of the hip, which is especially useful for visualizing osteonecrosis in the femoral head even when it may be difficult to see in an anterior-posterior view. **(B)** *Tomogram of the hip:* There is a crescent sign (open arrow). The extent of osteonecrosis and the rim of sclerotic healing are more clearly seen than in the plain radiograph. **(C)** *Follow-up plain radiograph:* Progressive collapse of the femoral head has eventually led to flattening of the superior articular surface and the rapid development of osteoarthritis in the joint.

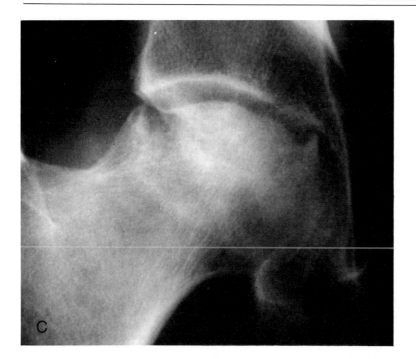

osteonecrosis or death of bone in the subarticular or epiphyseal areas, whereas bone infarction is usually reserved for osteonecrosis of the metaphyseal and diaphyseal areas. Bone death is caused by impaired or arrested blood flow due to the physical disruption, intraluminal occlusion, or external compression of arteries, capillaries, sinusoids, or veins. The most common causes of ischemic necrosis are exogenous steroids, traumatic interruption of the vascular supply, alcoholism, hemoglobinopathies, Gaucher's disease, irradiation, dysbaric injuries, and idiopathic states.

The first stage in osteonecrosis is cellular death within the bone. This can be seen with a biopsy specimen, but causes no change in the radiographic appearance of the bone. There is no radiographic evidence of a change in dead bone until the repair process appears many weeks or months after the death of the osteocytes. An inflammatory response to breakdown products from dying and dead cells is initiated, with a proliferation of capillaries and mesenchymal cells and an increase in blood flow to the adjacent area of viable bone. Radiographically this appears as osteopenia in the viable bone; the dead bone remains unchanged in density. After a period of time the dead bone will be more dense than the viable surrounding bone since it does not share the hyperemia and resulting osteoporosis of the viable bone. A transitional zone between the dead and normal bone develops and is an area of repair in which dead tissues are being actively resorbed. New living bone is first laid down on the dead trabecular bone, which is subsequently resorbed and replaced by new trabeculae. In the femoral head, which is the most important site of osteonecrosis, the transitional zone also extends into the subchondral area. The transitional zone is weak because of bone resorption, and the subchondral area may ultimately not be strong enough to support weight bearing. In such a case a subchondral fracture called a crescent sign (Fig. 5-47 A and B) will first occur, and with continued weight bearing the fracture fragment will collapse or settle, causing flattening of the femoral head. Eventually, changes of severe degenerative arthritis develop in the affected joint because of the deformity of the femoral head. The collapse of affected bone may not occur in other, non-weight-bearing bones (Fig. 5-47C). The repair process takes many months or years, and may stagnate for no apparent reason before it is complete.

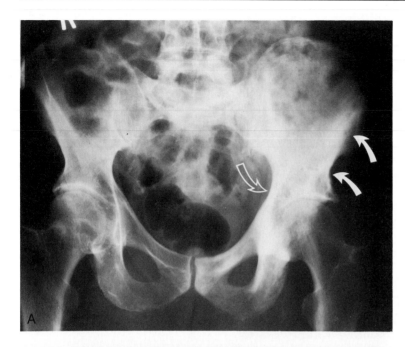

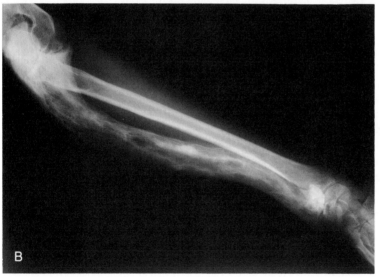

Fig. 5-48 Paget's disease.
History. This 79-year-old man had pelvic pain.
Findings. *Plain radiograph:* **(A)** This is the mixed stage of Paget's disease of the left hemipelvis, with most severe involvement in the iliac bone. Compare the thickened bone traveculae (arrows) and the bony sclerosis of the left innominate bone with those on the normal right side of the pelvis. The left innominate bone has enlarged modestly in most areas as compared to the right bone if the corresponding bone diameter is measured. **(B)** The forearm of the same patient demonstrates a more destructive phase of the mixed lytic-sclerotic stage of Paget's disease in the ulna. There is extensive bowing and expansion of the bone, loss of the normally clear distinction between the cortex and medullary cavity, and overgrowth of the bone length, causing interference with normal function of the wrist and a consequent osteoarthritis. There is no area of the bone which is not involved. Compare the ulna with the normal bone of the adjacent radius. This type of distribution of Paget's disease allows its differentiation from metastatic disease.

IS THIS PAGET'S DISEASE OR METASTASIS FROM PROSTATE CARCINOMA?

Paget's disease is of unknown etiology and rarely seen in patients under age 40, but occurs with a progressively increasing incidence thereafter. It causes an increase of severalfold in the bone turnover rate and an abnormal remodeling of bone. Early in the disease bone resorption is the most prominent feature, with large areas of bone lysis or destruction. The areas most often involved include the skull, spine, pelvis, and long bones, although no bone is exempt. In tubular bones the osteolysis begins almost exclusively at one end and progresses toward the opposite end. The advancing edge of osteolysis forms a V-shaped or flame-shaped lucency which is clearly differentiated from adjacent normal bone. The bone attempts to repair itself, but the abnormal bone that is produced results in an intermediate stage with a mixture of lytic and sclerotic areas (Fig. 5-48 A and B). This repair with abnormal bone results in coarsening of the trabeculae, an enlarged diameter of the bone, cortical thickening, and eventually a loss of clear differentiation between the cortex and medullary cavity of long bones. In the late stage of Paget's disease osteolysis is absent, and only an increased bone density or osteosclerosis remains. Despite its density, the bone is much weaker and softer than normal bone, and may easily fracture or bow (Fig. 5-48B).

Patients with Paget's disease may develop skeletal, neuromuscular, or cardiac complications. The skeletal complications include fractures, the bowing of long bones, increasing kyphosis, and protrusio acetabuli. Platybasia and vertebral-body fractures occur and cause bone impingement on the spinal cord, with neurologic deficits resulting in muscle weakness, incontinence, and even paralysis. The increased blood flow to the abnormal pagetic bone may cause a high-output congestive heart failure.

The early lytic stage of Paget's disease may be confused with other destructive lesions including metastases. Extension of the disease process to the end of a bone and the sharply defined, flame-shaped advancing osteolysis should distinguish it from lesions of other etiology. Clinicians frequently bring osteosclerotic cases of Paget's disease to the radiologist to confirm that it is not metastatic disease. The coarsened trabeculae, enlargement of bone, bowing of long bones, extension of the involvement to the ends of long bones, and confinement of the disease to one hemipelvis or unilaterally to a long bone are seen only in Paget's disease, and allow its differentiation from sclerotic metastases.

SUGGESTED READINGS

1. Bonakdar-pour A, Gaines VD: The radiology of osteomyelitis. Orthop Clin North Am 14:21–38, 1983
2. Dahlin DC: Bone Tumors. 3rd Ed. Charles C Thomas, Springfield, IL, 1978
3. Forrester DM, Brown JC, Nesson JW: The Radiology of Joint Disease. 2nd Ed. WB Saunders, Philadelphia, 1978
4. Glimcher MJ, Kenzora JE: The biology of osteonecrosis of the human femoral head and its clinical implications. Clin Orthop Rel Res 138:284–309, 139:283–312, 140:273–312, 1979
5. Jowsey J: Metabolic Diseases of Bone. WB Saunders, Philadelphia, 1977
6. Juhl JH: Essentials of Roentgen Interpretation. 4th Ed. Harper & Row, Philadelphia, 1981
7. Kricun ME: Radiographic evaluation of solitary bone lesions. Orthop Clin North Am 14:39–64, 1983
8. Murray RO, Jacobson HG: The Radiology of Skeletal Disorders. 2nd Ed. Churchill Livingstone, New York, 1977
9. Resnick R, Niwayama G: Diagnosis of Bone and Joint Disorders. WB Saunders, Philadelphia, 1981
10. Rockwood CA, Green DP: Fractures. JB Lippincott, Philadelphia, 1975
11. Rogers LF: Radiology of Skeletal Trauma. Churchill Livingstone, New York, 1982
12. Wilner D: Bone Tumors. WB Saunders, Philadelphia, 1982

6

Radiology of the Cardiovascular System

Lee Sider

The chest radiograph is often the first and certainly the most familiar view of the heart. It provides information on gross cardiac enlargement, abnormal cardiac calcifications (valvular, coronary artery, aneurysmal), gross deviations in cardiac contour associated with definite chamber or vessel enlargement (aortic aneurysm), the presence of congestive heart failure, and the status of the pulmonary vascularity (left-to-right shunting lesions or right-to-left shunting lesions).[1]

The cardiac anatomy is easily understood from the frontal and lateral views of the chest. The frontal or posterior-anterior (PA) film shows the right heart border to be formed mainly by the right atrium and the left heart border to be formed mainly by the left ventricle (Fig. 6-1). The right ventricle lies anteriorly and forms the anterior cardiac border as seen on the lateral film. The posterior heart border on the lateral film is made up of the more superior left atrium and more inferior left ventricle (Fig. 6-2).

A gross determination of heart size can be made on the frontal film. The greatest horizontal diameter of the heart is compared to the greatest horizontal diameter of the thoracic cavity (Fig. 6-3). The diameter of the normal-sized heart is less than half the measured diameter of the thoracic cavity. If the transverse diameter of the heart is greater than half, this suggests cardiac enlargement (cardiomegaly). Besides there being an increase in the overall heart size, the configuration or shape of the heart may change, signifying ventricular hypertrophy. The different chambers of the heart can individually enlarge or hypertrophy under different hemodynamic stresses, leading to specific alterations of the different heart borders. This is

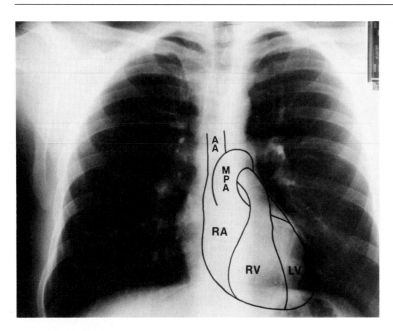

Fig. 6-1 Chamber location in a PA chest radiograph. The right atrium (RA) forms the right heart border. The right ventricle (RV) makes up the bulk of the cardiac shadow and lies anteriorly. A portion of the left ventricle (LV) projects slightly anteriorly to form the left heart border. Also note the position of the main pulmonary artery (MPA) and ascending aorta (AA).

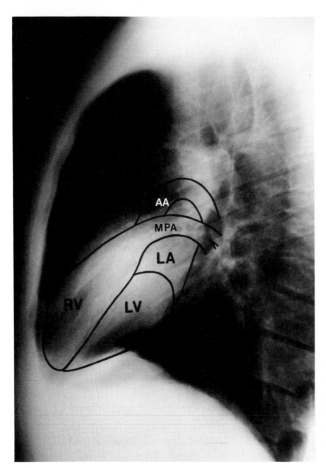

Fig. 6-2 Chamber location in a lateral chest radiograph. The right ventricle (RV) forms the anterior cardiac border. The left atrium (LA) and left ventricle (LV) form the posterior cardiac borders. The left ventricle forms the inferior base of the heart. Also note the postion of the main pulmonary artery (MPA) and ascending aorta (AA).

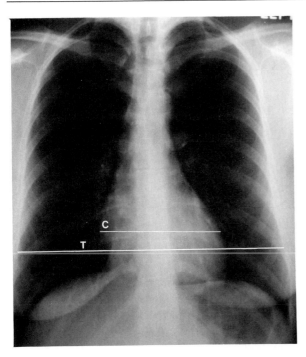

Fig. 6-3 Cardiac size determination. The cardiac diameter (C) is less than half the thoracic diameter (T), signifying a normal-sized heart.

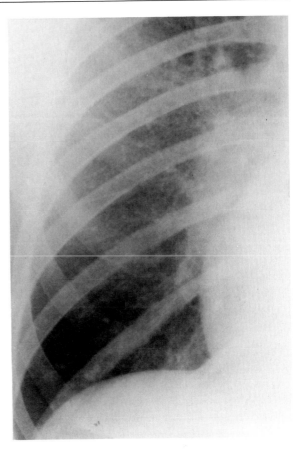

Fig. 6-4 Prominence of pulmonary vascularity, passive. This view of the right lung field shows a hazy prominence of the pulmonary vascularity as the pulmonary veins engorge in congestive heart failure.

appreciated in mitral valvular disease, in which there is predominant enlargement of the left atrium[2] (see Fig. 6-15 A and B).

The term "pulmonary vessels" refers to both the pulmonary veins and pulmonary arteries. Prominence of the pulmonary venous system is seen in congestive heart failure as the result of a secondary increase in venous pressure as the left ventricle fails. The engorged pulmonary veins are classically described as being hazy and indistinct in their outline (Fig. 6-4). On the other hand, pulmonary arterial prominence results from the preferential flow of blood into the lower pressure pulmonary arterial circulation from the higher pressure systemic circulation, usually as a result of intracardiac congenital lesions (left-to-right shunts). These left-to-right shunts result in an increase in the total volume of blood flowing through the lungs. The pulmonary arteries are dilated and appear prominent centrally and well into the periphery of the lungs; the dilated arteries remain sharp and distinct[3] (Fig. 6-5). The difference in pulmonary vessel appearance may be helpful in distinguishing

venous from arterial engorgement in a good-quality examination. A decrease in the amount of blood flow to the pulmonary arteries due to an outflow obstruction of the right ventricle and associated septal defect results in a generalized hyperlucency of the lungs as only a small amount of blood reaches the pulmonary arteries, with the preponderance instead shunted to the left side of the heart (right-to-left shunt). Pulmonary hypertension results in a chest-radiographic appearance of scanty peripheral pulmonary vascularity, producing hyperlucent lungs along with dilated central pulmonary arterial segments (Fig. 2-54).

The aorta is clearly imaged on the chest radiograph. Thoracic aneurysms, aortic tortuousity, and congeni-

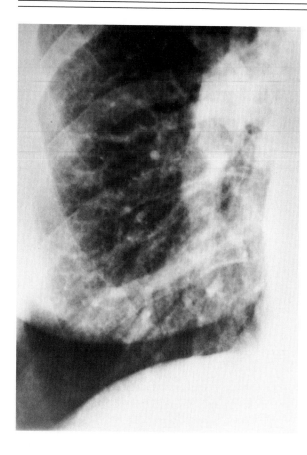

Fig. 6-5 Prominence of pulmonary vascularity, active. Although the pulmonary arteries are prominent, they remain distinct and individually defined in this patient with a left-to-right shunt (VSD).

tal anomalies (right-sided aortic arch) are easily detected by chest radiography.

Lastly, the bony anatomy, as seen on the chest radiograph, can often aid in the diagnosis of a cardiovascular anomaly. The ribs may be notched (coarctation of the aorta, Fig. 6-23), missing, or amputated, with the last indicating a previous thoracotomy for cardiac repair.

The cardiac anatomy, aorta, and pulmonary arteries are clearly visualized as a result of the axial orientation of CT (Fig. 6-6). Computed tomography is very helpful in studying the aorta for the presence and extent of aneurysms or dissecting hematomas. Pericardial effusions and pericardial thickening can also often be detected by CT scanning.

Echocardiography is done in either a one- or two-dimensional format, termed M mode or 2-D echocardiography, respectively. Echocardiography allows excellent evaluation of atrial or ventricular size and valvular integrity and motion, and permits the detection of even small amounts of pericardial fluid. Echo-

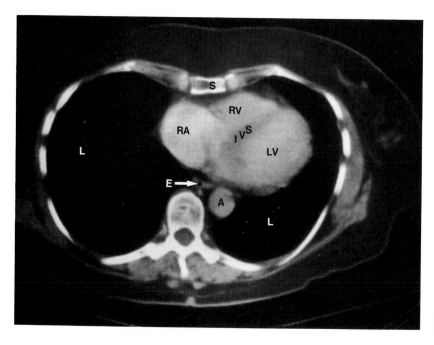

Fig. 6-6 Normal CT scan through the heart. RA = right atrium, RV = right ventricle, LV = left ventricle, A = descending aorta, E = esophagus, L = lung fields, S = sternum, IVS = interventricular septum.

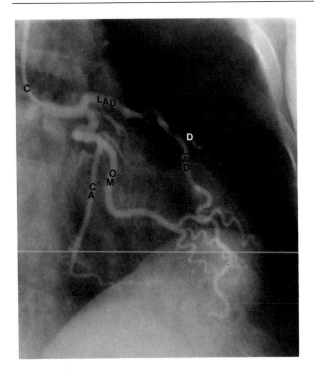

Fig. 6-7 Normal cardiac catheterization, left coronary artery. The tip of the catheter is in the main trunk of the left coronary artery in this oblique view. C = catheter in the aorta, LAD = left anterior descending artery, D = diagonal artery, OM = obtuse marginal artery, CA = circumflex artery.

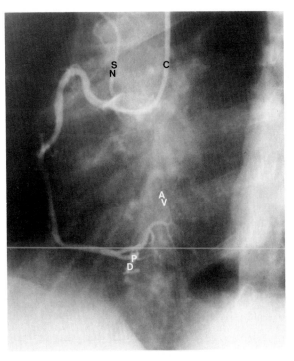

Fig. 6-8 Normal cardiac catheterization, right coronary artery. The tip of the catheter is in the main trunk of the Right coronary artery in this oblique view. C = catheter in the aorta, SN = branch to the sinus node, PD = posterior descending artery, AV = atrioventricular nodal artery.

cardiography is, however, beyond the scope of this text and will not be presented in much detail.

Angiography of the heart has long been the most specific and sensitive means of evaluating various forms of cardiac disease. Also called cardiac catheterization, it consists of two examinations. Under fluoroscopic control a catheter is positioned from its entry into the femoral artery or vein, or an arm vessel, into a chamber of the heart. An injection of a large bolus of iodinated contrast medium is made. The images of the contrast-filled chambers are recorded throughout the cardiac cycle on special cine-film, which provides a format similar to that of a motion picture. Subsequent viewing of the film sequence in a motion picture format results in information on cardiac dynamics (ejection fraction), wall motion, valvular function (stenosis or insufficiency), and the nature and severity of a suspected congenital heart disease.

The second part of a cardiac catheterization is the selective catheterization and injection of iodinated contrast medium into the left or right main coronary artery to detect and quantify the extent of coronary artery disease. The coronary arteries arise from the proximal ascending aorta. The left coronary artery branches into two major divisions: the left anterior descending and the circumflex arteries. The left anterior descending artery lies in a groove between the left and right ventricular chambers. The circumflex artery travels to the posterior wall of the heart in a groove that separates the left atrium and left ventricle (Fig. 6-7). The right coronary artery passes between the right atrium and ventricle to supply the posterior portion of the heart. In 70 percent of cases the right coronary artery gives rise to the posterior descending artery to supply the posterior portion of the interventricular septum (Fig. 6-8).

Most recently magnetic resonance has been utilized to allow views of the heart and aorta in many different projections. MR gives information on chamber size, the presence of congenital anomilies and intra-chamber masses or blood clots.

Angiography of the aorta is the most sensitive method for studying this great vessel for the severity of atherosclerotic disease and in suspected instances of aortic aneurysm or dissection. Angiography of the aorta is also generally performed before a selective catheterization of the individual abdominal arteries, in order to obtain an overview of the abdominal anatomy (Fig. 6-9).

Peripheral vascular narrowing or occlusion from atherosclertic disease, or less commonly from embolic disease, is best studied by peripheral angiography. After the introduction of the angiographic catheter, iodinated contrast medium is injected into the distal aorta. The flow of contrast medium is followed and recorded on x-ray film as the medium is carried by the blood from the distal aorta to the distal branches of the femoral artery, popliteal artery, and eventually to the

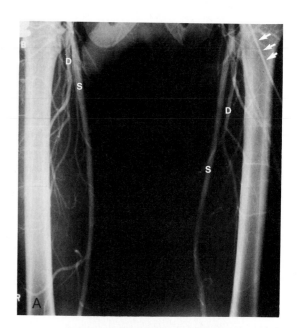

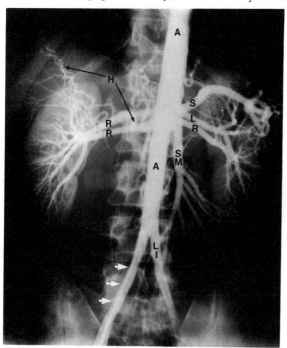

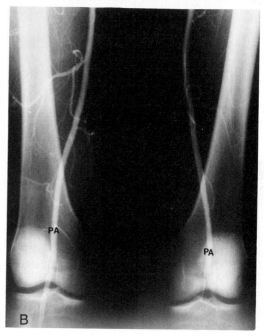

Fig. 6-9 Normal aortogram. The aorta is visualized with iodinated contrast medium introduced via a catheter that enters the right femoral artery and passes into the iliac artery and finally the aorta (arrows). LI = left iliac artery, A = aorta, S = splenic artery, H = hepatic artery, RR = two right renal arteries, LR = two left renal arteries, SM = superior mesenteric artery.

Fig. 6-10 Normal lower extremity angiogram.
Findings. *Peripheral Angiogram:* **(A)** An initial view at the level of the hips and thighs demonstrates the normal superficial (S) and deep (D) femoral arteries. The catheter that is entering the left superficial artery is also identified (arrows). **(B)** At the level of the knees there is opacification of the popliteal arteries (PA).

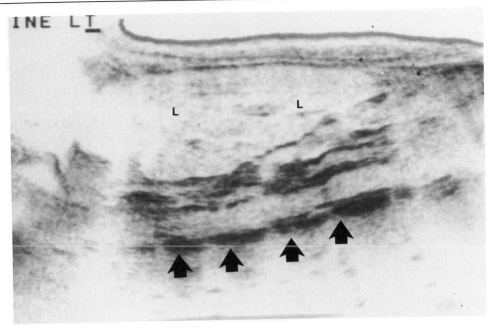

Fig. 6-11 Normal aorta, ultrasound. Longitudinal view of the left side of the abdomen, including a view of the liver (L), shows the posteriorly lying aorta with its thick muscular wall (arrows).

arteries of the lower leg and foot (Fig. 6-10 A and B).

Ultrasound is a noninvasive procedure that can quickly confirm a suspected aortic aneurysm. The patent lumen of the aorta, as well as any adherent clot, are well imaged (Fig. 6-11).

Nuclear medicine studies are playing a growing role in the evaluation of cardiovascular disease. There are three basic examinations in common use. Intravenous thallium has been coupled with the familiar stress electrocardiogram (ECG) to increase the sensi-

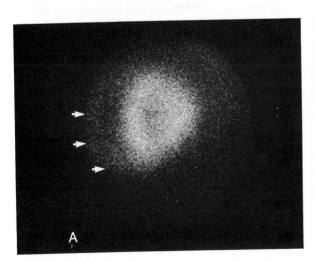
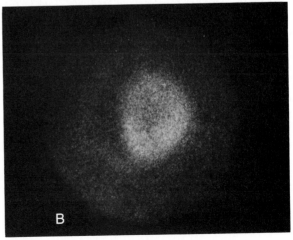

Fig. 6-12 Normal thallium stress test. **(A)** Initial stress vies show an intense uptake of thallium, predominantly in the doughnut shape of the left ventricle. A slight right ventricular activity is also noted (arrows). **(B)** Rest views obtained a few hours later show less intense but homogeneous activity about the left ventricle.

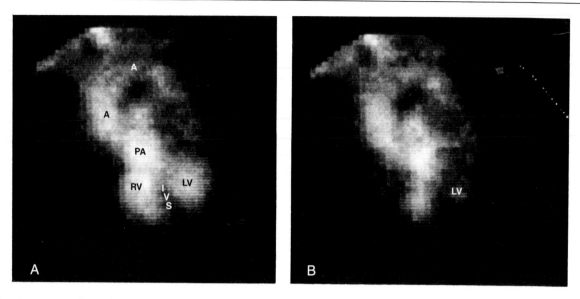

Fig. 6-13 Normal gated-pool ventriculogram. **(A)** Diastole of the heart, with activity filling the chambers of the heart. LV = left ventricle, RV = right ventricle, IVS = interventricular septum, A = aorta, PA = pulmonary artery. **(B)** Note that during systole the left ventricle (LV) contracts diffusely, squeezing out all of its contents, both blood and radiopharmecutical.

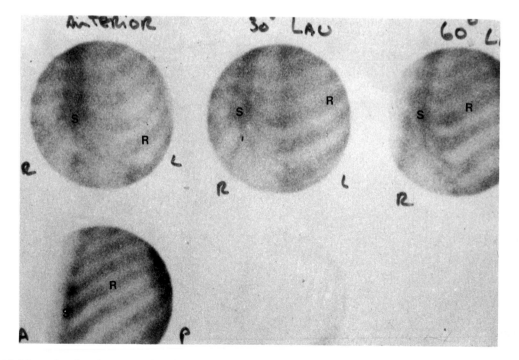

Fig. 6-14 Normal technetium pyrophosphate myocardial scan. Multiple projections over the side of the chest show activity in the ribs (R) and sternum (S), but no activity over the heart. (Courtesy of Dr. Stewart Spies.)

tivity and specificity of this examination as well as to allow accurate identification of the location of an ischemic portion of the heart (Fig. 6-12 A and B). A gated pool study allows a noninvasive alternative to cardiac catheterization in order to quantitate the ejection fraction and detect abnormal wall motion. The patient's red blood cells are removed, tagged with radioactive technetium in the laboratory, and then reintroduced intravenously. With the aid of a computer and ECG, the heart is imaged at various points during the cardiac cycle (Fig. 6-13 A and B), and the images are played back in a continuous motion-picture-like format. Technetium pyrophosphate is a radiopharmaceutical used to detect recent myocardial infarctions (MIs) when the patient's symptoms, ECG or laboratory values are confusing or contradictory (Fig. 6-14).

CLINICAL PRESENTATION: CARDIOMEGALY (ALGORITHM 6-1)

One of the most familiar examples of cardiovascular disease in medicine is an enlarged heart on a chest radiograph. Congestive heart failure, one of the most common causes of an enlarged heart, has been previously discussed. The enlarged heart of ischemic heart disease with or without accompanying congestive heart failure will be discussed in the next section. The other etiologies are varied and are presented below.

HYPERTENSION

The heart enlarges in response to longstanding hypertension as a result of an increased workload forced on the left ventricle. There is predominant enlargement of the left ventricle, resulting in an inferiorly oriented elongation of the apex of the heart. In hypertension, the aortic knob may enlarge while the aorta becomes increasingly tortuous.

MITRAL VALVULAR DISEASE

Rheumatic fever is a disease that predominantly affects connective tissues and blood vessels. The heart is frequently the only organ that has any residual or permanent damage. The incidence of rheumatic heart disease has been steadily declining in the last 30 years, making it much less common than ischemic or hypertensive heart disease.

Acutely, rheumatic fever affects children and is often mild or obscure in its cardiac symptomatology. However, an acute carditis may appear. The radiograph in cases of acute carditis may initially demonstrate a symmetrical enlargement of the heart, but with no evidence of pulmonary edema.

The acute carditis usually subsides, with no significant alteration of ventricular myocardial function. Valvular alterations, however, are very common sequlae. The mitral valve is the most commonly affected valve (60 percent of cases) followed by aortic valve (10 percent), a combination of aortic valve and mitral valve (30 percent), and finally the tricuspid valve (5 percent).[4]

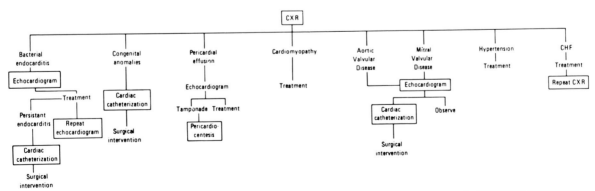

CLINICAL PRESENTATION: CARDIOMEGALY

Algorithm 6-1

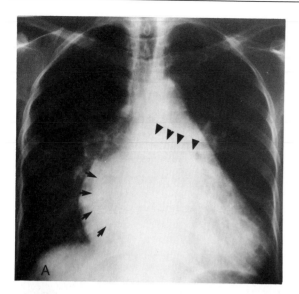

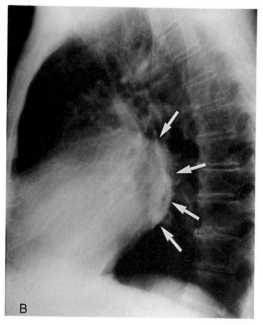

Fig. 6-15 Mitral valve disease.
History. This 47-year-old woman had had rheumatic fever as a child.
Findings. (A) *Frontal chest radiograph:* The heart is enlarged, with a straightening of the left heart border. A suggestion of a double density is seen through the heart from an enlarged left atrium (arrows). The left mainstem bronchus is elevated (arrowheads). The pulmonary circulation is engorged from chronic congestive heart failure. **(B)** *Lateral chest radiograph:* The enlarged chamber is identified in a superior and posterior position—the expected location of the left atrium (arrows).

Mitral stenosis is the most common valvular lesion resulting from prior rheumatic fever. The valve opening becomes narrowed or stenosed by scar tissue, leaving a small, slitlike opening. The valve leaflet itself thickens, resulting in its abnormal movement and incomplete closure. This combination leads to a reduction in the total amount of blood that can leave the left atrium for the left ventricle. This relative obstruction in turn results in increased pressure and subsequent enlargement of the nonmuscular left atrium. Eventually, this increased pressure extends to the pulmonary veins, with the development of chronic pulmonary venous congestion.

On the chest radiograph the heart shows the classic changes of significant left atrial enlargement along with a normal-sized left ventricle. The enlarged left atrium casts a shadow seen through the heart on the frontal film and leading to a "double density." The enlarged left atrium also causes the tracheal bifurcation to be widened as it lifts the neighboring left mainstem bronchus superiorly (Fig. 6-15A). The left atrial appendage may be displaced and dilated, and can be seen as a prominent bulge of the left cardiac border, lying inferior to the pulmonary artery. The lateral film confirms the left atrial enlargement by demonstrating the posteriorly and superiorly dilated left atrium (Fig. 6-15B). Calcification of the diseased mitral valve can frequently also be detected. The aortic knob may be barely visible as a reduced volume of blood reaches the left ventricle and is subsequently delivered to the aorta. The pulmonary veins are in a state of chronic engorgement, which may eventually result in the laying down of hemosiderin in the interstitial supporting network, with a secondary fibrosis. This fibrosis appears in the form of fine-granular opacities in the mid- and lower lung fields.

Echocardiography and angiography are used for further evaluation, especially if surgery is required. The postoperative chest radiograph may demonstrate a regression of the chronic failure pattern and some decrease in heart size. A prosthetic mitral valve can be identified in its expected location.

Along with the mitral stenosis, mitral insufficiency is another frequent sequel of rheumatic heart disease. The insufficiency may also be present following the rupture of a chorda tendinea or with papillary muscle dysfunction following an MI.

The chest radiograph shows a markedly dilated left atrium as the left ventricular blood regurgitates into

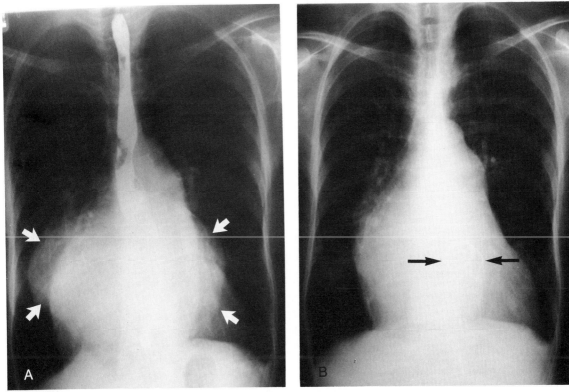

Fig. 6-16 Mitral insufficiency.
History. This 64-year-old woman had known and longstanding mitral insufficiency.
Findings. **(A)** *Chest radiograph:* The left atrium is markedly enlarged and is projected beyond both borders of the heart (arrows). There is barium in the esophagus, demonstrating the secondary pressure on the proximally located esophagus from the dilated left atrium. The left ventricle is also enlarged. **(B)** *Chest radiograph:* Three months later, after mitral valve replacement, the left atrium has diminished significantly in size. The prosthetic valve is in place (arrows).

the left atrium during systole, resulting in an increased atrial volume. In mitral insufficiency, as opposed to mitral stenosis, the left ventricle also enlarges as it receives an initially large blood volume from the dilated left atrium during diastole. The pulmonary vascularity is not engorged. There is usually no significant obstruction to the entry of blood into the left ventricle. Subsequently, there is no pressure elevation in the left atrium or pulmonary veins (Fig. 6-16 A and B).

Views of the left ventricle obtained at the time of cardiac catheterization confirm the diagnosis of mitral regurgitation. There is visualized a jet of contrast medium from the left ventricle into the dilated left

atrium during systole, through an incompetent seal of the diseased mitral valve.

AORTIC VALVULAR DISEASE

Aortic stenosis may arise from congenital anomalies (bicuspid valve) or be acquired later in life. When it is secondary to rheumatic fever there is always associated mitral valvular disease. Atherosclerosis may also result in aortic stenosis.

The heart, on the chest radiograph, is usually of normal size, since the muscular left ventricle thickens instead of dilates (like the left atrium) in response to obstruction of blood flow through the narrowed aor-

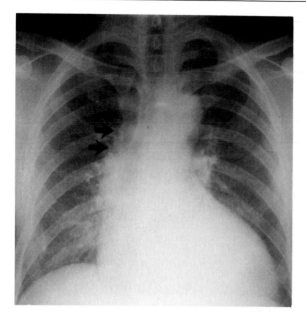

Fig. 6-17 Aortic stenosis.
History. This 54-year-old man had congenital aortic stenosis.
Findings. *Chest radiograph:* The left ventricle is enlarged. There is some widening of the right mediastinal border from poststenotic dilatation of the ascending aorta (arrows). There are also superimposed changes of mild congestive heart failure.

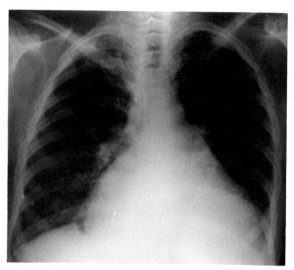

Fig. 6-18 Cardiomyopathy.
History. This 54-year-old woman was receiving chemotherapy with Adriamycin for carcinoma of the colon. A chest radiograph 3 months earlier had been normal.
Findings. *Chest radiograph:* The heart is enlarged and "floppy" in appearance. There is pulmonary venous congestion from a superimposed congestive heart failure.

tic valve. The most proximal portion of the ascending aorta may dilate as blood flow through the valve becomes turbulent and disorganized. This is called poststenotic dilatation of the aorta (Fig. 6-17). Calcification of the stenosed aortic valve is seen in 85 percent of cases.[5]

CARDIOMYOPATHY

The causes of cardiomyopathy are varied, but all lead to the same hemodynamic and subsequent radiographic changes. The etiologies may be divided into those causing primary myocardial impairment (postpartum cardiomyopathy, alcoholic cardiomyopathy); infectious involvement of the myocardium (e.g., by Coxsackie virus); infiltrative processes (amyloidosis, glycogen storage disease); endocrine imbalances (hyperthyroidism, Cushing's disease); and neuromuscular disorders (muscular dystrophy).

The chest film shows a markedly dilated heart with predominantly left ventricular and left atrial enlarge-

ment. The left ventricle becomes an ineffective pump, leading to secondary congestive heart failure and pulmonary edema (Fig. 6-18). The aorta is often small since the cardiac output from the left ventricle is reduced.[6]

PERICARDITIS/PERICARDIAL EFFUSION

Pericardial effusions also have various etiologies. The fluid can be a transudate (as in congestive heart failure), an exudate (as in infectious disease), or sanginous (as in metastatic disease). Both the rate at which the pericardial fluid accumulates and the total amount of pericardial effusion determine the severity of the symptoms. Chest pain and a friction rub constitute the milder symptoms, while large effusions may lead to congestive heart failure and shock.

The chest radiograph shows enlargement of the cardiac silhouette after the accumulation of 200 cc of effusion fluid. The heart appears enlarged, and has

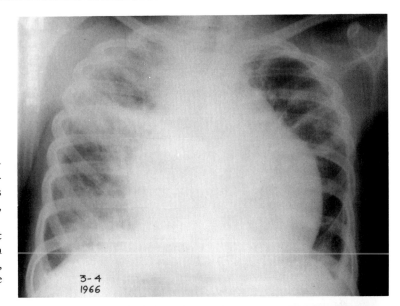

Fig. 6-19 Pericardial effusion.
History. This 68-year-old man with carcinoma of the colon presented with a progressive shortness of breath. A previous chest radiograph, done 3 months earlier, had been normal.
Findings. *Chest radiograph:* The heart size is markedly enlarged. In addition there is pulmonary venous congestion, consistent with a secondary congestive heart failure.

been described as having a "water bottle" shape (Fig. 6-19). The chest radiograph is often diagnostic when a grossly enlarged heart appears following the finding of a normal-sized heart on a previous study. Congestive heart failure may be noticeably absent.

The echocardiogram remains the most sensitive and specific examination for the detection or confirmation of a pericardial effusion. As little as 60 cc of effusion need be present to be detected by echocardiography.

With large effusions or rapidly accumulating moderate effusions there may be impairment of systemic venous return to the right atrium. This leads to a diminished cardiac output, hypotension, and finally circulatory shock. This is termed cardiac tamponade. The chest radiograph may be normal and show no change in the shape of the cardiac silhouette if the accumulation of pericardial fluid is rapid. Cardiac tamponade is frequently seen following penetrating trauma such as a stab wound.

Constrictive pericarditis produces a scarred pericardium that results in restriction of the normal heart movements. Tuberculosis remains the most common etiology for this condition. The chest radiograph may show pericardial calcifications in over half of all cases (Fig. 6-20). The shape of the cardiac silhouette is normal in half of cases, with mild to moderate cardiac

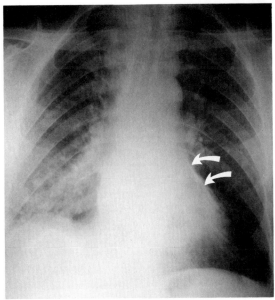

Fig. 6-20 Constrictive pericarditis.
History. This 52-year-old man had a previous history of tuberculosis.
Findings. *Chest radiograph:* There is calcification of the left side of the pericardium. The pulmonary venous system is engorged from a superimposed congestive heart failure.

enlargement present in the remainder. The left atrium is frequently the most prominent chamber, along with pulmonary venous congestion and dilatation of the superior vena cava, all resulting from incomplete distensibility of the pericardium covered left and right ventricles.[7]

CONGENITAL ANOMALIES

Entire books are dedicated to congenital anomalies of the heart. Most are discovered at birth or in the infant years, and corrective surgery is performed. Since this text is mainly descriptive of radiology of adults, mention will be made only of the common cardiac anomalies.

ATRIAL SEPTAL DEFECT

Atrial septal defects (ASDs) are by far the most common of the congenital cardiac lesions. Any portion of the septum that separates the left and right atrium may be absent. Hemodynamically, blood enters the left atrium upon returning from the pulmonary veins and can bypass its normal course through the high-pressure left ventricle and systemic arterial system in favor of the low-pressure right ventricle and pulmonary arterial system. The blood now travels from pul-

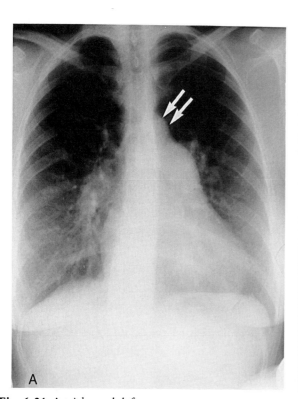
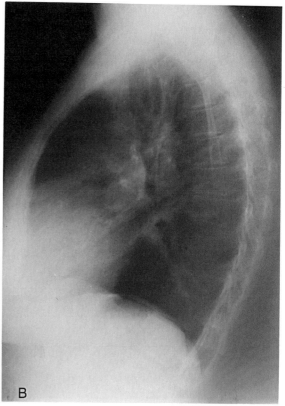

Fig. 6-21 Artrial septal defect.
History. This 21-year-old woman had congenital heart disease of an unclear type.
Findings. (A) *Frontal chest radiograph:* The heart is enlarged, with an upward tilt of the apex signifying predominantly right ventricular enlargement. The central pulmonary arteries and peripheral pulmonary arteries are engorged and sharply defined as a result of the left-to-right shunt. In addition, the aortic knob is small (arrows). **(B)** *Lateral chest radiograph:* The lack of left atrial or ventricular involvement is confirmed as these posterior chambers remain of normal size. Right ventricular enlargement is causing the cardiomegaly.

monary veins to the left atrium, right atrium, right ventricle, and pulmonary arteries, and finally returns to the pulmonary veins to start the cycle over again. The larger the defect, the more blood that is shunted. The chamber enlargement pattern as seen on the chest radiograph correlates with the hemodynamics of the condition. The left atrium and ventricle are small, since much of the returning blood from the engorged pulmonary circulation bypasses the chambers on the left side. The right atrium and ventricle enlarge to handle the excess shunted blood. The central main pulmonary arteries enlarge significantly in response to the excess flow to the lungs. The peripheral pulmonary circulation also engorges, thus becoming increasingly prominent on the chest radiograph (Fig. 6-21 A and B). The engorged pulmonary arteries remain sharply defined (Fig. 6-5), in contrast to the smudged pulmonary veins of congestive heart failure (Fig. 6-4).

Angiography is necessary to define which portion of the septum is absent, to determine the amount of the blood shunted, and to detect any accompanying congenital anomalies The jet of contrast medium through the atrial septum may be visualized on the angiogram.

VENTRICULAR SEPTAL DEFECT

In a ventricular septal defect (VSD) the blood travels from the left ventricle to the right ventricle through a defect in the intraventricular septum. The right atrium does not participate in the shunt, and in VSD is therefore of normal size, distinguishing this condition from an ASD. The chest radiograph shows left

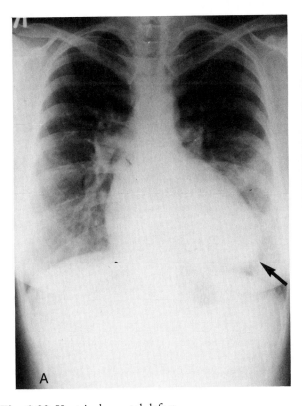
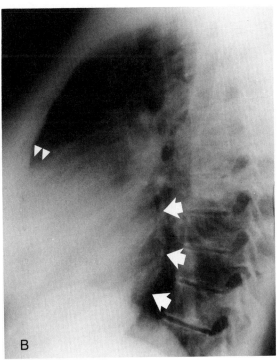

Fig. 6-22 Ventricular septal defect.
History. This 25-year-old woman had a heart murmur.
Findings. (A) *Frontal chest radiograph:* Left atrial and ventricular enlargement leads to a prominent and inferiorly oriented cardiac apex (arrow). The right heart border remains normal, since the right atrium is not involved in this anomaly. The pulmonary arteries are engorged but remain sharp in their outline. **(B)** *Lateral chest radiograph:* Left atrial and ventricular enlargement is confirmed by the posterior predominence of the heart (arrows). In addition, the retrosternal space is filled in by the enlarged, anteriorly lying right ventricle (arrowheads).

atrial, left ventricular, and right ventricular enlargement, again with sharply defined engorgement of the central and peripheral pulmonary arteries as a result of the left (left ventricle)-to-right (right ventricle) shunt (Fig. 6-22 A and B).

COARCTATION OF THE AORTA

In coarctation of the aorta there is narrowing involving a segment of the proximal portion of the descending aorta. This narrowed segment leads to decreased blood flow and decreased blood pressure to the lower extremities. The upper extremities demonstrate an increase in blood pressure. Arteries surrounding the coarctation enlarge to help supply blood to the lower regions of the body; these collateral vessels consist of the intercostal arteries, internal mammary arteries, and the arteries that course around the scapula.

The chest radiograph may show classic changes involving the aorta and ribs. The cardiac changes are minimal, with some left ventricular enlargement. The portion of the descending aorta above the coarctation is dilated. A notch representing the coarctation is often identified. The portion of aorta distal to the coarctation also dilates, from the disorganized and turbulent blood flow. The lateral border of the aorta thus forms a "figure-3 sign" representing the dilated prestenotic segment, coarctation, and dilated post-stenotic segment. The PA view of the chest may show notching of the ribs on their inferior surface, from secondarily enlarged and pulsating collateral intercostal arteries (Fig. 6-23A). A dilated internal mammary artery may be seen as a soft-tissue density behind and parallel to the sternum on the lateral film.

Angiography clearly defines the presence and severity of the coarctation (Fig. 6-23B). It also identifies the collateral circulation and reveals any accompanying congenital anomalies. Recent sources state that angiography is unnecessary in cases of coarctation with the classic symptomatology and the typical chest radiographic appearance of this condition.[8]

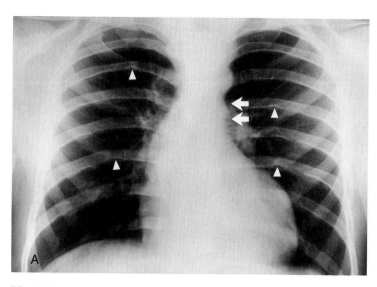

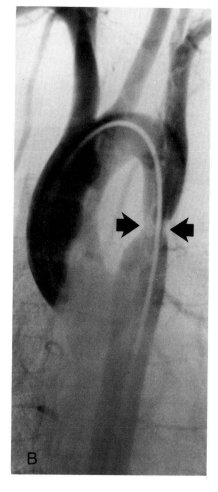

Fig. 6-23 Coarctation of the arota.
History. This 18-year-old man had a history of "congentital heart disease."
Findings. (A) *Chest radiograph:* There is notching of the ribs seen bilaterally, and mainly involving the fifth to ninth ribs (arrowheads). The notched aorta with a "figure-3" configuration is also appreciated (arrows). **(B)** *Angiogram:* A subtraction angiogram shows narrowing of a proximal portion of the descending aorta (arrows).

IDIOPATHIC HYPERTROPHIC SUBAORTIC STENOSIS

Idiopathic hypertrophic subaortic stenosis (IHSS) is a congenital anomaly that does not appear to be hemodynamically significant until the adult years. There is thickening of the muscles of the left ventricular outflow tract, predominantly involving the interventricular septum. This thickening is associated with an alteration of the mitral valve and secondary insufficiency.

The chest radiograph shows enlargement of the left ventricle alone, or with accompanying enlargement of the left atrium from a secondarily incompetent mitral valve. There may be some poststenotic dilatation of the proximal ascending aorta, but less severe than is present in simple aortic valvular stenosis.

Either angiography or echocardiography can confirm the diagnosis of IHSS when this condition is clinically suspected.

BACTERIAL ENDOCARDITIS

Bacterial endocarditis is an infection of the valves of the heart and is often associated with either congenital or acquired valvular defects. A recent dental extraction, ureteral instrumentation, tonsillectomy, acute respiratory infection, or gynecologic procedure often precedes a mild endocarditis of a previously diseased or deformed valve. A more fulminant course of bacterial endocarditis, in which there are no underlying valvular defects, is seen in IV drug abusers. This acute fulminant form of the disease leads to rapid destruction of the valves. Bacterial endocarditis can also develop about a suture or prosthetic valve following cardiac surgery. The prosthetic valve may require removal if antibiotic therapy cannot terminate the infection.[9] The findings of fever, splenomegaly, and a new or changing cardiac murmur should suggest the diagnosis of bacterial endocarditis.

The chest radiograph is generally of little benefit if the cardiac shadow is normal or shows evidence of previous valvular heart disease. If valvular destruction does occur, the heart may quickly and massively dilate, with a superimposed, fulminant congestive heart failure. If the valves on the right side are infected, septic emboli may appear in the lungs as one or more patches of nodular infiltrates which frequently cavitate.

Echocardiography is the best method for confirming a diagnosis of simple bacterial endocarditis. Any secondary valvular destruction or dysfunction requires prompt angiography and surgical correction.

CLINICAL PRESENTATION: CHEST PAIN (ALGORITHM 6-2)

CORONARY ARTERY DISEASE: ANGINA

Coronary artery disease and ischemic heart disease define a disease spectrum that most often results from an absolute reduction in blood flow to portions of the heart caused by the obstruction of large coronary arteries by atherosclerotic plaque.[10] The location of the plaque as well as the degree of luminal narrowing of the coronary artery determine whether the lesion results in an ischemia severe enough to lead to angina. The more proximally an obstructing atherosclerotic plaque is located, the more muscle mass is rendered ischemic and the more severe is the patient's ischemia and disability.

In patients with angina of recent onset or progressive or unrelenting angina, a baseline chest radiograph is obtained. The chest radiograph serves as a basis for comparison of future chest radiographs (to detect a changing heart size), and is useful for detecting such complications of coronary artery disease as congestive heart failure. An enlarged heart is indicative of longstanding ischemia and secondary myocardial damage and dilatation. In cases of suspected angina or unclear symptomatology, a stress ECG is obtained to establish the diagnosis of ischemic heart disease if the latter is present. Recently, the simple stress ECG or treadmill examination has been coupled with the intravenous administration of thallium-201 at the point of peak exercise. The thallium increases the sensitivity of the stress test, especially for detecting single-vessel occlusion. The thallium stress test also provides useful information in patients whose ECGs are not easily interpreted because of left bundle-branch blocks or arrhythmias, and in patients who do not achieve maximum heart rates because of fatigue or shortness of breath that would make the simple stress test otherwise less valuable. If a thallium stress test is normal, the chances of significant coronary artery disease is low. The false-negative rate is under 10 percent.[11]

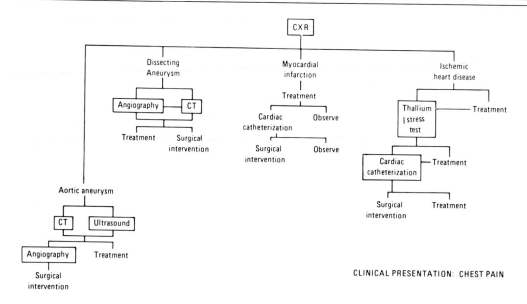

CLINICAL PRESENTATION: CHEST PAIN

Algorithm 6-2

An initial image is obtained immediately after exercise. In a patient with significant ischemic heart disease, a cold defect or absence of activity is seen in the normally homogeneous appearance of the heart (Fig. 6-24). This indicates that a segment of the heart is not receiving an adequate blood supply to fulfill its metabolic requirements during exercise. Different projections help pinpoint the location of the ischemic wall and so give information on which vessel is diseased. A delayed image of the heart is obtained several hours after this initial exercise image. With ischemic heart disease there is subsequent filling in of the pre-vious cold defect seen at peak exercise, as the blood supply to the heart reaches equilibrium in the resting state (Fig. 6-24B). This combination of a defect in the immediate postexercise thallium images and its filling in on resting images is virtually specific for ischemic heart disease.

The detection of secondary abnormalities in wall motion and a quantitation of the approximate ejection fraction can be done with the nuclear medicine gated cardiac blood-pool study or more invasive cardiac catheterization. Wall abnormalities can result from ischemia, myocardial infarction, or an aneurysm. Ab-

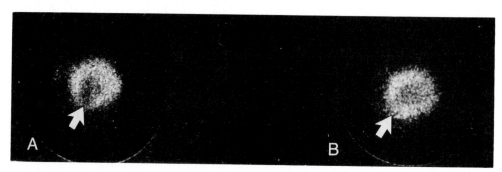

Fig. 6-24 Ischemic heart disease.
History. This 57-year-old man had dyspnea of new onset with exertion.
Findings. *Thallium stress test:* **(A)** Exercise. Images obtained immediately after exercise show a cold area or defect of the normal ring of activity (arrow). **(B)** At rest. Images obtained 2 hours later show that this previously cold defect has disappeared (arrow) and the ring or doughnut is now intact. (Courtesy of Dr. Steward Spies.)

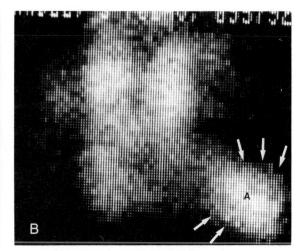

Fig. 6-25 Dyskinetic wall motion.
History. This 72-year-old man had had an MI 3 months earlier and had continued dyspnea with excertion.
Findings. *Gated ventriculogram:* **(A)** The left ventricle is somewhat enlarged in its distented state of diastole. **(B)** The systolic image demonstrates the apex of the left ventricle ballooning out (arrows) while the remainder of the ventricular wall contracts. The apex is said to be dyskinetic. This represents an aneurysm (A). (Courtesy of Dr. Steward Spies.)

normal wall motion may be segmental or diffusely involve the entire left ventricle. A segment of myocardium that moves out while the normal portions of the heart are moving inward during systole — as is seen when an aneurysm is present — is called a dyskinetic segment (Fig. 6-25 A and B). If a segment of myocardium remains motionless or contracts to a lesser degree than the normal portions of the heart, it is referred to as akinetic or hypokinetic, respectively.

Coronary arteriography is an invasive procedure but remains the only way to directly visualize atherosclerotic narrowing or occlusion of the coronary arteries. The indications for this procedure are angina in patients who are candidates for bypass surgery, known cardiac disease (post MI), continued heart failure following an MI, an abnormal treadmill test, and following coronary artery bypass surgery in some cases.[12] The location of the atherosclerotic narrowing, degree of the narrowing, and length of vessel involved are all important in determining the significance of a lesion. Most agree that a narrowing of 50 to 75 percent is clinically significant (Fig. 6-26).

The ventriculogram accompanying cardiac catheterization allows the most accurate determination of the ejection fraction, dyskinetic wall motion, presence or absence of an aneurysm, and secondary valvular dysfunction. The heart is observed for a number of cycles and pressure measurements are obtained that help generate the functional data.

The chest radiograph immediately following coronary artery bypass surgery or other cardiac surgery is an important and complicated film. It is valuable for checking the locations of the various tubes and catheters. The postoperative film following routine post cardiac surgery shows some mediastinal widening with overlying metallic sutures bridging the sternotomy site. There is frequently a small, left-sided pleural effusion as well as some atelectasis involving the left lower lung field. This atelectasis may persist for several days postoperatively. An endotrachial tube, Swan-Ganz catheter, epicardial pacemaker wires, and mediastinal drainage tubes are present. Surgical clips identify the course of the bypass graft. Round markers may be present that identify the new opening of the bypass vessel from the aorta (Fig. 6-27). The postoperative chest radiograph is also valuable for detecting postoperative complications, such as progressive congestive heart failure, mediastinal widening from a

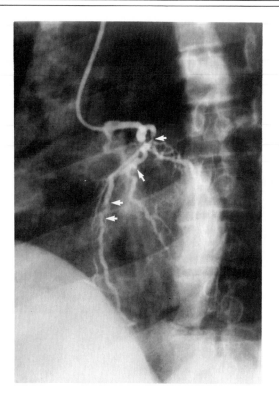

Fig. 6-26 Coronary artery disease.
History. Two cases of coronary artery disease.
Findings. *Cardiac catheterization:* There is nearly complete occlusion of the proximal portion of the anterior descending artery along with multiple levels of arterial irregularity (arrows), as consistent with severe coronary artery disease.

bleeding vessel, excessive pleural effusion, unrelenting atelectasis, or even dehiscence of the sternotomy.[13]

MYOCARDIAL INFARCTION

The clinical and laboratory identification of an acute myocardial infarction (MI) is usually straightforward. The patient with chest pain is admitted to a cardiac intensive care center where an initial baseline chest radiograph is obtained. The radiograph is usually normal immediately following the MI. Some degree of cardiac decompensation and failure occur later in over half of all infarct patients, and the chest radiograph shows dilatation of the heart and pulmonary venous congestion. Acute pulmonary edema may develop rapidly after an extensive myocardial infarction or after a smaller infarction in an already diseased ischemic heart.

In some cases the diagnosis of an acute MI is less clear and further testing is needed. For example, a patient may not present to the hospital for several days after experiencing chest pain, by which time the cardiac enzyme levels have returned to normal. In cases of left bundle-branch block or an acute MI near the site of a previous infarction, the ECG may be confusing.[14] The myocardial scan with technetium pyrophosphate has its maximum sensitivity in detecting acute MI at 48 to 72 hours, and is positive for up to 7 days after an acute infarction. The reported sensitivity of the myocardial scan is 80 to 100 percent in cases of

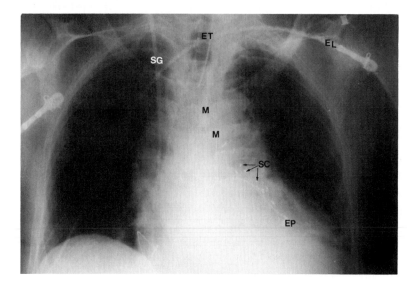

Fig. 6-27 Coronary artery bypass surgery, postoperative study.
History. This 67-year-old man was examined 2 days after a coronary artery bypass procedure.
Findings. *Chest radiograph:* An endotracheal tube (ET), Swan-Ganz catheter (SG), mediastinal chest tubes (M), and epicardial pacemaker (EP) are in place. The mediastinum is wide and there is a left pleural effusion. The surgical clips affixing the bypass graft are also identified (SC). An external cardiac lead is superimposed over the chest (EL).

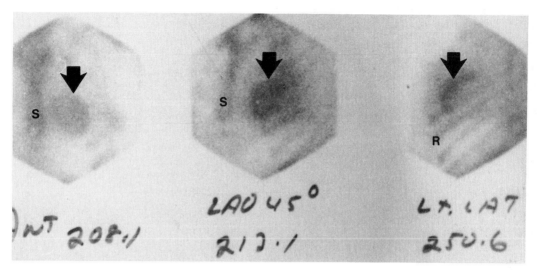

Fig. 6-28 Myocardial infarction.
History. This 67-year-old man had tight chest pain of new onset 2 days earlier and had become progressively short of breath. The ECG was abnormal but the cardiac enzymes were nonconfirmatory.
Findings. *Myocardial Scan:* There is diffuse uptake throughout the heart, indicating widespread myocardial damage (arrows). Normal activity is seen in the ribs (R) and sternum (S). (Courtesy of Dr. Stewart Spies.)

transmural infarction.[14] In an acute MI, the scan demonstrates an abnormal area of activity over the expected location in the heart. This abnormal myocardial activity projects between the ribs and sternum (Fig. 6-28). Multiple views are again obtained in order to localize the involved wall. By 3 weeks, the myocardial scan usually returns to normal.

Later complications of acute MI include aneurysm of the left ventricle and the postmyocardial syndrome. Aneurysms may appear shortly after an MI, arising from the softened, necrotic myocardium. They can also occur several months after an MI from a bulge of the fibrous myocardial scar. The chest radiograph shows a bulge or unusual prominence of the left ventricular border (Fig. 6-29). The nuclear medicine gated-pool study or contrast ventriculogram can reveal the abnormal shape of the ventricle as well as the dyskinetic movement of the aneurysm.

The postmyocardial infarction syndrome or Dressler's syndrome occurs within days to several months following an MI. It is believed to be secondary to an autoimmune pericarditis. The chest radiograph shows bilateral pleural effusion with the effusion on the left side usually greater than that on the right. Infiltrates may be found in the left base or both lung bases. A pericardial effusion causes enlargement of the

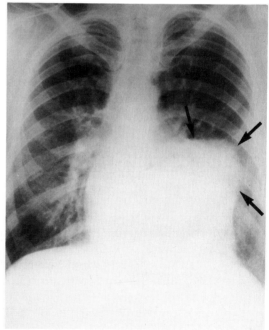

Fig. 6-29 Ventricular aneurysm.
History. This 72-year-old man had recurrent shortness of breath 4 months after an MI.
Findings. *Chest radiograph:* There is an obvious bulge of the left heart border (arrows) that was not present on previous chest radiographs.

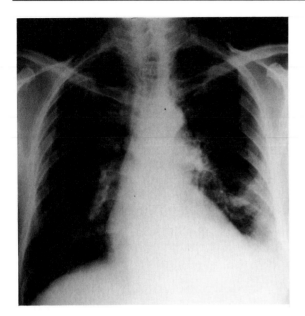

Fig. 6-30 Dressler's syndrome.
History. This 72-year-old man was seen 3 weeks after a MI, with fever and shortness of breath.
Findings. *Chest radiograph:* The heart is enlarged and significantly larger than in a previous study done 2 weeks earier. There is a left pleural effusion with mild pulmonary venous congestion consistent with mild congestive heart failure.

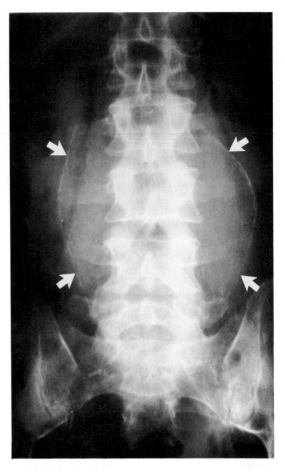

Fig. 6-31. Aortic aneurysm.
History. This 59-year-old man had persistent back pain. An intravenous pyelogram (IVP) was ordered to rule out chronic pyelonephritis.
Findings. *Preliminary Film from an IVP:* There is a 13-cm calcified aneurysm involving the distal aorta. The calcified wall is easily identified (arrows).

cardiac shadow (Fig. 6-30). The chest radiograph may take days to months to return to normal.[15]

ATHEROSCLEROSIS/AORTIC ANEURYSM

Aortic aneurysms are most often the result of extensive atherosclerosis and are most commonly found in the abdominal portion of the aorta. Atherosclerosis of the aorta and other large arteries initially leads to elongation (Fig. 2-3) and irregular thickening of the vessel wall as it becomes coated with atheromatous plaque. The plaque may then calcify. The diseased aorta may later aneurysmally dilate.

A calcified aorta or aneurysm is often detected on radiographs obtained for other reasons. If the diameter of the aorta is greater than 4 cm, the possibility for an aneurysm should be raised and a further workup initiated (Fig. 6-31).

The angiogram of a diseased aorta coated with atherosclerotic plaque demonstrates thickened, irregular walls and a narrowed lumen (Fig. 6-32). When an aneurysm has developed, there is an abrupt dilation of the aorta (Fig. 6-33A). The size of the opacified lumen of the aneurysm may be smaller than the actual diameter of the aneurysm, since the walls of the lesion are often coated with layers of clotted blood. The angiogram is helpful in determining which secondary arteries leading from the aorta (SMA, renal) are involved by the aneurysm, which makes corrective bypass surgery much more complicated or impossible.

Ultrasound and more recently CT give a more pre-

Fig. 6-32 Atherosclerosis of the abdominal aorta.
History. This 69-year-old man had claudication and almost nonexistent femoral pulses.
Findings. *Angiogram:* The angiogram has to be done via a trans-lumbar approach owing to the extensive atherosclerotic disease involving the patient's femoral arteries, which prevented the passage of a catheter. A long needle and catheter were directed through the patients back and through the posterior wall of the aorta with flouroscopic control (arrows). The aorta and iliac arteries are tortuous and irregular from the extensive atherosclerotic plaque (arrowheads).

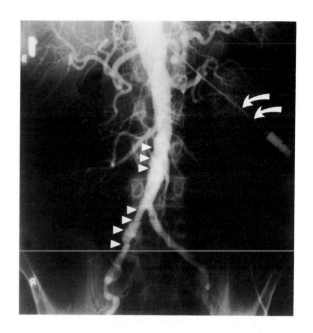

Fig. 6-33 Aortic aneurysm.
History. The 74-year-old man had progressive back pain and a new large mass felt on the left side of the abdomen.
Findings. (A) *Angiogram:* An angiogram shows the tortuous aorta and accompanying aneurysm. Only the patent lumen is opacified and imaged. **(B)** *CT scan:* A section below the level of the kidneys demonstrates a huge aneurysm filling the left side of the abdomen. Clotted blood has collected along the wall of the aneurysm in a laminated fashion (arrows). The patent lumen appears white after the administration of intravenous contrast medium (A).

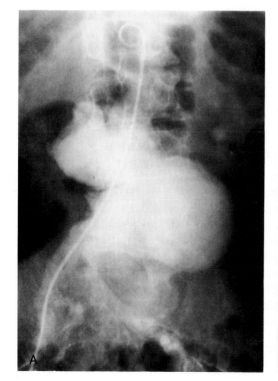

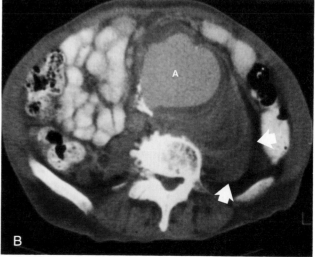

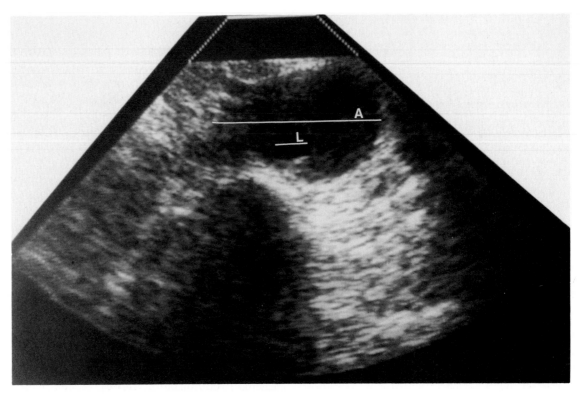

Fig. 6-34 Aortic aneurysm.
History. This 67-year-old woman had a pulsitile abdominal mass on a routine physical examination.
Findings. *US scan:* There is a 8-cm aneurysm seen in this longitudinal view of the distal aorta. The patent lumen (L) measures 2.6 cm with clotted blood filling the remainder of the aneurysm (A).

cise idea of the true size of an aneurysm since they image the wall of this lesion, whether or not there is a patent lumen, and any accumulated clotted blood (Figs. 6-33 B and 6-34).

DISSECTING HEMATOMAS (ANEURYSMS)

A dissection of the aorta starts in the proximal regions of the aorta in over 75 percent of cases. Dissections are associated with hypertension, atherosclerotic disease, pregnancy, coarctation of the aorta, Marfan syndrome, and valvular aortic stenosis. Following a rip in the intimal layer of the lumen of the aorta, blood dissects into the wall of the vessel, forming a hematoma. The dissection extends a variable distance through the aortic wall and results in the obstruction

of many of the major secondary arterial branches along its way.[16]

The chest radiograph may suggest the diagnosis of a dissecting hematoma with progressive widening of the aortic shadow or mediastinum in 70 percent of cases. Angiography is usually done for a definitive diagnosis. The angiogram shows the aorta segmented into a true and false lumen (Fig. 6-35), with the false lumen the new space created by the dissecting hematoma. The false lumen compresses and narrows the now irregular true lumen. The false lumen may opacify with contrast medium at the same time that the true lumen is opacified, or shortly thereafter. The intimal flap is seen as a thin septum dividing the true and false lumina. If the dissection involves the aortic valve, a secondary aortic regurgitation occurs.

Many reports acknowledge CT as a noninvasive

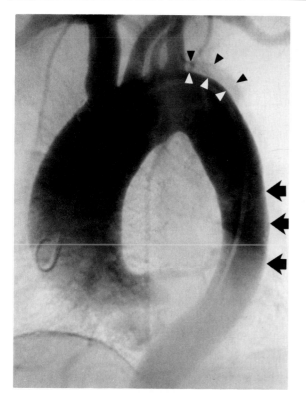

Fig. 6-35 Dissecting hematoma (aneurysm).
History. This 63-year-old man had intolerable chest pain.
Findings. *Angiogram:* The tip of the catheter is in the ascending aorta. Starting at the left subclavian artery there is narrowing of the true lumen of the descending aorta. The lateral wall of this portion of the aorta is irregular (arrows). In addition, portions of the false lumen can be visualized over the compressed true lumen (arrowheads).

means for diagnosing or reasonably excluding an aortic dissection, obviating the need for an angiogram in many cases. The cross-sectional views afforded by CT easily demonstrate the increased diameter of the aorta. With contrast-medium administration the true lumen opacifies quickly but appears deformed and narrowed as on the angiogram. The false lumen shows delayed opacification since it consists of clotted blood. The intimal flap separating the true and false lumina can frequently be appreciated on the CT scan as well. If surgery is contemplated, angiography is required in order to assess the precise involvement of the aortic branch vessels and to determine the exact sites of entry and termination of the dissection.

CLINICAL PRESENTATION: PAINFUL/COLD EXTREMITY (ALGORITHM 6-3)

PERIPHERAL ARTHEROSCLEROSIS

Atherosclerotic plaque formation, an inevitable sequel to aging, commonly leads to narrowing or occlusion of the major vessels of the lower extremity. The plaques in the peripheral arteries also frequently calcify, as previously discussed.

A plain radiograph of the leg may show irregular linear or curvilinear patches of calcification scattered throughout the area of the peripheral arteries. Calcification in the smaller vessels of the lower leg and foot

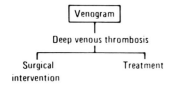

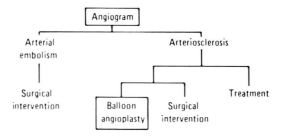

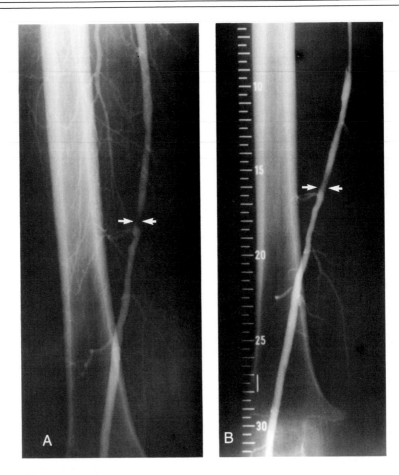

Fig. 6-36 Peripheral atherosclerosis.
History. This 78-year-old woman had progressive claudication of the right leg.
Findings. **(A)** *Preangioplasty angiogram:* There is tight narrowing of the femoral artery from an atherosclerotic plaque (arrows). **(B)** *Postangioplasty Angiogram:* The lesion has been reduced and the patent lumen of the artery is no longer narrowed (arrows).

is seen frequently in patients with the early atherosclerosis that is present in diabetics.

Angiography shows the now familiar diffuse, irregular luminal narrowing. Complete obstruction of a large artery results in an extensive collateral circulation that seeks to supply the distal arteries. The angiogram is required before a bypass procedure to evaluate the status of the more distal circulation.

In recent years, angioplasty has been successful in treating certain narrowed artherosclerotic lesions, obviating the need for bypass surgery. A special angiographic catheter with an inflatable balloon at the tip is inflated and then deflated at the area of narrowing. This results in a controlled splitting of the vessel wall and opening of the previously narrowed vessel (Fig. 6-36 A and B).

ARTERIAL EMBOLISM

Emboli to the peripheral arteries can result in acute and severe pain in a cold extremity. The emboli are usually cardiac in origin, stemming from endocarditis, atrial fibrillation, or a myocardial infarction. More proximal atherosclerotic plaque from the aorta may also dislodge and form distal emboli.[18]

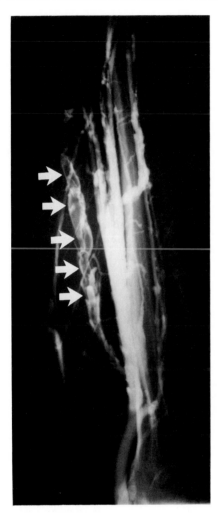

Fig. 6-37 Deep venous thrombosis.
History. This patient was a 55-year-old male quadriplegic.
Findings. *Venogram:* There are lobular filling defects in the posterior tibial vein representing blood clots. Contrast medium outlines the blood clots (arrows).

Angiography is required for the diagnosis of an embolism. It shows an abrupt termination of the occluded artery, with few collateral vessels yet formed. Prompt surgical correction is required.

THROMBOPHLEBITIS

Thrombi or blood clots are frequently found in the superficial or deep veins of the lower extremities. Superficial thrombosis occurs when a blood clot forms in the greater saphenous vein and results in a reddened, edematous, and tender leg. When the patient complains of local deep tenderness and swelling, a blood clot in the deep venous system must be suspected. The deep venous system can be categorized into three areas of thrombophlebitic involvement: the small veins of the calf, the femoropopliteal segment, and the iliofemoral area. The iliofemoral area is the most dangerous, since blood clots here have the greatest potential for dislodging and becoming fatal pulmonary emboli.[19] The causes of venous thrombus formation are potentially many, and include prolonged bed rest, severe illness, malignancy (pancreas, lung, GI tract), estrogen administration, congestive heart failure, post partum effects, and orthopedic injury.

The most accurate way to confirm a suspected deep venous thrombosis is through venography. With this, the location, extent, and number of thrombi can be detected. An iodinated contrast medium is injected into a superficial foot vein, with subsequent filling of the deep and superficial venous system. The blood clots appear as localized defects within the lumen (Fig. 6-37). The clots may completely obstruct the deep venous channels and result in an extensive collateral venous circulation that develops in order to bypass the obstruction.

REFERENCES

1. Cooley RN, Schreiber MH: Radiology of the Heart and Great Vessels. Williams & Wilkins, Baltimore, 1978, pp 7–9
2. Swishchuk LE: Plain Film Interpretation in Congenital Heart Disease. Williams & Wilkins, Baltimore, 1979, pp 30
3. Swishchuk LE: Plain Film Interpretation in Congenital Heart Disease. Williams & Wilkins, Baltimore, 1979, pp 17
4. Cooley RN, Schreiber MH: Radiology of the Heart and Great Vessels. William & Wilkins, Baltimore, 1978, pp 142–143
5. Teplick JG, Haskin ME: Roentgen Diagnosis. WB Saunders, Philadelphia, 1976, p 678
6. Gotsman MS, Vander Horst RL, Winship WS: The chest radiograph in primary myocardial disease. Radiology 99:1, 1971
7. Teplick JG, Haskin ME: Roentgen Diagnosis. WB Saunders, Philadelphia, 1976, p 711
8. Cooley RN, Schreiber MH: Radiology of the Heart

and Great Vessels. Williams & Wilkins, Baltimore, 1978, pp 215–216

9. Thorn GW, Adams RD, Braunwald E, et al: Harrison's Principles of Internal Medicine. McGraw Hill, New York, 1977, pp 797–800

10. Thorn GW, Adams RD, Braunwald E, et al: Harrison's Principles of Internal Medicine. McGraw Hill, New York, 1977, p 1261

11. Siegel BA, Alazraki NP, Alderson PO, et al: Nuclear Radiology (Second Series) Syllabus. American College of Radiology, Chicago, 1978, p 408

12. Cooley RN, Schreiber MH: Radiology of the Heart and Great Vessels. Williams & Wilkins, Baltimore, 1978, pp 446–447

13. Goodman LR, Putman CE: Intensive Care Radiology. Imaging of the Critically Ill. WB Saunders Company, Philadelphia, 1983, pp 135–139

14. Siegel BA, Alazraki NP, Alderson PO, et al: Nuclear Radiology (Second Series) Syllabus. American College of Radiology, Chicago, 1978, pp 122–123

15. Levin EJ, Bryk D: Dressler syndrome. Radiology 87:731, 1966

16. Baron MG: Dissecting aneurysm of the aorta. Circulation 43:933, 1971

17. Goldwin JD, Herfkens RJ, Skiolderbrand GG: Evaluation of dissections and aneurysms of the thoracic aorta by conventional and dynamic CT scanning. Radiology 139:655–660, 1981

18. Teplick JG, Haskin ME: Roentgen Diagnosis. WB Saunders, Philadelphia, 1976, p 750

19. Thorn GW, Adams RD, Braunwald E, et al: Harrison's Principles of Internal Medicine. McGraw Hill, New York, 1977, pp 1327–1328

7

Radiology of the Central Nervous System

Charles Lee
Lee Sider

The radiologic evaluation of the neurologic system will be divided anatomically into four regions: the brain, orbits, ears, and spine. The currently available imaging devices include skull radiography, tomography, angiography, computerized tomography (CT) with and without intravenous or intrathecal contrast agents, ultrasound, magnetic resonance imaging (MR), and myelography.

Skull radiography is a commonly ordered examination and represents the first study in the evaluation of the central nervous system. Views of the skull are obtained in various projections to optimize the visualization of the different components of the bony anatomy. The posterior-anterior (PA) view or frontal view, lateral view, and Towne view are demonstrated in Figure 7-1 A, B, and C. The normal bony landmarks should be identified when evaluating the skull. Their absence, destruction, or alteration may signify pathology. Other signs of pathology include abnormal calcifications and lucent lines representing fractures. Unfortunately the skull film is of limited use, since it reveals only bony changes or abnormal calcifications, and does not image soft-tissue densities or neural tissue.

Tomography allows one to image centrally located bony structures which would otherwise require radiographic views that are both difficult to obtain and interpret. Only those structures that lie in the tomographic plane of focus are sharply demonstrated, as the overlying bony structures are blurred out by the motion of the x-ray tube (Fig. 7-2). However, tomography is again useful only when there has been bony alteration or destruction. The soft-tissue structures are not visualized.

Myelography involves the introduction of an oil-based iodine-containing (Pantopaque) or water-based iodine-containing contrast agent (Amipaque) into the intrathecal space, most frequently via a lumbar punc-

251

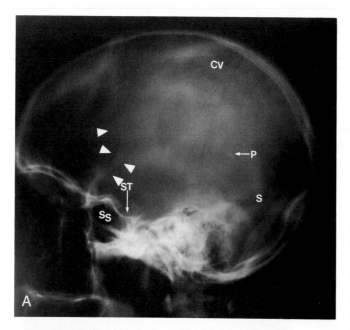

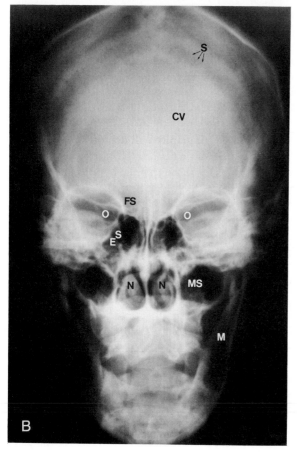

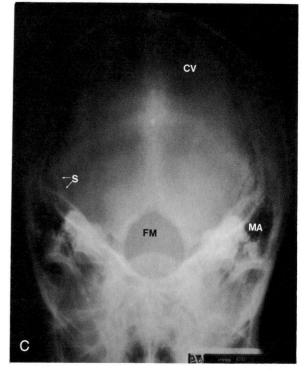

Fig. 7-1 Normal skull films. **(A)** Lateral view, **(B)** Frontal view, **(C)** Townes view. CV = cranial vault, S = suture, M = mandible, ST = sella turcica, P = calcified pineal, MA = mastoid air cells, O = orbits, SS = sphenoid sinus, FS = frontal sinus, ES = ethmoid sinus, MS = maxillary sinus, N = nasal turbinates, FM = foramen magnum, CN = cranial nerve exit foramina, arrowhead = vascular grooves.

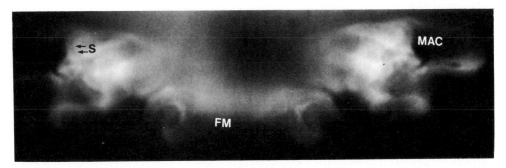

Fig. 7-2 Normal tomography of the internal auditory canals. Both internal auditory canals (IAC) are visualized in this frontal-plane tomogram. MAC = mastoid air cells within the petrous bone, FM = foramen magnum, S = semilunar canal.

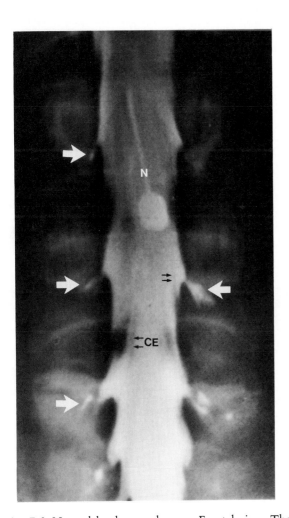

Fig. 7-3 Normal lumbar myelogram. Frontal view. The nerve roots (white arrows) are well delineated, without defects or amputation. N = spinal needle, CE = strands of cauda equina (black arrows).

ture (Fig. 7-3). This allows visualization of the spinal cord, and is used to detect cord-compressing extrinsic herniated discs, intrinsic spinal cord tumors, and inflammatory lesions of the arachnoid lining.

Angiography permits the visualization of vascular structures intracranially by the injection of an iodinated contrast agent into the arterial system coupled with rapid, sequential radiographic filming (Fig. 7-4 A, B, and C). Tumor localization can be done on the basis of the pattern of displacement of arterial and venous structures in the angiogram. The presence of a tumor blush or early-draining veins confirms the diagnosis of tumor. Computed tomography has replaced angiography in the early detection and localization of tumors, and can also differentiate a tumor from edema. Angiography will demonstrate only the total mass effect of both the edema plus the tumor. Nevertheless, the angiographic findings in certain types of tumor, such as meningioma, may be characteristic and at times pathognomonic when the CT findings are equivocal. Angiography retains a major role in the diagnosis of atherosclerosis occlusive disease, both of the extra- (Fig. 7-5) and intracranial arteries; in the diagnosis of arteriovenous malformations of the brain and their feeding and draining vessels; and in the diagnosis of intracranial aneurysms. It can demonstrate the parent vessel of the aneurysm and the anatomic relation of the aneurysm to the parent vessel (i.e., which way it points); which aneurysm has bled when several aneurysms are present; and whether or not secondary vasospasm is present. Angiography also demonstrates the resulting collateral circulation in cases of total occlusion of a vessel from atherosclerosis.

A recent technologic advancement in angiography

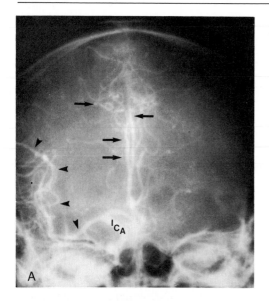

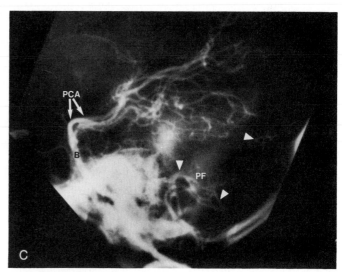

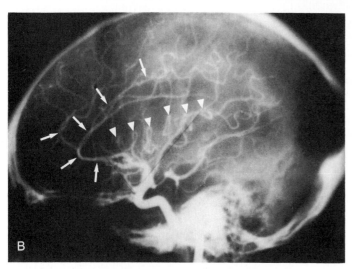

Fig. 7-4 Normal intracerebral angiogram. **(A)** Injection of contrast medium through a catheter placed in the right internal carotid artery shows both anterior cerebral arteries (ACA) (arrows) and the right middle carotid artery (MCA) (arrowheads). Note the midline course of the ACA. ICA = internal carotid artery. **(B)** Lateral view of area shown in A shows the distribution of the branches of the ACA (arrows) and the branches of the MCA (arrowheads). **(C)** After selective catheterization of the vertebral artery there is opacification of the posterior cerebral artery (PCA) (arrows) and arteries of the posterior fossa (PF) (arrowheads). B = basilar artery.

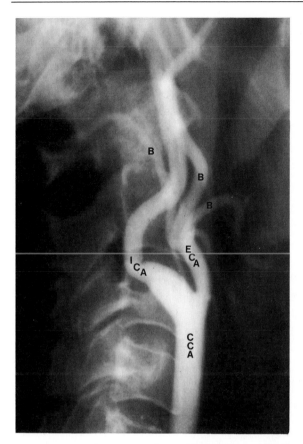

Fig. 7-5 Normal extracranial carotid angiogram. The tip of the catheter is in the common carotid artery. CCA = common carotid artery, ICA = internal carotid artery, ECA = external carotid artery, B = branches of external carotid artery.

has been the development of digital subtraction angiography (DSA). Subtraction itself has been a long-utilized photographic technique involving a mask (a negative print of the angiogram just before the contrast medium is visualized), which is superimposed over an angiographic film with the contrast medium in the vessel of interest. This technique literally "subtracts" all of the bony structures when a second print is made from the superimposed mask and angiogram film. The vascular structures can be clearly visualized without the superimposed density of the bone, and the contrast-filled vessels appear black (see Fig. 1-13). In DSA this same subtraction technique can be done electronically from a video or fluoroscopic screen, allowing the detection of low levels of arterial opacification from a venous injection of contrast-medium.

Theoretically DSA is a safe outpatient procedure, utilizing a venous route for arterial visualization—a technique that previously required an angiogram along with patient hospitalization and a resulting high cost. The catheter should be placed in the superior vena cava or right atrium in order to provide adequate arterial opacification (Fig. 7-6). However, the amount of contrast medium injected for venous DSA currently far exceeds the amounts used in conventional percutaneous transfemoral carotid arterial angiography. The most important limitation of DSA remains its lack of spatial resolution as compared to conventional angiography. As a result, the study often must be repeated with conventional angiography when examining the extracranial carotid arteries before surgical intervention. The main role of DSA is therefore for noninvasive screening in patients for whom surgical treatment is not planned, such as in a search for the cause of a TIA.

Computed tomography has revolutionized the study and diagnosis of diseases of the spine and brain.

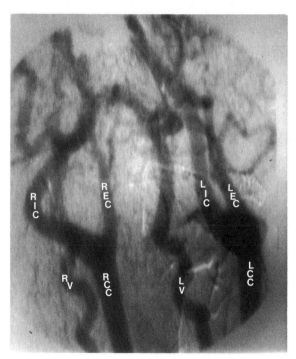

Fig. 7-6 Normal digital subtraction angiography (DSA) of the extracranial carotid arteries. After the intravenous injection of contrast material there is visualization of the carotid system. RCC = right common carotid artery, RIC = right internal carotid artery, REC = right external carotid artery, RV = right vertebral artery, LCC = left common carotid artery, LIC = left internal carotid artery, LEC = left external carotid artery, LV = left vertebral artery.

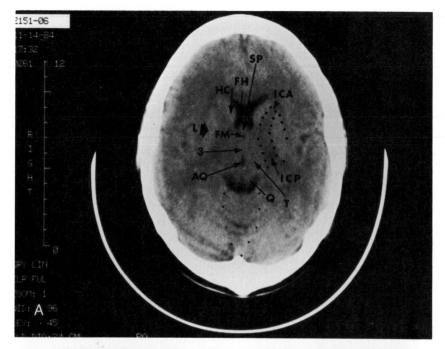

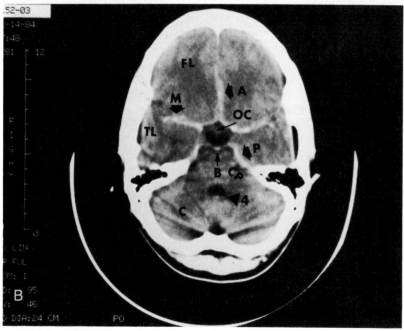

Fig. 7-7 (A) Normal CT scan of the brain, axial section. Preinfusion scan through the basal ganglia. Basal ganglia: HC = head of the caudate nucleus, SP = septum pellucidum, ICA = internal capsule (anterior limb), ICP = internal capsule (posterior limb), T = Thalamus, L = lentiform nuclei (globus pallidus and putamen), FH = frontal horn of the lateral ventricles, FM = foramen of Monroe, 3 = third ventricle, AQ = aqueduct, Q = quadrigeminal plate (cistern), Posterior dotted line = tentorium with cerebellum (posterior cranial fossa projecting through). **(B)** Normal CT scan of the brain, axial section. Postinfusion study at the level of the circle of Willis. (This is lower than the section shown in **A**). FL = frontal lobe/anterior cranial foss, TL = temporal lobe/middle cranial fossa, C = cerebellum/posterior cranial fossa, A = anterior cerebral arteries (bilateral), M = right middle cerebral artery, P = left posterior cerebral artery, B = basilar artery, OC = optic chiasm, CP = cerebello-pontine angle (CPA), 4 = fourth ventricle.

CT allows visualization of the brain, CSF filled ventricles and cisterns, and vascular structures, as well as the surrounding bony structures (Fig. 7-7 A and B). The ability to differentiate between tissues of slightly different radiographic densities allows one to see the gray and white matter, and particularly the gray outer cortex, basal ganglia, internal capsule, and radiating white matter tracts. Computed tomography can reveal recent hemorrhages, which appear white on the resulting image. Calcification also appears white on

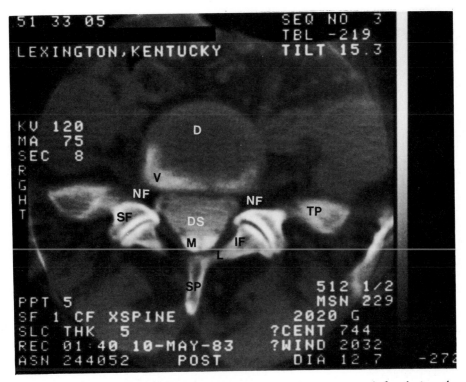

Fig. 7-8 Normal CT scan of the lumbar with Metrizamide. This CT section was scanned after the intrathecal administration of contrast material following a lumbar puncture. The section is through a vertebral disc. DS = dural sac, M = layering metrizamide in the dural sac, D = disk (L4/L5), V = portion of vertebral body (L4), TP = transverse process (L4), IF = inferior articulating facet (L4), L = lamina (L4), SP = spinous process (L4), SF = superior articulating facet (L5), NF = neural foramina.

the CT image, but can be differentiated from blood. Blood has a CT number measuring from 30 to 50 HU (Hounsfield units, the units of radiographic density measured in CT and named after the inventor of the technique), whereas calcium has numbers greater than 60 HU. Areas of edema (secondary to a tumor, infarct, demyelination, or necrosis), infarction, arachnoid cysts, and porencephalic regions appear as black or low-density areas. Tumors may even occasionally be separated into their types depending on their characteristic CT appearance. The ventricular size and thus hydrocephalus is easily detected without the morbidity associated with the previously utilized pneumoencephalography.

The visualization of anatomic structures and pathology of the brain on CT may be enhanced by the use of intravenous contrast agents. The vascular anatomy, such as that of the vertebrobasilar system, circle of Willis, main anterior and middle cerebral artery trunks, internal cerebral veins, vein of Galen, straight sinus, sagittal sinus, torcular Herophili, and sigmoid sinuses can be visualized routinely (Fig. 7-7 A and B). Aneurysms, arteriovenous malformations, and other vascular lesions are easily demonstrated. Computed tomography shows surrounding edema as separate from a tumor after the injection of intravenous contrast medium. In other pathologic states, such as subacute infarcts, tumors, meningitis, and multiple sclerosis, abnormal contrast enhancement is also seen. The etiology of vascular enhancement is twofold. In vascular lesions such as aneurysms, the enhancement is due to contrast medium within the lumen of the

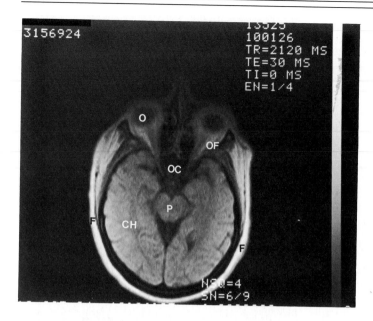

Fig. 7-9 Normal MR scan, axial section. Note how fat appears white and the bones of the calvarium and base of the skull are not imaged. The white around the calvarium is fat (F) that lines the brain coverings. O = orbits, OF = white orbital fat, OC = optic chiasm, P = pons, CH = cerebral hemispheres.

vascular anomalies. In tumors and infarcts the abnormal contrast enhancement is due to the breakdown of the blood-brain barrier and leakage of contrast medium through the vessels into the surrounding tissues.

Computed tomography is also applied with great success to evaluation of the spine and spinal cord. In the lumbar spine there is excellent identification of herniated discs. Epidural fat appears black on the CT scan and is plentiful in the lumbar region. The thecal (dural) sac and protruding disc material of soft-tissue density can be visualized against the natural contrast of the black fat. In order to visualize lesions of the spinal cord, especially in the fat-free areas of the cervical and thoracic spine, intrathecal water-soluble Metrizamide can be instilled into the subarachnoid spaces, usually via a lumbar puncture (Fig. 7-8). All spaces containing cerebral spinal fluid in the brain and spine appear white on subsequent CT images. This intrathecal contrast allows good visualization of the spinal cord for the detection of tumors.

Gray- and white-matter differentiation is far superior with MR than with CT. Bone is "invisible" on MR, as opposed to CT, and areas such as the posterior fossa and spinal cord can easily be seen without troublesome bone artifacts (Fig. 7-9). Furthermore, the ability to image not only in the transverse but also the sagittal and coronal planes without having to change the patient's orientation, such as in CT, gives MR a distinct advantage. Another feature of MR is its ability to demonstrate abnormal tissue without the need for a contrast agent.

A new technology, positron emission tomography (PET) scan, utilizes signals emitted from biochemically active compounds tagged with a radioactive particle which emits positrons. Such a scan requires a powerful linear accelerator to generate the radioactive particles. Areas of infarction and other pathologic states are now imaged on the basis of their biochemical abnormality.

CLINICAL PRESENTATION: LOSS OF CONSCIOUSNESS

Loss of consciousness due to trauma is probably the most common cause and the single most common reason for skull radiography in the emergency room. Calvarial and facial fractures are detected as lucent, straight lines in the dense bones (see Fig. 5-5). Accompanying air, dissecting under the skull next to the brain to create a pneumocephalus, is also easily seen on a plain skull radiograph. If there is an accompanying subdural hematoma one may see a shift of the normally calcified pineal gland to the contralateral side, as a result of the mass effect. Tumors and other causes of a mass effect may also cause a pineal shift. Most other pathologic states leading to loss of consciousness are not detected on plain skull radiographs. The most efficacious examination in cases of loss of consciousness in the absence of trauma would be a non-contrast-enhanced CT scan followed by intravenous contrast-medium administration if the non-contrast CT scan is negative. The most common causes of such unconsciousness include a stroke, an intracranial hemorrhage, or an inflammatory or systemic disorder.

UNCOMPLICATED STROKE

Stroke is due to interruption of the blood supply to the brain, either by a thrombotic or embolic event and resulting in a pale or red infarct, respectively. With thrombosis there is a slow, ongoing process of arterial occlusion. Since the blood supply to an area of the brain is cut off, the infarct appears pale. With emboli a clot temporarily occludes a vessel and then breaks into smaller fragments which propagate more distally. Reopening of the blood vessel as the clot resolves results in blood leaking from the damaged vessel and creating a parenchymal hemorrhage. This is called a hemorrhagic stroke or a red infarction. The red infarction will be discussed in the subsequent section on parenchymal hemorrhage.

Computed tomography is the method of choice for detecting an infarct and assessing whether or not there has been a secondary hemorrhage into the area of infarction. The first finding on CT in a case of simple infarction may not appear for 24 hours after the onset of symptoms. There is an ill-defined area of decreased density with a surrounding mass effect from edema. The mass effect produced by an infarct can usually be differentiated from the mass effect of brain tumor. Usually the edema of an infarct extends into both the gray and white matter, in contrast to the edema of a tumor, which remains confined to the white matter (Fig. 7-10 and see 7-31). The infarcted area becomes more sharply defined and lower in density as porencephalic changes from necrosis replace the initial area of edema. Furthermore, as the low-density area becomes better defined, the area of involvement remains within defined vascular territories. The area of the brain supplied by the anterior cerebral artery is a thin strip on either side of the interhemispheric fissure, about 1 to 1.5 cm wide. The border between the territory of the middle cerebral artery and the posterior cerebral artery is a straight line running directly posterior from the tip of the occipital (Fig. 7-10) horn of

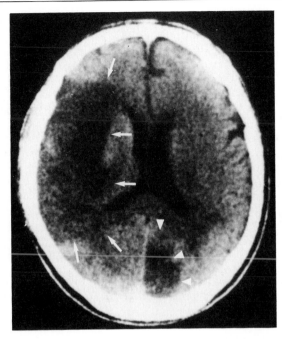

Fig. 7-10 Infarcts of the middle cerebral and posterior cerebral arteries.
History. This 80-year-old woman went into a sudden and deep coma.
Findings. *CT scan:* A low density replaces normal brain density in the classic distribution of the right middle cerebral artery (arrows) and left posterior cerebral artery (arrowheads) in this patient with multiple emboli from the heart to the brain. The low density involves both the white and gray layers of the brain.

the lateral ventricle. Tumor edema does not respect these vascular boundaries, and will cross over them. The mass effect from an infarct disappears within 1 week.

With the administration of contrast medium there may be enhancement of the infarct in the form of wavy lines of high density, indicating "gyral enhancement" from breakdown of the blood-brain barrier (Fig. 7-11). This abnormal contrast enhancement may persist for months, long after the edema has subsided.

One month after an initial infarction, the area of damaged brain appears as a region of low density approaching the black density of CSF. The necrotic brain has been replaced by CSF to produce porencephaly. There is an accompanying loss of brain volume, enlargement of the neighboring ventricle, and occasionally a shift of the midline structures toward

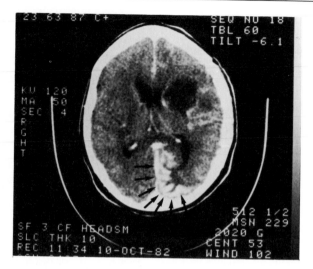

Fig. 7-11 Acute cerebral infarction.
History. This postoperative evaluation was done in a patient after the removal of a temporal-lobe glioma. He had a sudden onset of paralysis on the right side.
Findings. *CT scan:* A postinfusion study shows gyral serpinginous enhancement of the occipital lobe (arrows), indicating a new infarct from posterior cerebral artery occlusion.

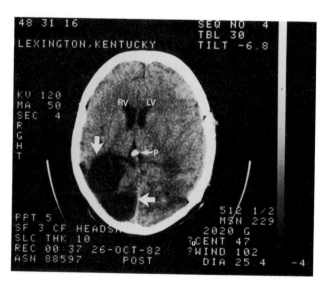

Fig. 7-12 Old cerebral infarction.
History. This 72-year-old man had a "massive stroke" 2 years earlier.
Findings. *CT scan:* The previous infarction has been replaced by low-density CSF and is now porencephalic (arrows). Note that the right lateral ventricle (RV) is also more dilated than the left (LV), which is another response to volume loss of the right brain substance. The ventricles are shifted to the right as well. P = calcified pineal gland, normal.

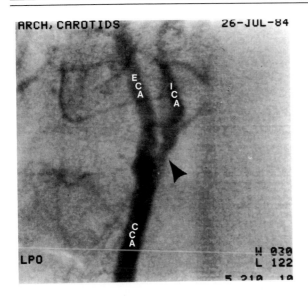

Fig. 7-13 Atherosclerosis of the carotid artery.
History. This 67-year-old man had recurrent TIAs.
Findings. *Digital subtraction angiography:* There is irregular narrowing of the wall of the left internal carotid artery (arrowhead) (ICA) from atherosclerotic plaque. CCA = common carotid artery, ECA = external carotid artery.

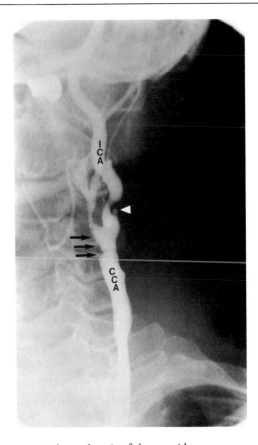

Fig. 7-14 Atherosclerosis of the carotid artery.
History. This 65-year-old man had recurrent "clumsiness" 6 months after a "mild stroke."
Findings. *Carotid angiogram:* There is irregular narrowing of the common carotid artery (CCA), most severe just before the bifurcation into its external and internal divisions (arrows). A large plaque causing significant narrowing is present at the origin of the internal carotid artery (ICA), with a central ulceration of this atherosclerotic plaque (arrowhead).

the affected side (Fig. 7-12). Magnetic resonance imaging demonstrates a stroke to even a better degree than CT, and may also allow its detection before 24 hours have elapsed.

Angiography plays a role in the evaluation of stroke only if definitive vascular surgery of the extracranial carotid arteries is planned. Not only is the anatomy of the stenotic cervical carotid artery studied (Figs. 7-13 and 7-14), but the intracranial circulation is also examined. If severe occlusive disease of the intracranial arteries is seen as with advanced atherosclerosis, extracranial carotid surgery may not be indicated.

PARENCHYMAL HEMORRHAGE

The etiologies of a hemorrhage into the brain parenchyma are many and include a hemorrhagic infarction, arteriovenous malformation, aneurysm, and trauma. All result in a spillage of blood into the brain substance that appears as a high-density area on the initial, non-contrast-enhanced CT image. Aneurysms will be discussed in a subsequent section.

HEMORRHAGIC INFARCTIONS

Hemorrhagic or red infarcts result primarily in parenchymal staining. The non-contrast-enhanced CT scan containing a hemorrhagic infarct shows a low-density area of edema extending into both the white and gray matter about a somewhat centrally located, high-density hemorrhage (Fig. 7-15). Abnormal gyral enhancement may also be present after contrast-medium administration, as discussed for non-hemorrhagic infarcts. An extension to the subarachnoid space may be present but is usually minimal.

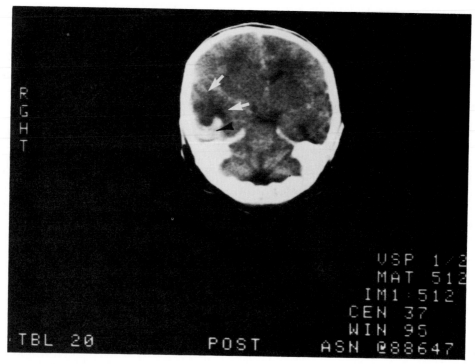

Fig. 7-15 Hemorrhagic infarct.
History. This neonate was irritable after a complicated delivery.
Findings. *CT scan:* There is a high-density collection of blood (arrowhead) with a surrounding low-density edema (arrows) in the right temporal lobe.

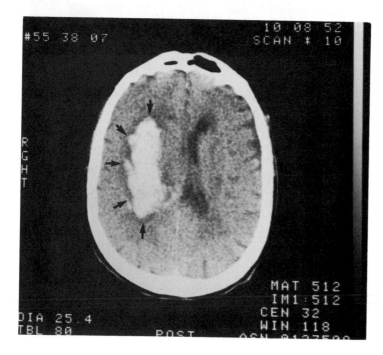

Fig. 7-16 Intracerebral hemorrhagic infarct of the basal ganglia.
History. This 61-year-old woman had poorly controlled hypertension and now had become unconscious.
Findings. *CT scan:* High-density blood (arrows) fills the expected location in the right basal ganglia.

Hemorrhagic infarcts of the basal ganglia caused by hypertension produce profound hemiparalysis and hemianesthesia due to compression of the corticospinal and spinothalamic tracts by the extravasated blood and edema. The CT scan shows a large high density lesion (blood) centered in the basal ganglia, often with associated penetration and spillage into the ventricular system (Fig. 7-16). Subarachnoid penetration can also occur. The surrounding mass effect may be quite prominent and responsible for a poor outcome, especially if the brainstem becomes further compressed by herniation of the temporal lobe.

As the blood in a parenchymal hemorrhage clots and the clot retracts with time, there is a squeezing out of serum. The high density blood in the CT scan resolves first at the edges, which then become indistinct. As the shrinkage progresses, there is a decrease in density of the hemorrhage, beginning peripherally. At 1 to 2 weeks after the initial hemorrhage one may observe a ringlike pattern of contrast enhancement. This is due to breakdown of the blood-brain barrier and leakage of contrast medium into the injured region.

ARTERIOVENOUS MALFORMATION

Arteriovenous malformations (AVM) are located in the brain parenchyma and therefore tend to produce parenchymal hemorrhages when they bleed. The initial noncontrast CT shows the typical high density collection of blood within the brain substance representing a hematoma. The contrast-enhanced CT scan is quite typical consisting of a tangled collection of serpiginous and dot-like vascular structures representing dilated arterial feeders and multiple dilated, draining venous channels.

If therapy is planned, formal angiography is necessary. Its main diagnostic role is to identify all arterial feeders (intracranial and extracranial) as well as the dilated venous channels. With new interventional methods, these AVMs may be reduced in size by embolization with Gelfoam, glues, and balloon catheter occlusion.

TRAUMATIC HEMORRHAGE

Traumatic injury produces subdural hematomas owing to tearing of the venous structures coursing through the subdural space. There is usually no accompanying skull fracture. Blood collects in the subdural space between the brain and dural lining. A non-contrast-enhanced CT scan is currently the method of first choice for examination of such suspected hematomas. The subdural collections of blood appear as crescentic, high-density collections adjacent to the inner table of the skull (Fig. 7-17). With time, as the hemoglobin or serum is resorbed, the subdural hematoma loses its high density, becomes isodense (the same as brain), and finally reaches a low density. The collection may then assume a more biconvex or lens shape. A pseudomembrane that may enhance with contrast-medium infusion forms along the inner aspect of the aging hematoma, separating it from the brain (Fig. 7-18 A and B).

An epidural hematoma is a frequent accompaniment of a skull fracture. The hematoma occurs from arterial damage. On the CT scan there is a high-density or white region with an initial biconvex or lens-

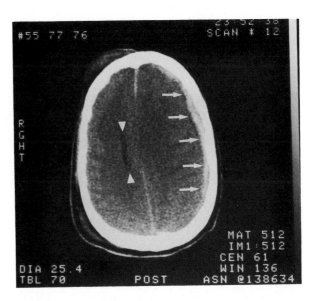

Fig. 7-17 Subdural hematoma.
History. This 21-year-old woman had a progressive headache following an automobile accident.
Findings. *CT scan:* A convex or crescentic collection of blood (arrows) is seen between the brain and calvarium. Also note the secondary flattening of the left lateral ventricle and shifting of the midline to the right from the mass effect of the subdural hematoma (arrowheads).

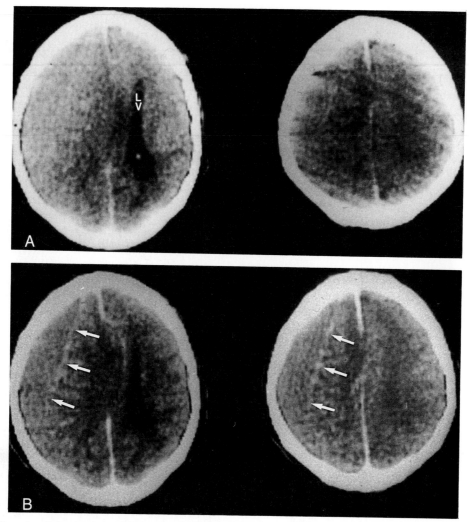

Fig. 7-18 Chronic subdural hematoma.
History. This 57-year-old man had continued neurologic symptoms a few weeks after an automobile accident.
Findings. *CT scan:* **(A)** A preinfusion scan shows obliteration of the right lateral ventricle and deviation of the left lateral ventricle (LV) further laterally. This implies a mass effect involving the right cerebral hemisphere. **(B)** A post infusion scan demonstrates the enhancing membrane of a chronic subdural hematoma (arrows). The hematoma is at the isodense stage at which it has the same density as the surrounding brain.

like appearance (Fig. 7-19A). Manipulation of the CT window settings to maximize bony detail often demonstrates the skull fracture adjacent to the epidural hematoma (Fig. 7-19B).

Computed tomography is probably more sensitive to vertically oriented fractures than is the plain skull radiograph, but fails if the fracture line is horizontal and therefore lies in the transverse or axial plane and overlapping CT cuts are not taken. Computed tomography is also the method of choice for the detection of suspected occipital or base of the skull fractures.

Other changes seen in CT scans and associated with head injury include those of a simple contusion,

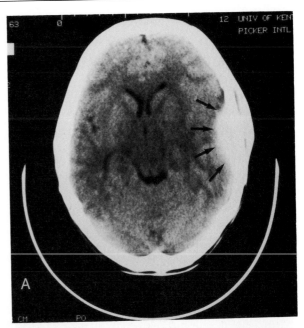

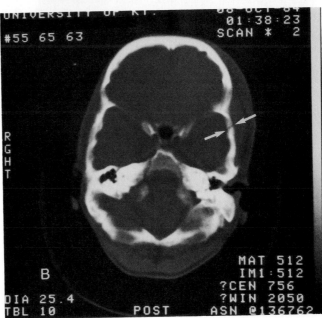

Fig. 7-19 Epidural hematoma.
History. This 31-year-old man had prolonged unconsciencousness after an automobile accident.
Findings. *CT scan:* **(A)** An axial projection demonstrates a double convex or lens-shaped, collection of high-density blood (arrows). **(B)** Same section as in **(A)**, but manipulation of the image to best visualize the bony skull demonstrates the associated skull fracture (arrows).

usually without an associated parenchymal hemorrhage. Contusions present as poorly defined zones of decreased density, usually patchy and less than 1 cm in size. These low-density areas may enhance minimally on CT. Larger zones of decreased density suggest a traumatic, non-hemorrhagic infarction, making it mandatory to rule out a vascular injury such as an intraparenchymal arterial tear or dissection. On the preinfusion scan, an associated hemorrhage (contusional hemorrhage or hemorrhagic contusion) again appears as a high-density collection with surrounding edema.

SUBARACHNOID HEMORRHAGE/ANEURYSM

Headache of severe onset, coupled with photophobia, a stiff neck, a sudden loss of consciousness, and a bloody spinal tap describe the clinical presentation of subarachnoid hemorrhage (SAH). This hemorrhage is most commonly due to a ruptured aneurysm, but may be secondary to a ruptured arteriovenous malformation, hemorrhagic infarct, tumor hemorrhage, or head trauma.

The non-contrast-enhanced CT scan demonstrates the subarachnoid collection of blood as a high-density pool just below the skull surface or outling the interhemispheric fissure and sulci (Fig. 7-20). The site of the ruptured aneurysm is often suggested by the distribution of the blood. Anterior communicating and posterior communicating aneurysms are the most common, and have about the same frequency of occurrence. The pattern of SAH in cases of these lesions would tend to be bilaterally symmetrically distributed because of the midline location of these aneurysms (Fig. 7-20 A and B). A unilateral SAH would favor an aneurysm of the middle cerebral artery bifurcation — the third most common location for a bleeding aneurysm. A focal high-density parenchymal hemorrhage further localizes the site of aneurysm rupture (Fig. 7-21). Intraventricular blood can also occur with a ruptured aneurysm and subarachnoid hemorrhage, with blood entering through the choroidal fissure

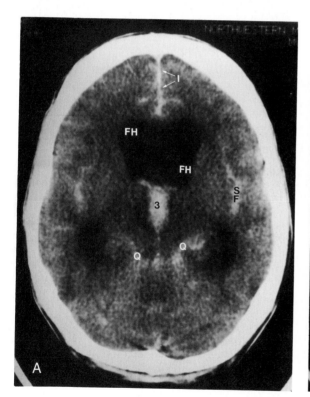 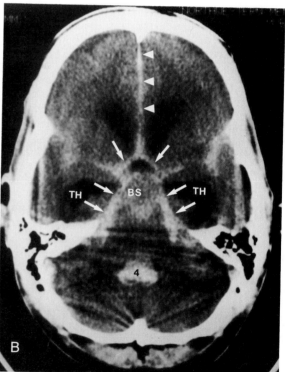

Fig. 7-20 Massive subarachnoid hemorrhage from an aneurysm of the posterior communicating artery.
History. This 55-year-old man was in a coma for unknown reasons.
Findings. *CT; non-contrast-enhanced section:* **(A)** Same level as Figure 7-7A. Blood, appearing white, fills the sylvian fissure (SF), third ventricle (3), quadrigeminal/cistern (Q), and interhemispheric fissure (I). Note that the frontal horns (FH) of the lateral ventricles are markedly dilated, representing hydrocephalus. **(B)** Same level as in Figure 7-7B. Blood collects about the brainstem (BS) in a location where only CSF is normally located (arrows). Blood also outlines the interhemispheric fissure (arrowheads). Note the dilated and blood-filled fourth ventricle (4). TH = dilated temporal horns of the lateral ventricles. At autopsy, an aneurysm of the posterior communicating artery was found.

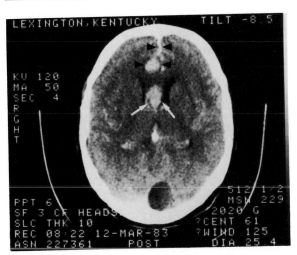

Fig. 7-21 Aneurysm of the anterior cerebral artery.
History. This 40-year-old woman presented in an acutely unresponsive state.
Findings. *CT scan:* There is a circular, high-density collection of blood in this postinfusion axial section, representing an aneurysm (arrows). In addition, a localized hematoma (this density was also present on the preinfusion scan) is present in the septum pellucidum and interhemispheric fissure, representing the subarachnoid extension of the hemorrhage (arrowheads). This localized collection of blood pinpoints the aneurysm to the anterior cerebral artery.

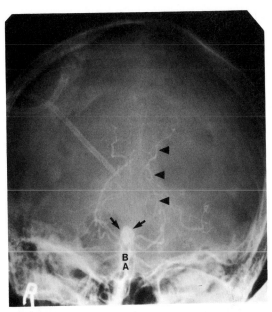

Fig. 7-22 Basilar artery aneurysm.
History. This 61-year-old man had severe headaches.
Findings. *Angiogram:* An aneurysm (arrows) is present on the tip of the basilar artery (BA). Note the very narrow caliber of the posterior arteries, indicating secondary vasospasm (arrowheads).

into the temporal horns and through the foramina of Luschka and Magendie in the fourth ventricle to fill all of the ventricles (Fig. 7-20).

An SAH can produce severe vasospasm 10 to 12 days after the bleeding episode, resulting in secondary areas of infarction. At that time the CT scan may show multiple, low-density acute infarctions, as previously described. Angiography shows a smooth narrowing of multiple intracranial arteries, consistent with vasospasm (Fig. 7-22).

INFLAMMATORY DISORDERS

Various infectious etiologies may be considered in the patient who loses consciousness and has a fever. Computed tomography may aid in making a more specific

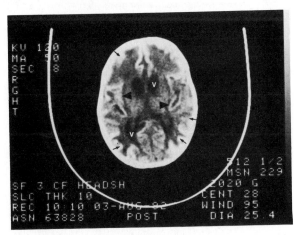

Fig. 7-23 Meningoencephalitis.
History. This 3-week-old male infant had a rigid neck and fever.
Findings. *CT scan:* There is marked enhancement of the meningeal coverings of the brain (arrows). The enhancement extends into the sylvian fissure (arrowheads). The brain substance is also of a somewhat higher than normal density for a neonate, with dilated ventricles (v), suggesting encephalitis.

diagnosis in cases of suspected inflammatory disorder.

Meningitis can present with a profound alteration in the state of consciousness. An intense, abnormal contrast enhancement following a cortical sulcal pattern suggests meningeal irritation and possibly meningitis (Fig. 7-23). However, subarachnoid hemorrhage from any etiology may also produce this intense meningeal enhancement.

Encephalitis may or may not produce CT effects. There may be some ill-defined areas of low density on the non-contrast-enhanced scan. If the encephalitis is quite severe it may appear as a low-density area of infarction with a mass effect. In adults with herpes encephalitis the ill-defined areas of low density, favoring the temporal lobe and uncus as seen on early CT scans, are almost diagnostic. Magnetic resonance imaging may be as or more sensitive than CT in encephalitis. Angiography infrequently may demonstrate an irregular tangle of vessels.

Either CT or MR should be used first in the evaluation of a suspected intracerebral abscess. The abscess cavity appears as an ill-defined, low-density area and exhibits a ringlike pattern with subsequent contrast-medium administration. The enhancing wall represents the pseudomembrane or capsule as the abscess walls off. It is usually thin and of uniform thickness and homogeneity (Fig. 7-24). If the wall is thick, nodular or irregular, a metastatic or primary tumor, is more likely, but an abscess cannot be entirely excluded. Other causes of an enhancing ringlike pattern on the CT scan include mature infarcts and resolving hematomas, as previously discussed.

The angiogram in cases of abscess may demonstrate a "capsular blush" or stain representing the abscess capsule. Again, a tumor may exhibit the same characteristics.

SYSTEMIC DISORDERS

Conditions such as diabetic ketoacidosis, hyper- or hypocalcemia, hypoxia, and septicemia may present with an alteration in acute mental status and even unconsciousness; however, the CT findings in such cases tend to be sparse. Other clinical and physical findings will help narrow the many diagnostic possibilities. Abnormal calcification of the basal ganglia

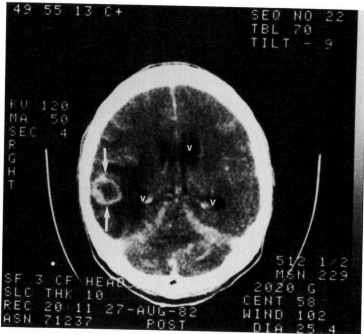

Fig. 7-24 Cerebral abscess.
History. This 29-year-old homosexual male had acquired immune deficiency syndrome (AIDS) and disseminated toxoplasmosis.
Findings. *CT scan:* There is a ring-enhancing lesion of the temporal lobe (arrow), with a surrounding low-density edema. v = lateral ventricles.

(i.e., seen on a CT scan of a patient under 40 years of age) — otherwise a normal finding with age — suggests a hypercalcemic state.

Angiography has very little to offer in systemic disorders except to rule out an unsuspected arteritis. Magnetic resonance imaging remains to be explored, but at present it better defines areas of abnormal storage depositions in the white matter than does CT.

CLINICAL PRESENTATION: FOCAL NEUROLOGIC DEFICITS

There are many processes that lead to focal neurologic deficit, including brain tumors, intracranial hemorrhage, infarctions, abscesses, central nervous system storage deposition diseases, and demyelinating/degenerative disorders of the white matter. The CT appearances of some of these entities have been described in the previous section.

NEOPLASMS

Tumors are a frequent cause of focal neurologic deficits. They are categorized either as primary brain tumors or metastatic involvements of the brain, frequently from primary carcinomas in the breast or lung. The primary brain tumors can be further divided into those that start within the brain parenchyma (intra-axial) and those originating from structures outside the brain but inside the bony skull (extra-axial). These include tumors of the meningeal coverings (meningiomas) or optic nerve (optic neuromas).

MENINGIOMA

Meningiomas are benign, slow-growing tumors that can arise from any meningeal surface. They have a propensity for the meningeal surfaces at the apex or top of the skull, olfactory groove, sellar region, sphenoid wings, and petrous ridge. Meningiomas incites a secondary thickening of the proximally situated bone that can be detected on the plain skull radiograph. This is called a hyperostosis (Fig. 7-25). The vascular grooves that criss-cross the skull may dilate as the tumor requires an increased blood supply. From 15 to 20 percent of meningiomas have internal calcifications.

The typical CT appearance of a meningioma is that of an isodense to slightly high density lesion with or without calcifications on precontrast scans. The lesion exhibits an intense, homogeneous pattern of

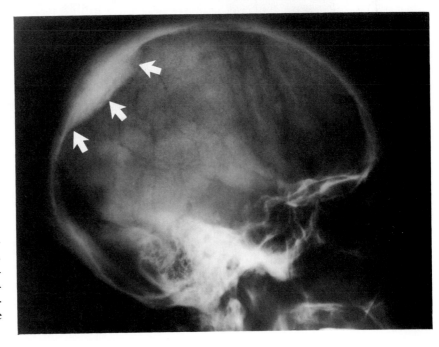

Fig. 7-25 Meningioma. **History.** This 42-year-old woman had unrelenting headaches. **Findings.** *Lateral skull radiograph:* There is obvious thickening (hyperostosis) of the superior and posterior aspects of the cranial vault (arrows).

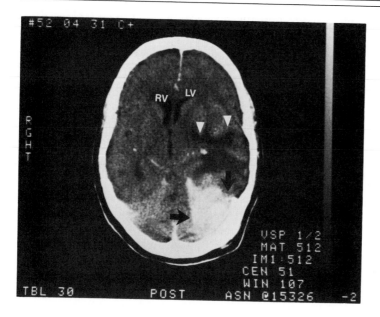

Fig. 7-26 Meningioma.
History. This 49-year-old woman had progressive difficulty walking.
Findings. *CT scan:* A postinfusion study shows a homogeneously enhancing tumor involving the middle and posterior cranial fossae (arrows). Additionally, surrounding edema of the left temporal lobe is causing a low-density area in the brain (arrowheads). Note the secondary compression of the left lateral ventricle (LV) from this edema, as compared to the normal right lateral ventricle (RV).

contrast enhancement that is virtually pathognomonic for a meningioma (Fig. 7-26).

BRAIN METASTASIS

Metastatic tumors are the most common intraaxial tumors in the adult population. The plain radiograph in such cases may show associated bony destruction of the skull (Fig. 7-27). There are no characteristic CT findings, except that the lesions are frequently multiple. Metastatic lesions usually have an irregular pattern of contrast enhancement, an associated extensive edema, and indistinct margins that suggest the invasiveness of these malignancies (Fig. 7-28).

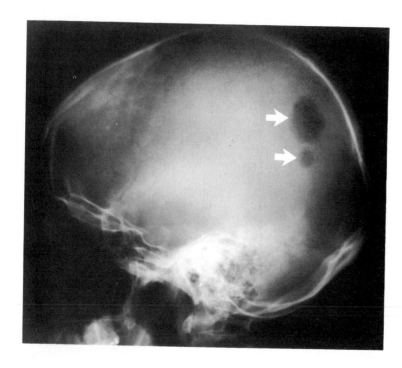

Fig. 7-27 Metastasis to the skull.
History. This 47-year-old woman had an 18-month history of breast carcinoma.
Findings. *Lateral skull radiograph:* This single view demonstrates two irregular lucent or lytic areas of metastasis (arrows) in the posterior cranial vault.

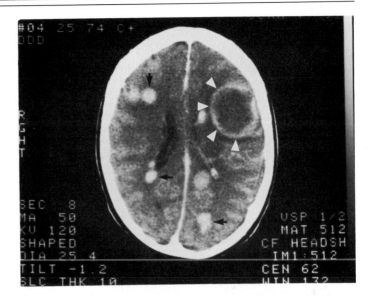

Fig. 7-28 Brain metastasis.
History. This 63-year-old man had newly discovered lung cancer.
Findings. *CT scan:* There are multiple dense deposits throughout the brain (arrows) in this postinfusion study. One metastatic deposit demonstrates ringlike enhancement of its wall and a necrotic, low-density center (arrowheads).

PRIMARY BRAIN TUMORS

Primary tumors of the brain or gliomas have appearances that vary according to their malignant potential. Computed tomography is useful in the staging of gliomas. Grade I gliomas are seen as ill-defined, low-density masses without significant contrast enhancement (Fig. 7-29). Grade II gliomas often have a low-density "cystic" appearance with ringlike contrast enhancement, and possibly a localized nodule on the wall (a mural nodule) that also enhances (Fig. 7-30). Grade III and IV gliomas (glioblastoma multiforme) are the most aggressive lesions, often being cavitary with an irregular and thick wall and exhibiting abnormal and bizarre contrast enhancement (Fig. 7-31).

Magnetic resonance imaging is as sensitive to tumors as CT. However, it may be difficult to distinguish edema from tumor mass with MR (Fig.

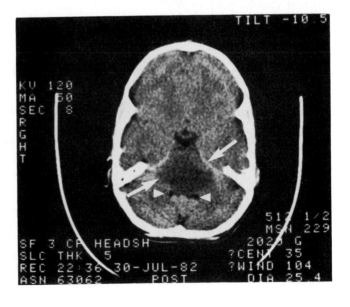

Fig. 7-29 Glioma of the brainstem.
History. This 47-year-old woman had extensive neurologic abnormalities on examination.
Findings. *CT scan:* There is a huge low-density mass (arrows) with consequent flattening and posterior displacement of the fourth ventricle (arrowheads).

7-32). Nor, to date, can tumors be reliably distinguished according to histologic type, as was hoped for MR.

Angiography has a much diminished role in the evaluation of tumors. It utilizes characteristic shifts of the normal vascular distribution to help localize the tumor mass (Fig. 7-33 A and B). This is no longer necessary with the advent of CT, which clearly localizes a tumor. The size of the tumor is also frequently overestimated with angiography, since surrounding edema adds to the vascular shift. Tumor vessels have a classic bizarre and tortuous appearance along with early venous shunting.

DEMYELINATING DISEASE

Demyelinating diseases such as multiple sclerosis are another source of focal deficits. The CT appearance of demyelinating disorders varies. The most typical pattern is that of a low-density plaque with abnormal contrast enhancement during the active phase of the disease. A mass effect can also be identified. Older plaques are well defined but do not enhance with the administration of contrast medium. These plaques typically line the ventricles in a periventricular distribution. Magnetic resonance imaging is proving to be more sensitive to the alterations of multiple sclerosis than is CT, but much work remains to be done (Fig. 7-34).

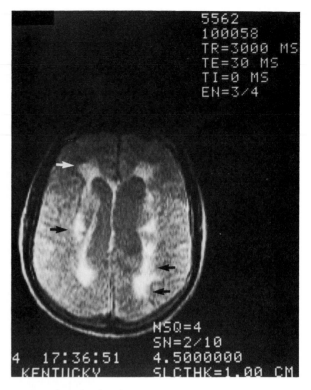

Fig. 7-34 Multiple sclerosis.
History. This 50-year-old woman had a long history of multiple sclerosis, now causing acute symptoms.
Findings. *Magnetic resonance image:* There are multiple areas of bright plaques (arrows) situated about the lateral ventricles. These represent an active demylination of the periventricular white matter.

CLINICAL PRESENTATION: SEVERE HEADACHES

The majority of patients with severe headaches have negative CT scans, but many important etiologies must be considered, diagnosed, and treated in such cases, often with great speed. Migraine headaches are common, and CT or angiography are unrevealing in this condition. Another possible cause of severe headache is a ruptured aneurysm with a subsequent subarachnoid hemorrhage. This, as previously discussed, is quickly diagnosed with CT. Hydrocephalus is a third cause of severe headaches and is today best evaluated with CT.

HYDROCEPHALUS

Hydrocephalus is an important cause of severe headache, particularly in childen. The ventricular size is age dependent (Fig. 7-35); the older one is the larger the ventricles become as the surrounding brain atrophies and the ventricles expand to fill the created void (Fig. 7-36). On the CT scan hydrocephalus appears as a dilatation of the ventricle that is discordant with the patient's age. The causes of hydrocephalus are many, and can be categorized as obstructive or nonobstructive.

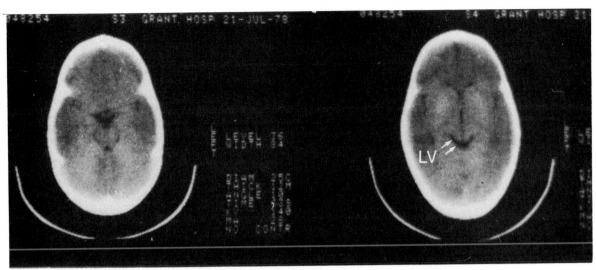

Fig. 7-35 Normal pediatric CT scan of the brain.
History. This 3-year-old boy presented after an automobile accident.
Findings. *CT scan:* The lateral ventricles (LV) have only a slit like width at this age.

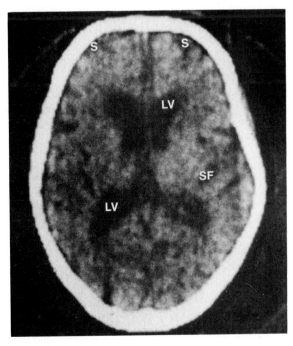

Fig. 7-36 Cerebral atrophy.
History. This 81-year-old man had dementia.
Findings. *CT scan:* The lateral ventricles are dilated (LV) and the brain sulci (S) and sylvian fissure (SF) are prominent, as the brain normally atrophies with age.

OBSTRUCTIVE HYDROCEPHALUS

Obstructive hydrocephalus results from a blockage of the flow of CSF at the level of any one of the four (two lateral, third, and fourth) cerebral ventricles. Tumors are an important cause of hydrocephalus. Depending on the location of the obstruction different combinations of the ventricular enlargement occur. If the obstruction is within the fourth ventricle or brainstem, the CT reveals dilatation of the lateral and third ventricles (Fig. 7-37). A tumor of the brainstem may also led to compression of the fourth ventricle. If the lesion is at the foramen of Monro the lateral ventricles enlarge while the third and fourth ventricles remain of normal size. If a lesion at the foramen of Monro is located more to one side, unilateral dilatation of one lateral ventricle may occur.

NONOBSTRUCTIVE HYDROCEPHALUS

Nonobstructive etiologies such as acute subarachnoid hemorrhage (Fig. 7-20), late subarachnoid hemorrhage with the development of arachnoid scarring, postinflammatory arachnoid scarring (meningitis), and thrombosis of the superior sagittal sinus may also result in hydrocephalus. In these pathologic states the

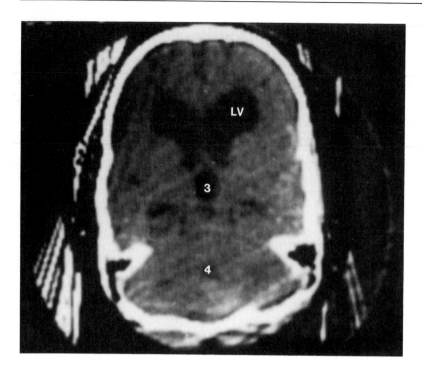

Fig. 7-37 Obstructive hydrocephalus.
History. This 7-year-old girl had lethargy and headaches.
Findings. *CT scan:* The lateral (LV) and third (3) ventricles are immensely dilated for a child. The fourth (4) ventricle is of normal size. This implies that the obstruction lies between the third and fourth ventricles. In this case the hydrocephalus is a result of narrowing of the sylvian aqueduct.

CSF cannot be absorbed by the arachnoid as is normal. A papilloma of the choroid plexus that overproduces CSF, leading to an increased CSF volume, also results in hydrocephalus.

CLINICAL PRESENTATION: ENDOCRINE DISTURBANCES

Patients may present with a variety of endocrine disturbances including amenorrhea and galactorrhea. The serum prolactin levels in such conditions may be elevated. It is first necessary to rule out end-organ disease such as with CT scanning of the adrenals. Once this is accomplished a central cause must be sought. A tumor of the pituitary gland, compression of the pituitary by an abnormal pocket of CSF, or hypothalmic infarction are the most common etiologies.

PITUITARY TUMOR

Chromophobe adenoma is the most common pituitary tumor in the adult. Computed tomography has replaced conventional tomography and plain radiography for evaluation of the sella turcica; it not only allows visualization of the bony sella, as do the earlier methods, but also clearly images the pituitary gland itself and accompanying tumor. The plain radiographic or tomographic evaluation of pituitary tumors is based on a secondary bony erosion or enlargement of the sella turcica (Fig. 7-38). The tumor must be fairly large to be detectable with these modalities, which are thus relatively insensitive to early masses.

In a case of chromophobe adenoma, CT clearly demonstrates the sellar enlargement and accompanying bony destruction of the sella. The adenoma itself is usually slightly more dense than the normal pituitary, and may extend well above the sella turcica. With the administration of contrast medium there is intense, uniform contrast enhancement, with the tumor sharply defined (Fig. 7-39). Magnetic resonance imaging also clearly demonstrates the pituitary enlargement (Fig. 7-40). In addition, the multiplane ability of MR can detect secondary optic-nerve compression better than can CT.

EMPTY SELLA SYNDROME

Cerebrospinal fluid and accompanying dura can herniate into the sella turcica from an incompetent cover-

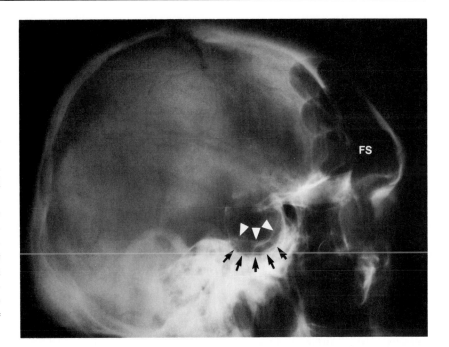

Fig. 7-38 Chromaphobe adenoma.

History. This 39-year-old woman had visual disturbances and irregular menstruation.

Findings. *Lateral skull radiograph:* The sella turcia is tremendously enlarged from the intrasellar tumor. Note the double floor appearance of the floor of the sella as the tumor grows assymmetrically, eroding the sellar boundaries (arrows, arrowheads). FS = frontal sinus.

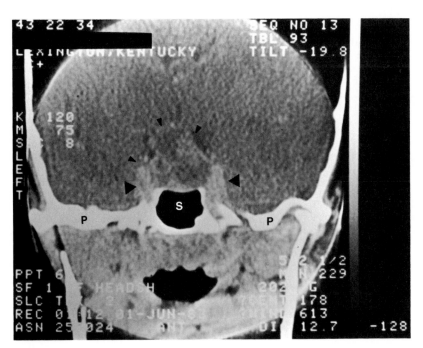

Fig. 7-39 Pituitary tumor.

History. This 41-year-old woman had "double vision."

Findings. *CT scan:* A low-density lesion extends from the sella turcia superiorly. The capsule of the tumor enhances with contrast medium (small arrowheads). The normal cavernous sinuses, are also enhanced (large arrowheads) in this postinfusion study. S = sphenoid sinus, P = petrous bone.

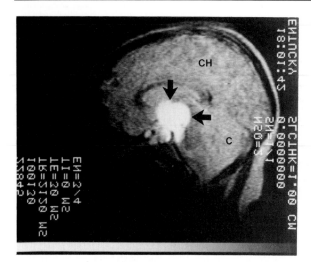

Fig. 7-40 Pituitary tumor.
History. This 39-year-old man had visual disturbances.
Findings. *Magnetic resonanic image:* A sagital image shows the dense white pituitary tumor with an extensive suprasellar component (arrows). CH = cerebral hemispheres, C = cerebellum.

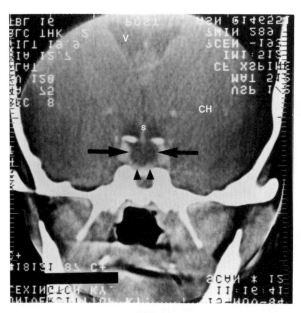

Fig. 7-41 Empty sella syndrome.
History. This 47-year-old woman had menstrual irregularities.
Findings. *CT scan:* A coronal view demonstrates low-density (black) CSF in the sella turcia (arrow). The flattened pituitary gland is barely discernible (arrowheads) on the sella floor. S = pituitary stalk, CH = cerebral hemisphere, V = lateral ventricles.

ing of the sella by the diaphragma sellae. As a result the pituitary gland becomes flattened posteriorly against the inner wall of the sella. There is resulting pituitary insufficiency. On CT the water density of CSF is seen filling the sella. Coronal sections can identify the compressed pituitary gland (Fig. 7-41). Magnetic resonance imaging is also proving helpful in making the diagnosis of empty sella syndrome.

HYPOTHALAMIC INFARCTION

The hypothalamus is located on either side of the third ventricle. Either a tumor or infarction involving this region can produce dysfunction of the hypothalamus and a secondary endocrine imbalance. The CT appearance of infarcts in the basal ganglia or hypothalamus has already been described (Fig. 7-16).

CLINICAL PRESENTATION: PROPTOSIS

The causes of proptosis are many, including thyroid ophthalamopathy, orbital pseudotumor, retrobulbar hematoma and tumors of the optic nerve, sheath, or lacrimal glands. Carotid cavernous (CC) fistula, vascular lesions such as varices or hemangiomas, orbital cellulitis, and encephalocele are less common and are beyond the scope of this text. Computed tomography affords excellent images of the orbit and orbital muscles as they form the orbital cone. The orbital cone is appreciated on CT with the orbit as the base and the extraocular muscles joining to form the apex. The optic nerve is also well visualized. The normal periorbital fat clearly outlines the anatomy by providing a low-density background for the soft-tissue structures (Fig. 7-42).

THYROID OPHTHALAMOPATHY

Thyroid ophthalamopathy usually presents with bilateral proptosis, but can manifest with unilateral symptoms. The CT scan demonstrates symmetrical enlargement and thickening of the extraocular muscles, with the medial and inferior rectii muscles most consistently involved (Fig. 7-43).

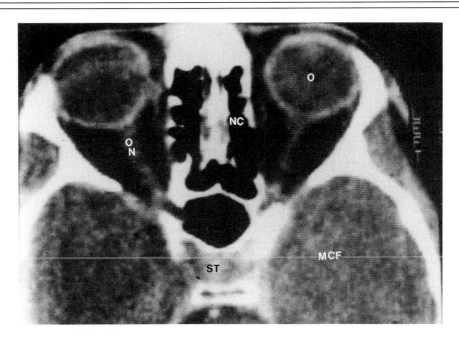

Fig. 7-42 Normal Orbits, CT. Section through the midportion of the orbits. ON = optic nerve, O = orbit, NC = nasal cavity, MCF = middle cranial fossa, ST = sella turcica.

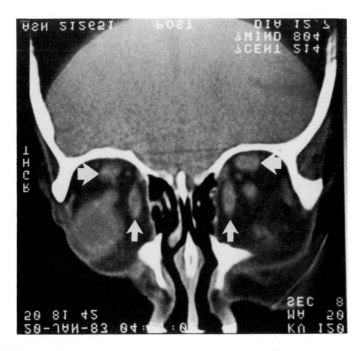

Fig. 7-43 Thyroid ophthalamopathy.
History. This 42-year-old woman had a progressive tremor, heat intolerance, and "bulging" eyes.
Findings. *CT scan:* A coronal section through the orbits demonstrate enlargement of both the superior and medial rectii muscles (arrows).

PSEUDOTUMOR

The next most common cause of proptosis is pseudo-tumor, an inflammatory disorder of uncertain etiology. This disorder is often confirmed by its rapid response to steroids. On CT a mass is seen near the apex of the orbital cone and which may blend indistinguishably with the extraocular muscles (Fig. 7-44). Although there may be some accompanying swelling of the extraocular muscles in pseudotumor, it does not usually involve the entire length of the muscle, as with thyroid disease.

OPTIC-NERVE GLIOMA

An optic-nerve glioma can also produce proptosis. The CT scan shows assymetric enlargement of the optic nerve, which may exhibit abnormal contrast enhancement. The involvement may be bilateral (Fig. 7-45).

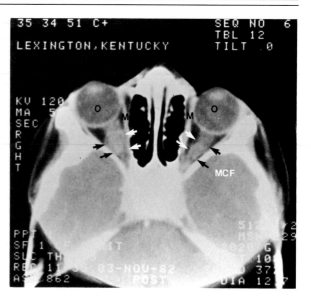

Fig. 7-45 Optic glioma.
History. This 39-year-old man had progressive proptosis and loss of vision.
Findings. *CT scan:* An axial scan through the orbits shows bulky nodular enlargement of both optic nerves (arrows). O = orbits, MCF = middle cranial fossa, M = medial rectus muscle.

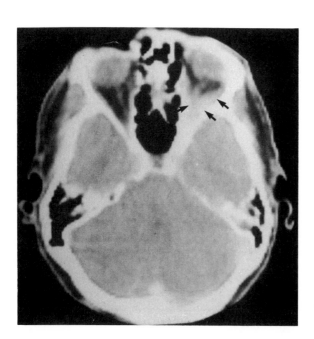

Fig. 7-44 Orbital pseudotumor.
History. This 43-year-old man had pain and blurred vision.
Findings. *CT scan:* A soft-tissue mass fills the posterior portion of the orbital cone on the left (arrows).

RETROBULBAR HEMATOMA

Retrobulbar hematoma is related to bony trauma or penetrating injury. A plain radiograph of the skull is obtained initially in cases of facial trauma to detect facial or orbital fractures and any residual foreign body.

A CT scan should be done in cases of suspected retrobulbar hematoma. It can provide information about whether the hematoma is intra- or extraconal (i.e., within the orbital cone or not). Computed tomography is also much better than plain radiography for the detection of residual foreign objects and can additionally demonstrate any hemorrhage within the globe as a result of a penetrating injury or foreign body. Moreover, CT is ideal for detecting accompanying orbital fractures, since its axial orientation is often perpendicular to the fracture (Fig. 7-46).

Tomography is as good as CT for delineating the bony anatomy in facial fractures, but does not demonstrate hemorrhages or other soft-tissue injuries, and so is less useful.

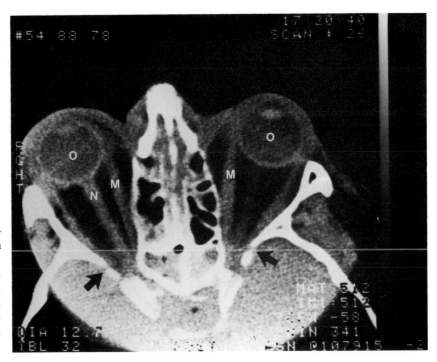

Fig. 7-46 Orbital fractures. **History.** This 27-year-old woman complained of blurred vision after an automobile accident. **Findings.** *CT scan:* There are bilateral fractures through the lateral orbital walls (arrows). The orbits are spared any secondary damage. N = optic nerve, M = extraocular muscles, O = orbits.

CLINICAL PRESENTATION: LOSS OF HEARING

Loss of hearing can be separated into conduction or neurosensory defects. In a conduction abnormality there is impedance to or obstruction of the passage of sound waves to the cochlea, where the mechanical motion of the sound wave is translated into electrical activity for transferance to the brain. This obstruction can occur at various levels. There may be obstruction at the level of the external auditory canal, either due to a foreign object, a soft tissue tumor, or secondary swelling from an ear infection. Likewise, the propagation of sound waves may be halted with trauma and injury to the tympanic membrane or disruption of the ossicular chain of the middle ear. A neurosensory defect is related to interruption of the translated electrical signal from the cochlea to the brain, and occurs primarily with abnormalities of the acoustic nerve. An acoustic nerve neuroma is a familiar neurosensory cause of hearing impairment.

Anatomic imaging of the ear is today best performed with CT. A CT scan with slices spaced at 2 to 3 mm in both axial and coronal projections provides the best anatomic detail of the external, middle, and internal ear structures. The course of the facial and acoustic nerves, and the ossicular chain, vestibule, ampulla, cochlea, and semicircular canals can all be demonstrated with high-resolution CT.

Tomography had traditionally been the means for studying the middle ear and internal auditory canal. The petrous bone anatomy is well demonstrated tomographically when 1 mm-spaced slices are used (Fig. 7-2), but tomography does not demonstrate the soft tissues structures well and has largely been replaced by CT.

Magnetic resonance imaging does not reveal bone, and as a result is not hampered by bone-produced artifacts, as is CT. Therefore, MR can delineate the cranial nerves better than CT, and may replace CT when more experience with it is gained.

CONDUCTIVE DEFECTS

The external auditory canal and tympanic membrane are readily accessible and so are better evaluated with the otoscope. Tearing of the tympanic membrane is thus best visualized by otoscopy.

TRAUMA

Disruption of the ossicular chain as a result of trauma is equally well demonstrated by tomography and CT. On CT the normal anatomic relationships between the ossicles are disrupted. Ossicular disruption can occur alone, but is more often associated with a longitudinal petrous-bone fracture (oriented along the long axis of the petrous bone), which is well seen on a CT scan. This longitudinal fracture is also associated with facial nerve injury, since the fracture may intersect with the bony canal of the facial nerve.

CHOLESTEATOMA

A cholesteatoma causes a hearing loss because of a build up of keratinized squamous epithelium in the middle ear cavity. Early in the formation of a cholesteotoma, CT can demonstrate retraction of the tympanic membrane as well as a small cholesteatoma adherent to the membrane. With growth of the cholesteatoma CT clearly shows an expanding soft-tissue mass — the cholesteatoma — as well as extensive secondary bone destruction with displacement of the ossicular chain. Tomography again does not show the soft-tissue mass but clearly reveals the secondary bone destruction.

NEUROSENSORY DEFECTS

ACOUSTIC NEUROMA

Acoustic neuromas produce a neurosensory hearing loss which may also be associated with a facial-nerve deficit due to facial-nerve compression. By the time an acoustic neuroma presents clinically, it is often a large mass. The tumor normally grows outward from the internal auditory canal, eroding the medial inner boundary of the latter. This bony erosion can be detected by tomography (Fig. 7-47)

Computed tomography has replaced tomography as the initial mode of evaulation for acoustic neuromas. With an air cisternogram (Fig. 7-48), it can reveal small tumors localized within the internal auditory canal that present only with symptoms of facial-nerve compression. In this technique air is introduced through a spinal tap, after which the patient is turned so that, the air is trapped in the internal auditory canal. This allows individual visualization of the cranial nerves VII and VIII. With a larger tumor there is an isodense soft-tissue mass in the cerebrellopontine angle, seen lying next to the internal auditory canal in the CT scan. The fourth ventricle of the midbrain is displaced posteriorly and to the contralateral side (Fig. 7-49). Manipulating the CT windows to optimize bony detail allows one to visualize secondary erosion and widening of the inner boundary of the internal auditory canal.

Angiography can also be used to diagnose acoustic neuromas, but may underestimate the actual size of

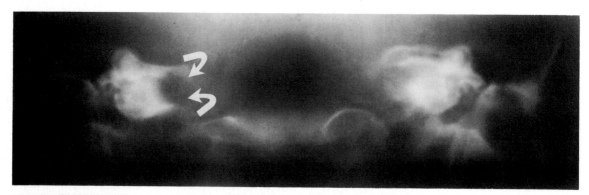

Fig. 7-47 Acoustic neuroma.
History. This 56-year-old man had a progressive hearing loss in the right ear.
Findings. *Tomogram:* The right internal auditory canal is markedly dilated (arrows) in comparison to the left.

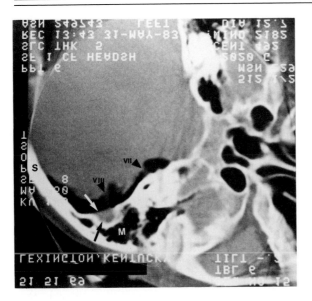

Fig. 7-48 Acoustic neuroma.
History. This 51-year-old woman had a unilateral hearing loss. The conventional CT scan was reported normal.
Findings. *Air Cisternogram CT:* After the introduction of air through a spinal tap, a mass in the internal auditory canal is demonstrated as it prevents the air from entering the canal (arrow). Cranial nerves VII and VIII are also identified. M = mastoid air cells, S = skull.

these tumors. It is no longer utilized now that CT and, more recently, MR have become available.

CLINICAL PRESENTATION: BACK PAIN/RADICULAR PAIN

One of the most common complaints in the United States is that of back pain, and often its radiation down a leg or arm. By far and away the most common etiology of this pain is muscle strain, which is usually relieved by conservative management. If the pain persists or is unrelenting, a more aggressive workup is warranted.

Radiographs of the spine should initially be obtained whenever a lesion involving the spinal cord or spine is suspected. These films may show the classic changes of degenerative arthritis that appear with aging. There is narrowing of the spaces between the vertebral bodies as the disc material degenerates. Other changes of degenerative arthritis include the appearance of osteophytes or bony bridges linking neighboring vertebral bodies. These osteophytes may extend posteriorly, compressing the exiting nerve roots and causing a radicular-type pain. The spine

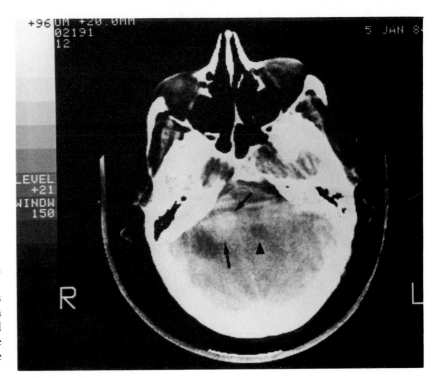

Fig. 7-49 Acoustic neuroma.
History. This 49-year-old man had a progressive hearing loss.
Findings. *CT scan:* A large mass is enhanced in this postinfusion view at the level of the internal auditory canal (arrow). The fourth ventricle is displaced to the left (arrowhead).

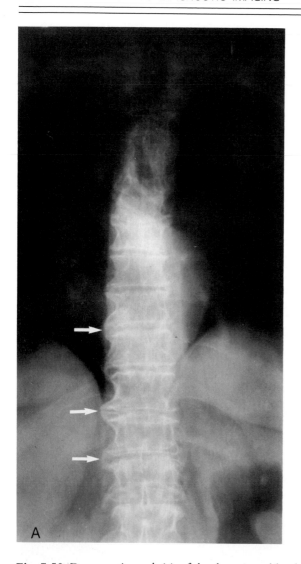

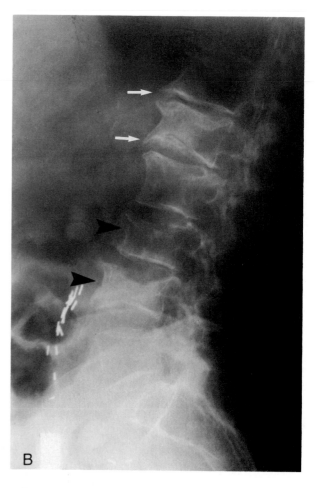

Fig. 7-50 Degenerative arthritis of the thoracic and lumbar spine.
History. This 71-year-old woman had progressively worsening back pain.
Findings. *Lumbar spine radiographs:* The frontal projection of the lower thoracic and upper lumbar spine **(A)** and lateral projection of the lumbar sacral spine **(B)** demonstrate large bridging osteophytes anteriorly (arrows) as well as multiple compression fractures of the vertebral bodies (arrowheads). In addition, all of the bones are somewhat osteoporotic.

often appears somewhat more lucent from the osteo-porosis of old age, and may frequently collapse, lead-ing to wedge-shaped compression deformities (Fig. 7-50 A and B). Metastatic disease to the vertebral bones may also be detected on plain spine radiographs. The pedicle is frequently the first site involved by a lesion of the spine or cord, with loss of its definition

seen best on a frontal view of the spine (Fig. 7-51A). With more extensive involvement the entire verte-bral body is overrun by a lytic (lucent) or blastic (dense) process typical of the primary tumor of origin (Fig. 7-51 B). A herniated disc often shows no abnor-malities on the plain film, since soft-tissue disc mate-rial is not identified.

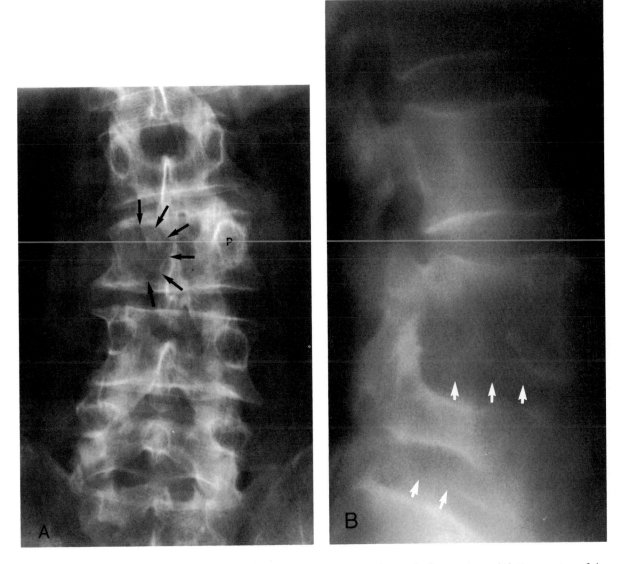

Fig. 7-51 Metastatic disease of the spine. Two cases of metastatic spinal spread of a neoplasm. **(A)** Destruction of the pedicle of L3 signifies early metastatic spread to the spine (arrows). P = normal pedicle in the left side. This was from a lung carcinoma. **(B)** A tomogram of the lumbar spine shows destruction of two vertebral bodies. The lower bony borders are not identifiable (arrows). This was the same patient as in Figure 7-55, with lung carcinoma.

The next step in the evaluation of back or radicular pain is either myelography, CT, or more recently, MR, depending on the clinical symptomatology. Any mass involving the spinal cord can be localized to one of three spaces. First, it can be entirely outside the dural sheath (extradural) and smoothly flatten the entire dural contents (Fig. 7-52A). Two common examples of such masses are herniated discs and metastasis to the bony spine. Second a mass may be within the

dural sheath (intradural) but not part of the spinal cord (extramedullary) (Fig. 7-52B). A neurofibroma of an exiting nerve root and meningioma are the most common examples of this type of mass. The third and last possibility is a mass that involves the spinal cord itself (intradural and intramedullary) (Fig. 7-52C). Two examples of this are a spinal cord glioma and localized dilatation of the central canal of the spinal cord (hydromyelia). These three mass locations are

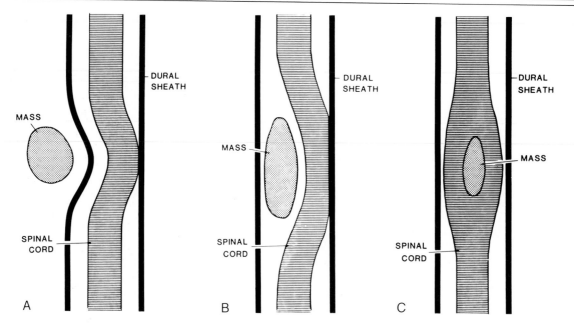

Fig. 7-52 Mass location in the spinal canal. **(A)** Extradural. The mass lies outside the dural sheath, smoothly indenting the dura and spinal cord. **(B)** Intradural but extramedullary. The mass lies within the dural sheath but outside the spinal cord. The spinal cord is pushed to one side and compressed by the mass. **(C)** Intradural and intramedullary. The mass lies within the spinal cord, causing a local widening of the cord.

easily detected with myelography and CT, and help in obtaining the proper diagnosis.

EXTRADURAL MASS

HERNIATED INTERVERTEBRAL DISC

The radiologic approach to a suspected disc herniation of the lumbar spine depends on the expected clinical management. If analgesics, rest, and conservative management are to be the probable forms of treatment, plain CT should be the imaging modality of first choice. If the patient's symptoms are severe and surgery is planned, then a Metrizamide-lumbar myelogram should be done, perhaps followed immediately, by Metrixamide-enhanced CT scan. A CT scan with intrathecal Metrizamide has a higher accuracy rate than does either a Metrizamide-myelogram or a plain CT scan.

Myelography is a time-tested modality for the detection of herniated discs. The extradural disc material indents the otherwise smooth column of contrast medium (Fig. 7-53). In more subtle cases there is frequently only non-filling of one of the exiting nerve roots by the Metrizamide, also from extrinsic compression by the protruding disc material (Fig. 7-54A).

The CT scan demonstrates protrusion of the soft-tissue-density disc material focally into the spinal canal, with compression of the nerve root or displacement of the dural sac containing the spinal cord. This is an extradural defect, since the compression of the cord originates from a source outside the enclosures of the dural sac. The CT scan may also demonstrate accompanying bony osteophytes that can further compromise the spinal canal. With the use of the intrathecal Metrizamide, the CSF-filled dural sac is easily detected (Fig. 7-54B).

METASTASIS

Metastasis to the bones of the spine are common in a number of malignancies such as breast, lung, and prostate carcinomas. Often this bony involvement can

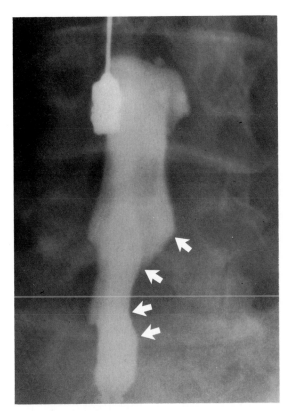

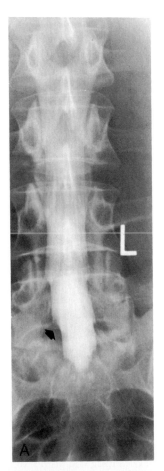

Fig. 7-53 Herniated disc.
History. This 32-year-old man had shooting leg pain of acute onset after a day of heavy lifting.
Findings. *Myelogram:* Note how there is obvious smooth narrowing of the left side of the contrast-filled dural sac at the level of the intervertebral space (arrows). This signifies the etiology, a herniated disc, which lies outside the dural sac. Compare this to Figures 7-56b and 7-57a.

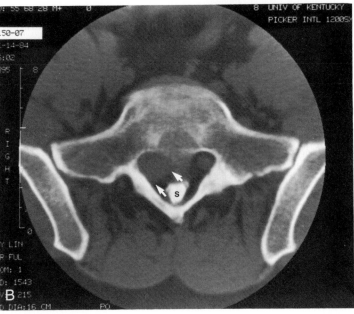

Fig. 7-54 Herniated disc.
History. This 37-year-old man had radicular pain.
Findings. (A) *Myelogram:* A Metrizamide-enhanced study shows a subtle amputated right L5/S1 nerve root (arrow) from compression of a herniated disc. **(B)** *CT scan:* A subsequent CT scan easily confirms the presence of a herniated disc (arrows). The Metrizamide-filled dural sac is identified (S).

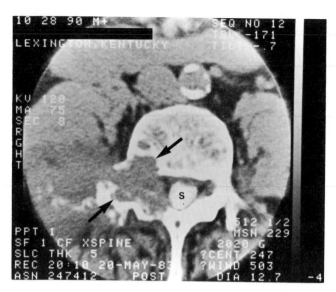

Fig. 7-55 Metastasis to the spine.
History. This 59-year-old woman had newly diagnosed lung cancer and back pain.
Findings. *Computed tomography scan:* There is destruction of the right pedicle and a portion of the vertebral body by a soft-tissue mass (arrows). This mass is encroaching on the spinl sac. Metrizamide (white) has been injected into the dural sac (S).

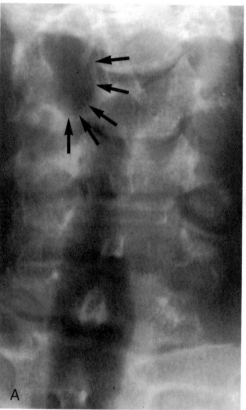

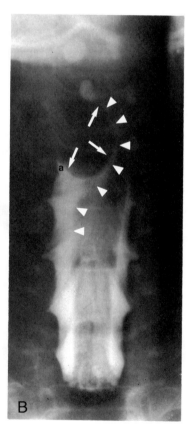

Fig. 7-56 Neurofibromatosis.
History. This 29-year-old man had neurofibromatosis and a progressive right-arm neuropathy.
Findings. (A) *Cervical spine radiograph:* A single frontal view of the cervical spine shows erosion of the neural foramina between the fourth and third vertebral bodies (arrows). The erosion is smooth, suggesting a slow-growing benign lesion.
(B) *Myelogram:* The neurofibroma lies within the dural sheath (intradural) but outside the spinal cord (extramedullary) (arrows). Note how the cord is pushed to the far wall of the dura and compressed by the tumor (arrowheads), and how the contrast medium outlines the tumor with an acute angle (a). These are classic findings in cases of intradural extramedullary tumor. Compare this to Figures 7-53 and 7-57a.

lead to extrinsic or extradural compression of the dural sac. This may simulate a herniated disc both in its symptoms and in its radiographic appearance.

The myelogram shows the extrinsic compression, which is often not at an intervertebral level, such as is seen with a herniated disc. The impingement on the cord usually coincides with visualized bony destruction, also allowing its differentiation from a herniated disc. The CT scan clearly demonstrates the destruction of the vertebral body, along with the secondary compromise of the spinal cord extradurally (Fig. 7-55).

INTRADURAL MASS

Primary tumors of the spinal cord or nerve roots present a unique radiographic appearance on plain radiographs, CT scans, and myelograms. The cord abnormality and deficit in these cases occur from within the dural wrapping.

In slow-growing tumors of the cord or nerve roots there may be secondary erosion or scalloping of the posterior surface of the vertebral body or neural forminia from continued local pressure. This is often detected on a plain radiograph of the spine (Fig. 7-56).

EXTRAMEDULLARY: NEUROFIBROMA

In extramedullary but intradural tumors such as neurofibroma, there is deviation of the spinal cord away from one dural wall as myelographic contrast medium

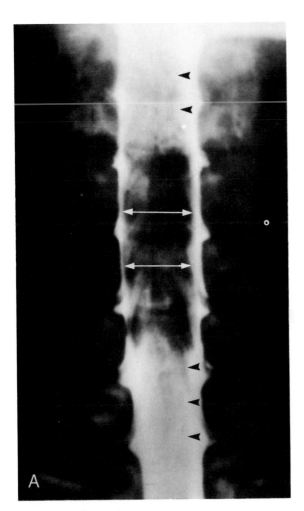

Fig. 7-57 Hydromyelia.
History. This 30-year-old woman had progressive neurologic deficits (same patient as in Figure 1-52).
Findings. (A) *Myelogram:* The normal cord (arrowheads) quickly dilates with the dilated central canal (arrows). At surgery, a glioma of the spinal cord was found, obstructing the canal and causing its dilation. Compare this to Figures 7-53 and 7-56b. **(B)** *Magnetic resonance image:* The axial scan confirms the dilated canal (arrows).

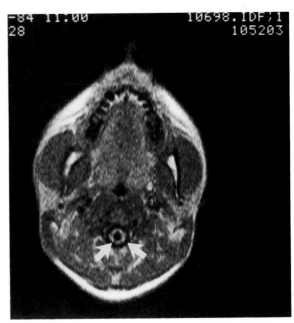

outlines the tumor (Fig. 7-56B). Computed tomography may confirm the presence of a mass.

INTRAMEDULLARY: HYDROMYELIA

In a primary process of the spinal cord the myelogram shows widening of the contents contained within the dural sheath. The cord itself appears locally widened and not pushed to the side, as previously discussed for neurofibroma (Fig. 7-56B). The CT scan confirms a widening of the dural contents, but the cord itself may be difficult to image. Magnetic resonance imaging has a distinct advantage over CT in actually and clearly imaging the cord apart from the surrounding soft tissues. Again, since bone is invisible on MR, axial, coronal, and even sagittal views can be obtained without artifacts. Also, MR clearly reveals widening of the cord from a dilated central canal or tumor (Fig. 7-57B), and may be able to reveal an early, subtle

tumor of the cord before it has even expanded the cord, by revealing changes in cord homogeneity.

REFERENCES

1. Ramsey RG: Neuroradiology with Computed Tomography. WB Saunders, Philadelphia, 1981
2. Lee SH, Rao KCU: Cranial Computed Tomography. McGraw Hill, New York, 1983
3. Obsorn AG: Introduction to Cerebral Angiography. Harper & Row, Philadelphia, 1980
4. Taveras JM, Wood E: Diagnostic Neuroradiology. Williams & Wilkins, Baltimore, 1981
5. Shapiro R: Myelography. Year Book Medical Publishers, Chicago, 1984
6. Rogers, LF, Meschen, I, Potter GL, et al: Disorders of the Head and Neck (II) Syllabus. American College of Radiology, Chicago, 1977
7. Peterson HO, Kieffer SA: Introduction to Neuroradiology. Harper & Row, New York, 1972

Index

Page numbers followed by f represent figures; page numbers followed by t represent tables.

Abdominal aorta, atherosclerosis of, 245f
Abscess
  cerebral, 268f
  pancreatic, 169
  pulmonary, 75–76, 76f
  renal, 19f, 121–122, 122f
  urinary, 130
Absorption, x-ray, 3–6, 4–6f
Achalasia, 171–172, 172f
Acoustic neuroma, 282f, 283f
Acquired immune deficiency syndrome, pneumonia in, 55f, 56
Adenocarcinoma, lung. See Lung, adenocarcinoma of.
Adenoma
  bronchial, 73–74, 74f
  hyperparathyroidism due to, 204
  pituitary, 276, 277f
  villous, 147–148, 148f
Adenomatous polyp, 147f
Adenopathy, pulmonary. See Hilar adenopathy.
Age, bone tumors and, 201–202
Air bronchogram, 52f
Air cisternogram, in acoustic neuroma, 282, 283f
Air contrast study
  of colon cancer, 148f
  of lower gastrointestinal tract, 144f
  of ulcerative colitis, 176–177f, 177
Airspace disease. See Alveolar disease.
Airway obstruction, 46–49
Alveolar cell carcinoma. See Lung, alveolar cell carcinoma.
Alveolar disease, 46, 51f, 52f
  alveolar cell carcinoma. See Lung, alveolar cell carcinoma.
  pneumonia, 52f, 53f, 55f
  proteinosis, 57
  pulmonary edema
    cardiac, 50f, 51f, 50–52
    noncardiac, 52
  pulmonary hemorrhage, 56
  tuberculosis, 53–55f, 54–55
Alveolar proteinosis, 57

Aneurysm
  aortic, 37, 244–246, 244–246f
  atherosclerosis and, 244–246f
  cerebral, 266f, 267f
  dissecting hematoma, 246–247, 247f
  intracranial, 253
  myocardial infarction and, 243f
  ventricular, 243, 243f
Angina
  coronary arteriography in. See Angiography, angina.
  diagnosis of, 239–242, 240–242f
Angiodysplasia, 145, 145f
Angiography
  digital subtraction. See Digital subtraction angiography.
  nuclear medicine, 34, 35f
  of angina, 241, 242f
  of angiodysplasia, 145f
  of aorta, 228f
  of aortic aneurysm, 244–246, 245f
  of central nervous system, 253–255, 254f, 255f
  of cerebral infarction, 261f
  of congenital heart defects, 236–239, 238f
  of dissecting hematoma, 246–247, 247f
  of gastrointestinal hemorrhage, 150
  of gliomas, 273f, 274
  of heart, 227f
  of kidney, 89f
  of lung, 44, 46f
  of pulmonary embolism, 64–65, 65f
  of renal abscess, 122
  of renal vein thrombosis, 97
  of renovascular hypertension, 112f, 113f
  peripheral, 228f
Angiomyolipoma, renal, 102, 103f
Ankylosing spondylitis, 214f
Aorta
  abdominal, 245f
  angiography of, 228f
  mediastinum location of, 40f
  technetium scan of, 34, 35f
  tortuous, 40, 41f
  ultrasound of, 229f

Aorta *(Continued)*
  x-ray of, 225–226
Aortic aneurysm, atherosclerosis and, 244–246f
Aortic coarctation, 238f, 238
Aortic stenosis, 233–234, 234f
Aortic valve disease, 233–234, 234f
Aphthous ulcer, Crohn's disease and, 178, 179f
Arteriogram, 8f
Arteriography, *See* Angiography.
Arteriovenous malformation, 77, 263
Arthritis
  degenerative, 215–217, 216f, 283–284, 284f
  diagnosis of, 210–217, 211–216f
  gouty, 217f
  psoriatic, 215f
  rheumatoid, 211–215f
  septic, 196f
Asbestosis, 62, 63f
Ascites, ultrasound of, 17, 19f
Aseptic necrosis, 217–219, 218–219f
Aspiration pneumonia, 53–54
Asthma, x-ray of, 46, 48f
Atelectasis, 67–70, 68f, 69f
Atherosclerosis
  aortic aneurysm and, 244–246f
  carotid artery, 261f
  peripheral, 247–248, 248f
  renovascular hypertension and, 111, 112f
Atomic number, x-ray and, 3–4
Atrial septal defect, 236–237, 236f
Atrium, mediastinal location of, 40f
Autonephrectomized kidney, 123f, 124
Avascular necrosis. *See* Aseptic necrosis.

Back pain, 283–290
  degenerative disease and, 283–284, 284f
  extradural mass and, 286–288f
  herniated discs and, 285
  hydromyelia and, 289f, 290
  intradural mass and, 289
  metastasis and, 284–285, 285f
  neurofibroma and, 288f, 289–290
Back-wall enhancement, ultrasound, 13
Bacterial endocarditis, 239
Balloon angioplasty, in renovascular hypertension, 113f,
    114
Barium
  in computed tomography, 26, 27f
  in upper gastrointestinal tract study, 134, 135f
  x-ray use of, 7–8, 8f
"Bat wing" pattern, 51f
Biliary obstruction, 153
Biliary sludge, 161, 161f
Biliary system, ultrasound use in, 20t
Biopsy, needle aspiration
  abdominal, 155, 155f
  transthoracic, 44, 46

Bladder
  carcinoma of, 109f, 110f, 109–110
  ultrasound of, 15f
Blood clot
  pulmonary, 63–65, 64f, 65f
  tibial vein, 249f
Blood flow, nuclear medicine and, 34, 35f
Bone
  blastic metastasis, 197–198, 198–199f
  computed tomography of, 23
  fracture, 184–189, 184–189f
  infection of, 192–197, 194–197f
  leukemia of, 202f
  lytic metastasis, 199
  metastasis, 197–200, 198–200f
    Paget's disease vs., 221
    technetium nuclide scan of, 33, 34f
  nuclide scan of, 183–184, 185f
  radiology of, 183–221
  stress fracture, 183–184, 184f
  tumors of, 200–204, 201–203f
    classification of, 204
  x-ray absorption in, 3, 6f
Bowel
  large. *See* Colon.
  small, anatomy of, 134, 135f
Brain
  computed tomography of, 256f
  glioma of, 271–273f
  magnetic resonance imaging of, 36–37, 37f
  meningioma of, 269f, 270f
  metastasis, 270f, 271f
Breast
  carcinoma of
    bone metastasis in, 134f
    gastric metastasis in, 142–144, 143f
  magnetic resonance imaging of, 37
Bronchiectasis, 70–71
Bronchitis, chronic, 48
Bronchoalveolar cell carcinoma. *See* Lung, alveolar cell
    carcinoma.
Bronchogenic carcinoma. *See* Lung, carcinoma of.
Bronchography, 46
Bronchopneumonia, 52–53
Bronchus, anatomy of, 42
Brown tumor, hyperparathyroidism and, 205–206,
    206f

Calcium
  deficiency of, 204
  parathormone and, 204
Calculus
  pyelonephritis and, 123–124
  staghorn, 102, 105f
  urinary, 102, 104–107f, 105–107
Callus, in fracture healing, 190f, 191–192
Camera, gamma, 32f

Candidiasis
  esophagitis, 175f
  gastric erosion in, 137
Caplan's syndrome, 60
Carbuncle, renal, 121–122, 122f
Cardiac tamponade, 235
Cardiomegaly
  algorithm for, 231
  aortic valvular disease and, 233–234
  atrial septal defect and, 236–237, 236f
  bacterial endocarditis and, 239
  cardiomyopathy and, 234, 234f
  coarctation of aorta and, 238, 238f
  congenital abnormalities and, 236–239, 236–238f
  hypertension and, 231
  idiopathic hypertrophic subaortic stenosis and, 239
  mitral valvular disease and, 231–233, 232f, 233f
  pericardial effusions and, 234–236, 235f
  pericarditis and, 234–236
  rheumatic fever and, 231
  tuberculosis and, 235
  ventricular septal defect and, 237–238, 237f
Cardiomyopathy, cardiomegaly due to, 234, 234f
Cardiovascular system
  computed tomography use in, 30t
  magnetic resonance imaging of, 37–38
  nuclear medicine in, 35t
  radiology of, 223–250
  ultrasound use in, 20t
Carditis, rheumatic fever and, 231
Carotid artery, atherosclerosis of, 261f
Catheterization, cardiac, 227f
Central nervous system
  magnetic resonance imaging of, 37
  nuclear medicine and, 35t
  radiology of, 251–290
Cerebral abscess, 268f
Cerebral atrophy, 274, 275f
Cerebral hemorrhage, 261–265, 262–265f
Cerebral infarction, 259f, 260f
Chest
  anatomy of, 39–42, 223, 224f
  computed tomography of, 23f, 30t
  frontal film of, 39, 40f
  lateral film of, 41, 41f
  nuclear medicine and, 35t
  radiology of 4–5, 5f, 39–83
  ultrasound use in, 20t
Chest pain
  algorithm for, 240
  aneurysm and
    aortic, 244–246, 244–246f
    dissecting, 246–247, 247f
    ventricular, 243, 243f
  angina and, 239–242
  aortic aneurysm and, 244–246, 244–246f
  atherosclerosis and, 244–246, 245f

coronary artery disease and, 239–242, 242f
  dissecting hematomas and, 246–247, 247f
  Dressler's syndrome and, 243, 244f
  ischemic heart disease and, 239–242, 240f
  myocardial infarction and, 242–244, 243f
  postmyocardial infarction syndrome and, 243, 244f
  ventricular aneurysm and, 243, 243f
Cholangiography. *See* Percutaneous transhepatic cholangiography.
Cholangiopancreatography. *See* Endoscopic retrograde cholangiopancreatography.
Cholecystitis, acute, 163–164, 163f
Cholecystogram, oral. *See* Oral cholecystogram.
Cholescintigraphy, of gallbladder, 163f
Cholesteatoma, 282
Chondrocalcinosis, hyperparathyroidism and, 206
Chondrosarcoma, 203f
Chromophobe adenoma, 276, 277f
Cisternogram. *See* Air cisternogram.
Coarctation, aortic, 238, 238f
Coin lesion, pulmonary, 74
Cold extremities. *See* Extremity, painful/cold.
Cold spot, 33, 34f
Collagen vascular disease, 60, 60f
Colon
  angiodysplasia of, 145
  carcinoma of, 148f
    colitis and, 177–178
    computed tomography of, 28, 29f
  diverticulosis of, 145, 146f
  inflammation of, 176–178f, 177–178
  polyps, 147, 147f
Complex pattern, ultrasound, 17
Compression fracture, 184, 186f
Computed tomography
  artifacts, 28, 30f
  history of, 2
  in liver metastasis, 157f
  indications for, 30–31t
  of acoustic neuroma, 282, 283f
  of arteriovenous malformation, 263
  of atelectasis, 69f
  of bladder tumors, 110f
  of bone metastasis, 199–200, 200f
  of brain tumors, 269–272f
  of central nervous system, 255–258, 256f, 257f
  of cerebral hematoma, 263–265f
  of cerebral infarction, 259f, 260f
  of ear, 281
  of endocrine disorders, 276–278, 277f, 278f
  of gallbladder, 153f
  of gallstones, 161–162, 162f
  of hemorrhagic infarction, 262f, 263
  of herniated intervertebral disc, 286, 287f
  of hydrocephalus, 274–276, 275f, 276f
  of kidney, 87, 88f
  of lung, 43, 45f

Computed tomography *(Continued)*
    of obstructive jaundice, 153, 154–155f
    of pancreatic cancer, 169–171, 170f
    of pancreatic pseudocyst, 167, 168f
    of pancreatitis, 166–167f
    of polycystic kidney disease, 114, 115f
    of pyelonephritis, 94f, 96
    of renal abscess, 122
    of renal cell carcinoma, 98–100, 99f
    of renal cyst, 119
    of renal hematoma, 108f
    of renal vein thrombosis, 96f, 97
    of subarachnoid hemorrhage, 266f, 267f
    physics of, 21f
Congenital heart defects, 236–239, 236–238f
    aortic coarctation, 238, 238f
    atrial septal defect, 236–237, 236f
    bacterial endocarditis, 239
    idiopathic hypertrophic subaortic stenosis, 239
    ventricular septal defect, 237–238, 237f
Congestive heart failure, 50–52, 51f
Consciousness, loss of, 258–269
    inflammatory disorders and, 267–268
    parenchymal hemorrhage and, 261–265
    ruptured aneurysm and, 266–267
    stroke and, 259–261
    subarachnoid hemorrhage and, 266f
    systemic disorders and, 268–269
Contrast agent
    computed tomography, 26, 27f
    x-ray, 7–8, 8f, 9f
Contusion, cerebral, 264–265
Coronary artery bypass, 242f
Coronary artery disease, 239–242, 242f
Crohn's disease, 178–179, 179f, 180f
    gastric erosion in, 137
Crystal, piezoelectric, 11f
Cyst
    bronchogenic, 76f
    liver, 157–158
    renal, 118–120, 119f, 120f
        computed tomography of, 25f
        peripelvic, 120
        puncture, 91, 119–120
        ultrasound of, 13–15, 14f
Cystic glioma, 271, 272f, 273f
Cystitis, urinary, 109
Cystography, urinary tract, 89–90
Cystourethrography, 89–90

Deep venous thrombosis, 249, 249f
Degenerative arthritis, 215–217, 216f, 283–284, 284f
Demineralization
    fracture healing and, 190f, 191
    osteomyelitis and, 194–196, 195f

Demyelinating disease, 274f
Density
    computed tomography use of, 22
    x-ray and, 3–4
Diaphragm, anatomy of, 41
Diarrhea
    algorithm for, 176
    Crohn's disease and, 178–180, 178–180f
    granulomatous ileocolitis and, 178–180
    regional interitis and, 178–180
    toxic megacolon and, 178, 178f
    ulcerative colitis and, 176–178, 176–177f
Digital subtraction angiography
    aortic, 91f
    central nervous system, 255f
    history of, 2
    in renovascular hypertension, 111–113, 112f
    renal, 91f
Dislocation
    joint, 192, 193f
    rheumatoid arthritis and, 213
Dissecting hematoma, 246–247, 247f
Diverticulitis, 146f
Diverticulosis, 145–146, 146f
Dressler syndrome, myocardial infarction and, 243–244, 244f
Drug use, gastric erosion due to, 137
Duodenal ulcer, 136–137f
Dysphagia
    achalasia and, 171–172, 172f
    algorithm for, 171
    Candida esophagitis and, 175, 175f
    esophageal cancer and, 172–173, 173f
    metastatic disease and, 175
    peptic esophagitis and, 173–174, 174f
    scleroderma and, 174–175, 174f
Dyspnea
    algorithm for, 47
    alveolar proteinosis and, 57
    asbestosis and, 62, 63f
    aspiration pneumonia and, 53–54
    asthma and, 46–48
    atelectasis and, 67–70, 68f
    bacterial pneumonia and, 52–53
    bronchitis and, 48
    bronchogenic carcinoma and, 67
    collagen vascular disease and, 60
    diffuse lung disease, interstitial pattern, 57–62
    emphysema and, 49
    granulomatous disease and, 57–59
    inhalational diseases and, 61–62, 62f, 63f
    lung metastasis and, 60–61, 61f
    obstructive airway disease and, 46–49
    parenchymal lung disease, alveolar pattern, 50–57
    pleural effusions and, 60, 66–67, 67f
    pneumonia and, 52–56

pneumothorax and, 65–66
progressive massive fibrosis and, 61–62, 62f
pulmonary edema and
    cardiac, 50–52
    noncardiac, 52
pulmonary embolism and, 63–65, 64f, 65f
pulmonary fibrosis and, 59, 60
pulmonary hemorrhage and, 56
pulmonary neoplasia and, 56–57
rheumatoid arthritis and, 60
sarcoidosis and, 57–59, 58f, 59f
silicosis and, 61–62, 62f
squamous cell carcinoma and, 69f
tuberculosis and, 54–55
viral pneumonia and, 55–56
Dystrophic calcification, renal, 107f

Ear
    anatomy of, 253f, 281
    conductive defects of, 281–282
    neurosensory defects of, 282f, 283t
Echo pattern, ultrasound, 12–13
Echocardiography, 226–227
Edema, pulmonary, 50f, 51f
Electrocardiogram, thallium in, 229f, 231
Embolism
    arterial, 248–249
    pulmonary, 63–65, 64f, 65f
    stroke due to, 259
Embolization, gastrointestinal hemorrhage, 150
Emphysema, 49f
Empty sella syndrome, 276, 278f
Encephalitis, 268
Endocarditis, 239
Endocrine system, disorders of, 276–278
Endoscopic retrograde cholangiopancreatography, 164, 165f
    in pancreas cancer, 171
    in pancretitis, 169f
Epidural hematoma, 263–264, 265f
Epiphysis, fracture of, 188f, 189f
Erosion, gastric, 137–138, 138f
Esophagitis
    Candida in, 175f
    peptic, 173–173, 174f
Esophagram
    in achalasia, 172f
    in esophagitis, 173–175, 174f–175f
    in esophagus cancer, 173f
    in scleroderma, 174f, 175
Esophagus
    anatomy of, 134, 135f
    carcinoma of, 172–173, 173f
    dysphagia of, 171–175
    varices, 140–141f, 141

Extremity, painful/cold
    arterial embolism and, 248–249
    deep venous thrombosis and, 249, 249f
    peripheral atherosclerosis and, 247–248, 248f
    thrombophlebitis and, 249

Fat
    computed tomography of, 23
    x-ray absorption in, 5f
Fibroma, nonossifying, 203f
Fibromuscular dysplasia, renovascular hypertension and, 111, 113f
Film, x-ray, 4f
"Fish vertebra", osteoporosis and, 208, 210f
Fistula
    Crohn's disease and, 179, 180f
    diverticulosis and, 146
Fluid, ultrasound of, 13–15, 14f
Fluoroscopy, 8–9, 9f
    angiographic use of, 227
Focal neurologic deficit
    demyelinating disease and, 274
    neoplasms and, 269–274
Fracture
    diagnosis of, 184–189, 185–189f
    epiphyseal, 189f
    healing of, 189–192, 190–192f
    osteoporosis and, 208
    Paget's disease and, 188, 221
    pathologic, 188–189, 189f
    radiolucent line, 184–186
    Salter, 188f
    skull, 187f
    spiral, 184
    stress, 183–184, 184f
    torus, 188f
    vertebral body, 187f

Gallbladder
    acute cholecystitis, 163f
    computed tomography of, 153f
    diseases of, 158–163, 159–162f
    ultrasound of, 151–153, 153f
    wall, ultrasound of, 12, 12f
Gallstone, 159–162f
    ultrasound of, 12f
Gamma camera, 32f
Gantry, CT scanner, 21, 21f
Gas, ultrasound of, 13f
Gastric ulcer, 138–139f
Gastritis, erosive, 137–138, 138f
Gastrointestinal hemorrhage, 133–151
    brisk
        angiography in, 150
        lower, 145–146

Gastrointestinal hemorrhage *(Continued)*
    radionuclide imaging in, 149–150
    upper, 134–141
  diagnosis of, 149–151
  lower
    algorithm for, 144
    angiodysplasia and, 145, 145f
    brisk, 145–146
    colon cancer and, 148–149
    colonic polyps and, 147, 147f
    colorectal carcinoma and, 149
    diverticulosis and, 145–146, 146f
    polyps and, 147, 147f
    slow, 147–149
    villous adenoma and, 147–148, 148f
  slow
    lower, 147–149
    radionuclide imaging in, 151
    upper, 141–144
  upper
    algorithm for, 134
    brisk, 134–141
    duodenal ulcer and, 136–137, 136–137f
    erosive gastritis and, 137–138, 138f
    gastric erosions and, 137–138, 138f
    gastric metastasis and, 142–144, 143f
    gastric ulcer and,
      benign, 139–140, 139f
      malignant, 139f, 140
    lymphoma and, 142, 143f
    Mallory-Weiss syndrome and, 135, 141
    peptic ulcer disease and, 136, 137f
    slow, 141–144
    stomach cancer and, 141–142, 142f
    varices and, 140–141, 141f
Gastrointestinal system
  computed tomography use in, 31t
  nuclear medicine in, 36t
  radiology of, 133–181
  ultrasound use in, 20t
  x-ray of, 7–8, 8f
Gated-pool ventriculogram, 230f, 231
Genitalia, ultrasound use in, 21t
Giant cell tumor, bone, 201f
Glioglastoma multiforme, 271, 272f, 273f
Glioma, 271–273f
  optic nerve, 280f
Gout, 217f
Granulomatous ileocolitis, 178–180, 179–180f
Greenstick fracture, 188f
Gyral enhancement, in cerebral infarction, 259, 260f

Hamartoma, pulmonary, 74
Hampton's line, 140
Head, computed tomography use in, 30t

Headache, hydrocephalus and, 274–276, 275f, 276f
Hearing, loss of, 281–283
Heart
  anatomy of 223, 224f, 225f
  catheterization of, 227f
  computed tomography of, 226f
  frontal view of, 224f
  gated-pool ventriculogram, 230f
  lateral view of, 41, 224f
  magnetic resonance in, 38, 227–228
  nuclear medicine in, 229f, 230f, 231
  size determination, 223, 225f
  thallium stress test, 229f
Hemangioma, computed tomography of, 26, 28f
Hematemesis, in gastrointestinal hemorrhage, 134
Hematochezia, in gastrointestinal hemorrhage, 134
Hematogenous osteomyelitis, 193, 194f
Hematoma
  cerebral, 263–264, 263–265f
  dissecting, 246–247, 247f
  fracture and, 191
  renal, 107–108, 108f
  retrobulbar, 280
  urinary, 130
Hematuria
  algorithm for, 92–93
  angiomyolipoma and, 102, 103f
  benign neoplasms and, 102
  bladder cancer and, 109–110, 109–110f
  calculi and, 102–107
  cystitis and, 109
  hydronephrosis and, 105–106
  infections and, 93–96
  medullary sponge kidney and, 106f, 107
  neoplasms and, 97–102
  nephrolithiasis and, 102–107, 106f
  papillary necrosis and, 97, 98f, 99f
  pyelonephritis and
    acute, 93–94, 94f
    chronic, 94–96, 95f
  renal cell carcinoma and, 97–100, 99–101f
  renal stone disease and, 104f
  renal trauma and, 107–109
  renal vein thrombosis and, 96–97, 96f
  transition cell carcinoma and, 100–102, 102f
  urethral diseases and, 109–110
Hemoptysis
  algorithm for, 70
  benign tumors and, 73–74
  bronchiectasis and, 70–71
  bronchogenic carcinoma and, 71–73
  hemorrhagic, 74
  inflammatory, 70–71
  neoplastic, 71–74
  traumatic, 74
  vascular diseases and, 74

Hemorrhage
  diverticulosis and, 145–146
  gastrointestinal. *See* Gastrointestinal hemorrhage.
  pulmonary, hemoptysis and, 74
Hemorrhagic infarction, 259, 261, 262f, 263
Hepatic duct, stone in, 154f
Hernia
  hiatal, esophagitis and, 173
  intervertebral disc, 286, 287f
Hilar anatomy, 41f
Hilar enlargement
  algorithm for, 77
  bilateral
    inhalational, 78
    lymphoma and, 78, 78f
    neoplastic, 78
    pulmonary artery, 78
    pulmonary hypertension and, 78–79, 79f
    sarcoidosis and, 59, 78
    silicosis and, 61, 78
  unilateral
    fungal infection and, 78
    histoplasmosis and, 78
    inflammatory, 77–78
    neoplastic, 77–78
    tuberculosis and, 78
Histiocytoma, malignant fibrous, 202f
Histiocytosis X, pneumothorax and, 65
Histoplasmosis, 78
Honeycomb lung, 60
Hot spot, 33, 34f
Hydrocephalus
  nonobstructive, 275–276
  obstructive, 275, 276f
Hydromyelia, 285, 289f, 290
Hydronephrosis
  ultrasound of, 87
  urinary calculi and, 102, 105–106
Hyperostosis, meningioma and, 269f
Hyperparathyroidism, diagnosis of, 204–206f
Hyperplastic polyp, 147
Hypertension
  algorithm for, 111
  cardiomegaly due to, 231
  pulmonary, x-ray of, 225
  renal
    chronic renal failure and, 114–115, 115f
    digital subtraction angiography in, 111–113
    end-stage renal disease and, 116f
    fibromuscular dysplasia and, 111
    parenchymal disease and, 114–116, 115f
    polycystic disease and, 114, 115f
    renal artery stenosis and, 111, 113
    renal infarction and, 116–118, 117f
Hypoechoic mass, 17, 18f, 19f
Hypothalamic infarction, 278

Idiopathic hypertrophic subaortic stenosis, 239
Ileitis, ulcerative colitis and, 177f
Ileocolitis, granulomatous, 178–180, 178–180f
Illeum, Crohn's disease of, 179f
Image intensifier, fluoroscope, 8–9, 9f
Imaging, introduction to, 1–38
Indeterminate ulcer, 140
Infarction
  hypothalamic, 278
  myocardial, 242–244, 243–244f
  renal, 116–118, 117f
Interitis, regional, 178–180, 178–180f
Interstitial lung disease, 46, 50f
  asbestosis and, 62, 63f
  collagen vascular disease, 60f
  congestive heart failure, 50f, 51f
  granulomatous disease, 57–59
  inhalation and, 51–62, 62f, 63f
  lung metastasis, 60–61, 61f
  pneumonia, 52–56
  progressive massive fibrosis, 61–62
  pulmonary fibrosis and, 59
  sarcoidosis, 57–59, 58f, 59f
  silicosis, 61–62, 62f
Interstitium, anatomy of, 46
Intervertebral disc, herniation of, 286, 287f
Intestine
  large. *See* Colon.
  small, 134, 135f
  x-ray absorption in, 5f, 6
Intradural mass, 289
Intravenous pyelogram, 8, 9f
  in acute tubular necrosis, 126f
  in benign prostrate hypertrophy, 124–125, 145f
  in chronic renal failure, 116f
  in papillary necrosis, 97, 98f
  in polycystic disease, 114, 115f
  in pyelonephritis, 93–95, 94f, 95f
  in renal cell carcinoma, 98, 99f
  in renal cyst, 118, 119f
  in renal infarction, 117f
  in renal tuberculosis, 123f, 124
  in renal vein thrombosis, 96f
Involucrum, 193, 195f
Iodine
  angiographic use of, 227
  computed tomography use of, 26, 27f
  renal use of, 90f, 91
  x-ray use of, 8f, 9f
Ischemic heart disease, thallium imaging of, 240f
Ischemic necrosis. *See* Aneptic necrosis.

Jaundice
  algorithm for, 152
  metastatic disease and, 156–158, 157f

Jaundice *(Continued)*
    nonobstructive, 155–156, 156f
    obstructive, 153–155, 153–155f
Joint
    dislocation vs. subluxation, 192
    radiology of, 183–221
Juxtarenal mass, 121

Kerley's B line, 50f
Kidney
    angiomyolipoma and, 102, 103f
    calcification in, 102, 104–107f, 105–107
    carcinoma of, 97–102, 99–102f
        computed tomography of, 26f
        ultrasound of, 17, 18f
    chronic failure, 114, 116f
    computed tomography use in, 30t
    cyst, 25f, 118–120
    duplicated collecting system in, 120–121
    dystrophic calcification of, 107, 107f
    fibrosis, ultrasound of, 17, 18f
    medullary sponge, 106f, 107
    nuclear medicine in, 35–36t
    technetium scan of, 34, 35f
    tomograph of, 10f
    transplant. *See* Renal transplant.
    trauma to, 107–109, 108f
    tuberculosis of, 123f, 124
    tumors of, 97–102
Kidney stone. *See* Calculus, urinary.

Larynx, computed tomography use in, 30t
Leukemia, 202f
Lingula, pulmonary, 41–42, 42f
Liver
    alcoholic, 23, 25f
    computed tomography use in, 31t
    magnetic resonance of, 38
    metastasis in, 156–158, 157f
        from liver cancer, 29f
        technetium scan of, 33, 34f
    nuclear medicine in, 156f
    tumor of, computed tomography of, 26, 28f, 29f
    ultrasound of, 15, 16f, 20t
Lobar nephronia, 94
Lobe, pulmonary, 42
Lumbar spine
    computed tomography of, 257f, 258
    degenerative arthritis of, 284f
Lung
    adenoma of, 73, 74f
    anatomy of, 42f
    benign tumors of, 73–74
    carcinoma of
        adenocarcinoma, 72f, 73

        alveolar cell carcinoma, 56f, 57f
        bronchogenic carcinoma, 63f
        hemoptysis in, 71–73f
        large cell carcinoma, 73
        oat cell carcinoma, 73, 73f
        "scar", 73
        small cell carcinoma, 73
        squamous cell carcinoma, 69f, 71f, 72f, 73
        x-ray of, 6f, 7
    computed tomography of, 23f
    hamartoma, 74
    major fissure of, 42f
    metastasis, 60–61, 61f
    minor fissure of, 42f
    pseudotumor of, 51f, 52
    solitary nodule, 74–77
        abscess and, 75–76, 76f
        arteriovenous malformation and, 77
        cyst and, 76f
        sequestration and, 77
    tomography of
        computed, 43, 45f
        conventional, 42–43, 43f, 44f
Lung scan, 44, 45f
    pulmonary embolism, 64, 65f
Lymph node. *See* Hilar enlargement.
Lymphocele, 129f
Lymphoma
    bilateral hilar enlargement and, 78f
    computed tomography of, 26, 27f
    gastric, 142, 143f
Lytic metastasis, bone, 197–200, 198–200f

Magnetic resonance imaging
    history of, 2
    of central nervous system, 37, 258f
    of chromophobe adenoma, 276, 278f
    of ear, 281
    of gliomas, 271, 273f, 274
    physics of, 36, 36f
Malignant melanoma, gastric metastasis and, 142–144, 143f
Mallory-Weiss syndrome, 141
Mediastinum
    anatomy of, 39–40, 40f, 79, 80f, 81
    computed tomography use in, 30t
    magnetic resonance of, 38
    mass in
        algorithm for, 79
        anterior, 80f, 81
        middle, 81f
        posterior, 82f
    x-ray absorption in, 4, 5f
Medullary sponge kidney, 106f, 107
Megacolon, toxic, ulcerative colitis and, 178, 178f

Meningioma, 269f, 270f
Meningitis, 267f
Metabolic arthritis, 210, 217f
Miliary tuberculosis, 54–55, 55f
Mitral insufficiency, 232–233, 233f
Mitral stenosis, 232f
Mitral valve disease, 231–233, 232f, 233f
Multiple sclerosis, 274f
Myelography
    of central nervous system, 2, 53f, 251, 253
    of herniated disc, 286–287f
Myocardial infarction, diagnosis of, 242–244, 243–244f
Myocardial scan, 242–243, 243f

Necrobiotic nodule, 60
Necrosis
    acute tubular, 125–126, 126f
        renal transplant and, 127–128, 128f
    aseptic, 217–219, 218–219f
    papillary, 97, 98f, 99f
Nephrocalcinosis, 106f
Nephrolithiasis, 102, 105f
Nephronia, lobar, 94
Nephrostomy, 90–91
Neurofibroma, 288f, 289–290
Neuroma, acoustic, 282f, 283f
Nonunion, fracture healing, 192f
Nuclear imaging
    history of, 2
    in acute tubular necrosis, 127–128, 128f
    in cholecystitis, 163f
    in cirrhosis, 156f
    in transplant evaluation, 126–127
    indications for, 35–36t
    of bone, 183–184, 185f
    of chronic renal failure, 116
    of gastrointestinal hemorrhage, 149f
        brisk, 149–150
        slow, 151
    of kidney, 90f, 91
    of liver metastasis, 156, 157f
    of lung, 44, 45f
    of renal trauma, 109
    of urinary calculi, 106
    physics of, 31–32

Oat cell carcinoma. *See* Lung, carcinoma of.
Obstetrics, ultrasound use in, 21t
Obstructive airway disease
    asthma, 46, 48f
    bronchitis, 48
    emphysema, 49f, 49
Obstructive jaundice, 153–155f
Oligemia
    emphysema and, 49

pulmonary embolism and, 64
Oliguria
    acute tubular necrosis and, 125–126
    algorithm for, 125
    benign prostatic hypertrophy and, 124–125, 125f
    renal failure, acute, 125–126
Optic nerve, glioma of, 280f
Oral cholecystogram, 159f, 160f
Orbit
    anatomy of, 278, 279f
    fracture of, 280, 281f
    pseudotumor of, 280f
Ossicular disruption, 282
Osteoarthritis. *See* Degenerative arthritis.
Osteodystrophy, osteomalacia due to, 206–207, 207f
Osteoid osteoma, 201f
Osteolysis, Paget's disease and, 220–221
Osteoma, 201f
Osteomalacia, renal osteodystrophy and, 206–207, 207f
Osteomyelitis
    diagnosis of, 192–194, 194–197f
    in children, 193–194, 194f
Osteonecrosis. *See* Aseptic necrosis.
Osteophyte, arthritis due to, 283, 284f
Osteoporosis
    diagnosis of, 207–208, 208f–210f
    rheumatoid arthritis and, 211f–212f, 212
Osteoscarcoma, 200, 201f
Osteosclerosis, Paget's disease and, 220f

Paget's disease, 220f
Pain
    back, 283–290
        extradural mass and, 286–288f
        hydromyelia and, 289f, 290
        intradural mass and, 289
        neurofibroma and, 288f, 289–290
    chest. *See* Chest pain.
    extremities. *See* Extremity, painful/cold
    right upper quadrant
        acute cholecystitis and, 163–164, 163f
        algorithm for, 158
        biliary colic and, 163
        biliary sludge and, 161, 161f
        echogenic bile and, 161
        gallbladder disease and, 158–164, 159–163f
        gallstones and, 160f, 161
        pancreas cancer and, 169–171, 170f
        pancreatic disease and, 164–171, 165–170f
        pancreatitis and, 165–166, 166f
        pseudocysts and, 167
Pancreas
    abscess of, 169
    carcinoma of, 169–171, 170f
        ultrasound of, 17, 19f

Pancreas *(Continued)*
  computed tomography of, 23, 24f, 31t
  disease of, 164–171
  mass in, 155f
  ultrasound of, 13f, 14f, 15, 20t
Pancreatic duct, obstruction of, 154f
Pancreatitis, 165–166, 166f–169f
  chronic, 169f
  complications of, 166–169, 168f
  computed tomography of, 23, 24f
  ultrasound of, 17f
Papillary necrosis, 97, 98f, 99f
Parathormone, effect on bone, 204
Pathologic fracture, 188–189, 189f
Pelvis
  computed tomography use in, 31t
  magnetic resonance of, 38
  ultrasound of, 15f, 20t
Peptic esophagitis, 173–174, 174f
Percutaneous transhepatic cholangiography, in biliary obstruction, 155f
Perforation, duodenal ulcer and, 136
Periarticular osteoporosis, rheumatoid arthritis and, 211f–212f, 212
Pericardial effusion, cardiomegaly due to, 234–235, 235f
Pericarditis, cardiomegaly due to, 235f
Periosteum
  calcification of, 195f
  osteomyelitis of, 193, 194f
Periostitis, osteomyelitis vs., 196
Peripelvic cyst, 120
Peripheral atherosclerosis, 247–248, 248f
Pertechnetate scan, gastrointestinal hemorrhage, 151f
Phlegmon, pancreatitis and, 167–169
Phosphorus, hyperparathyroidism and, 204–205
Pituitary gland, tumor of, 276, 277f, 278f
Pixel, CT scanner, 22f
Pleural effusion, 66–67, 67f
  heart failure and, 51f
Pneumatoceles, 53f
Pneumoconiosis, 60
Pneumocystis carinii pneumonia, 55f, 56
Pneumonia
  aspiration, 53–54
  bacterial, 52f, 53f
  viral, 55f
Pneumothorax, 65–66, 66f
Polycystic disease, renal, 114, 115f
Polyp
  adenomatous, 147f
  colonic, 147f
  gallbladder, 161, 162f
Portable chest x-ray, 39
Positron emission tomography, of central nervous system, 258
Positron scanning, 35

Postobstructive pneumonitis, 71f
Progressive massive fibrosis, silica and, 61, 62f
Proptosis
  optic nerve glioma and, 280, 280f
  pseudotumor and, 280, 280f
  retrobulbar hematoma and, 280, 281f
  thyroid ophthalamopathy and, 278, 279f
Prostate, benign hypertrophy of, 124–125, 125f
Proteinosis, alveolar, 57
Pseudocyst, pancreatitis and, 166–167, 168f
Pseudofracture, osteomalacia and, 207f
Pseudotumor, orbital, 280f
Psoriatic arthritis, 215f
Pulmonary artery
  mediastinum location of, 40f
  x-ray of, 225, 226f
Pulmonary edema
  cardiac, 50f, 51f, 50–52
  noncardiac, 52
Pulmonary embolism, 63–65, 64f, 65f
  angiography of, 44
Pulmonary hypertension
  bilateral hilar enlargement due to, 78–79, 79f
  x-ray of, 225
Pulmonary nodule, solitary. *See* Solitary pulmonary nodule.
Pyelogram, intravenous. *See* Intravenous pyelogram.
Pyelonephritis
  acute, 93–94, 94f
  chronic, 94–96, 95f
  xanthogranulomatous, 123–124
Pyonephrosis, 122–123
Pyuria
  algorithm for, 121
  carbuncle and, 121
  pyonephrosis and, 123–124
  renal abscess and, 121–122, 122f
  tuberculosis and, 124
  xanthogranulomatous pyelonephritis and, 123–124

Radioactivity, nuclear medicine, 31–32
Radiolucent line, fracture and, 184–186, 185f, 186f
Radionuclide imaging. *See* Nuclear imaging.
Radiopharmaceutical, definition of, 32
Real-time scanning, ultrasound, 11
Red blood cell pertechnetate scan, in gastrointestinal hemorrhage, 151f
Red infarction, 259, 261, 262f, 263
Reflux esophagitis, 173–174, 174f
Regional interitis, 178–180, 178–180f
Reiter's syndrome, 214–215, 215f
Renal abscess, 19f, 121–122, 122f
  acute, 121–122
  chronic, 123–124
Renal artery occlusion, 129

Renal artery stenosis, 111–114
Renal carbuncle, 121–122, 122f
  ultrasound of, 17, 19f
Renal cell carcinoma
  computed tomography of, 26f
  embolization of, 100, 101f
  hematuria in, 97–100, 99–101f
  staging of, 100
  ultrasound of, 17, 18f
Renal cyst, 118–120, 119f, 120f
  computed tomography of, 25f
  ultrasound of, 13–15, 14f
Renal failure
  acute, 125–126, 126f
    transplant and, 127–128, 128f
  chronic, 18f, 114, 116f
  hyperparathyroidism due to, 204–205
  ultrasound of, 17, 18f
Renal hypertension. *See* Hypertension, renal.
Renal infarction, 116–118, 117f
  therapeutic, 91
Renal mass
  algorithm for, 118
  duplicated collecting system and, 120–121
  juxtarenal mass and, 121
  simple cyst and, 118–120, 120f
Renal scan, in transplant evaluation, 126–127
Renal transplant
  acute tubular necrosis and, 127–128, 128f
  algorithm for, 127
  lymphocele and, postoperative, 129f
  perirenal abnormalities and, 129–130
  postoperative evaluation of, 126–127, 129f
  preoperative evaluation of, 126
  rejection of, 128–129, 128f
  urethral abnormalities and, 129–130
  vascular occlusion and, 129
Renal vein thrombosis, 96–97, 96f
Renin, renal vein levels of, 113–114
Renogram, 34, 90f, 91
  in renovascular hypertension, 114
Renovascular hypertension, 111–114, 112f, 113f
Reticulonodular pattern, 46, 59f
Retrobulbar hematoma, 280
Retrograde pyelography
  papillary necrosis, 97, 99f
Rheumatic fever, mitral valve disease due to, 231–232, 232f
Rheumatoid arthritis, 60f, 211f–215f
  variants of, 214f–215f
Rotation, fracture due to, 184
"Rugger jersey" spine, osteomalacia and, 206f, 207

"Salt and pepper" skull, in hyperparathyroidism, 205f
Salter fracture, 188f, 189f

Sarcoidosis, 57–59, 58f, 59f
  bilateral hilar enlargement and, 58f, 59
  fibrosis, 59f, 59
  interstitial pattern, 59
  reticulonodular pattern, 59
  nodules, 59
Scar carcinoma. *See* Lung, carcinoma of.
Scleroderma, 174f
Septic arthritis, 196f
Sequestration, pulmonary, 77
Shadowing, ultrasound, 12
Silhouette sign, in pneumonia, 52
Silicosis
  adenopathy, 61, 62f
  interstitial disease due to, 61–62, 62f
  progressive massive fibrosis, 61, 62f
  unilateral hilar enlargement and, 78
Single-contrast medium, in lower gastrointestinal tract, 144
Skeleton, radiology of, 183–221
Skip lesion, Crohn's disease and, 179
Skull
  fracture of, 187f
    healing, 192
  radiology of, 251, 252f
Small bowel
  anatomy of, 134, 135f
  computed tomography of, 24f, 28
Small cell carcinoma, pulmonary. *See* Lung, carcinoma of.
Sodium urate, gout due to, 217
Soft tissue swelling, osteomyelitis and, 194, 195f
Solitary pulmonary nodule
  abscess and, 75–76, 76f
  algorithm for, 75
  arteriovenous malformation and, 77
  bronchogenic cysts and, 76, 76f
  lung cancer and, 75f
  pulmonary sequestration and, 77
Sound wave, ultrasound use of, 10, 11f
Spinal cord
  computed tomography of, 30t, 257f, 258
  magnetic resonance of, 37
  mass in, 285, 286f
  metastasis of, 284, 285f, 286, 288f, 289
Spleen
  enlargement of, x-ray of, 7f
  nuclear medicine in, 156f
  ultrasound use in, 20t
Spondylitis, anklyosing, 214f
Spondyloarthropathy, seronegative, 214f–215f
Spontaneous pneumothorax, 65, 66f
Squamous cell carcinoma. *See* Lung, carcinoma of.
S-sign of Golden, 69f, 71
Staghorn calculus, urinary, 102, 105f
Stenosis
  aortic, 233–234, 234f

Stenosis (*Continued*)
    duodenal ulcer and, 136–137
    idiopathic hypertrophic subaortic, 239
    mitral valve, 232f
    renal artery, 111–114
Stomach
    anatomy of, 134, 135f
    carcinoma of, 141–142, 142f
    computed tomography of, 24f, 28
    erosion in, 137–138, 138f
    lymphoma of, 142, 143f
    metastasis in, 142, 143f, 144
    ulcer of, 138f–139f
    ultrasound of, 13f
    varices of, 140f–141f, 141
Stress fracture, 184f
Stroke, uncomplicated, 259f–261f
Subarachnoid hemorrhage, 266f, 267f
Subdiaphragmatic pleural effusion, 66–67, 67f
Subdural hematoma, 263f, 264f
Subluxation
    joint, 192
    rheumatoid arthritis and, 213
Subperiosteal resorption, in hyperparathyroidism, 204f,
    205
Sulfur colloid, technetium and, 32
Suture line, fracture vs., 186–187, 187f
Synovitis
    gout and, 217f
    rheumatoid arthritis and, 212

Technetium, half life of, 32
Technetium scan
    in cirrhosis, 156f
    in gastrointestinal hemorrhage, 149f
    in transplant evaluation, 127
    myocardial, 230f, 231
    renal, 90f, 91
Tendon, rheumatoid arthritis and, 211f, 213
Tension, fracture due to, 184
Tension pneumothorax, 66f
Thallium stress test, cardiac, 229f, 230
Thrombophlebitis, 249f
Thrombosis
    deep venous, 249f
    renal vein, 96f
    stroke due to, 259
Thyroid
    nuclear medicine in, 35t
    ophthalamopathy, 278, 279f
    technetium scan of, 32, 33f
Tomography, 9–10, 10f
    of bone, 184
    of central nervous sytem, 251, 253f

of ear, 253f, 281
of lung, 42–43, 43f, 44f
of osteomyelitis, 197f
of urinary tract, 85
Tophus, gout and, 217
Tortuous aorta, 40, 41f
Torus fracture, 188f
Toxic megacolon, ulcerative colitis and, 178, 178f
Trabecula, osteoporsis and, 208, 209f
Trachea, anatomy of, 42
Transcatheter arterial embolism, gastrointestinal hemor-
    rhage and, 150
Transitional cell carcinoma, papillary, 101–102
Transthoracic needle aspiration biopsy, 44, 46
Trauma
    cerebral, 263f–265f
    osteomyelitis due to, 196–197
    pulmonary, hemoptysis in, 74
    renal, 107–109, 108f
Tuberculoma, 55
Tuberculosis, 53–55f, 54–55
    genitourinary, 123f
    miliary, 54–55, 55f
    pericarditis due to, 235
    renal, 123f, 124
Tubular necrosis, renal, 125–126, 126f
    renal transplant and, 127–128, 128f

Ulcer, duodenal, 136f–137f
Ulcerative colitis, 176f–177f, 176–177
    complications of, 177–178, 178f
Ultrasound
    history of, 1–2
    in acute cholecystitis, 163
    in aortic aneurysm, 244–246, 246f
    in chronic renal failure, 116
    in gallbladder polyp, 161, 162f
    in gallstones, 160f–161f, 161
    in liver metastasis, 156–157
    in obstructive jaundice, 153, 154f
    in pancreas cancer, 171
    in pancreatic pseudocyst, 167, 168f
    in polycystic disease, 114, 115f
    in pyelonephritis, 94–95
    in renal cell carcinoma, 98, 100f
    indications for, 20–21f
    of female pelvis, 91
    of gallbladder, 151–153, 152f
    of lung, 46
    of renal abscess, 122f
    of renal cyst, 118–119, 120f
    of urinary tract, 85, 87f
    physics of, 10
Urinary tract, radiology of, 85–130
Urine, decreased output of. *See* Oliguria.

Urinoma, 130
Uropathy, obstructive, 130

Varices, gastroesphageal, 140f–141f
Vascular disease, pulmonary, hemoptysis in, 74
Vascular groove, fracture vs., 186–187, 187f
Vascular opacification, 8
Vasopressin infusion, in gastrointestinal hemorrhage, 150
Vena cava, superior
    mediastinal location of, 40f
Venography, renal vein thrombosis, 97
Venous thrombosis, deep, 249f
Ventricle, mediastinum location of, 40f
Ventricular septal defect, 237f
Ventriculogram
    angina, 241
    gated-pool, 230f, 231

Vertebra, fracture of, 187f
Villous adenoma, 147–148, 148f
Voxel, CT scanner, 22f

Xanthogranulomatsus pyelonephritis, 123–124
X-ray
    beam, 3f
    contrast agents, 7–8, 8f, 9f
    film, 4f
    history of, 1
    physics of, 2–3, 3f
    tissue absorption of, 3–6, 4f–6f

Zollinger-Ellison syndrome
    duodenal ulcer in, 136